Radiographic Pathology
for Technologists

Radiographic Pathology for Technologists

JAMES D. MACE, MBA, RT (R)

Senior Director—Professional Services
Riverside Methodist Hospitals
Columbus, Ohio

NINA KOWALCZYK, MS, RT (R)

Associate Director—Radiology
The Ohio State University Hospitals
Columbus, Ohio

Second Edition

with 331 illustrations

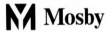 Mosby

St. Louis Baltimore Boston Chicago London Madrid Philadelphia Sydney Toronto

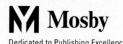
Mosby
Dedicated to Publishing Excellence

Editor: Don E. Ladig
Associate Developmental Editor: Lisa Potts
Project Manager: Carol Sullivan Wiseman
Designer: Jeanne Wolfgeher
Cover Designer: Betty Schulz

SECOND EDITION
Copyright © 1994 by Mosby–Year Book, Inc.

Previous edition copyrighted 1988

Printed in the United States of America

Composition by Carlisle Communications, LTD.
Printing/binding by R.R. Donnelley & Sons Company

Mosby–Year Book, Inc.
11830 Westline Industrial Drive
St. Louis, Missouri 63146

Library of Congress Cataloging in Publication Data
Mace, James D.
    Radiographic pathology for technologists / James D. Mace, Nina
Kowalczyk. — 2nd ed.
      p. cm.
    Includes bibliographical references and index.
    ISBN 0-8016-7059-4
    1. Diagnosis, Radioscopic. 2. Diagnostic imaging. 3. Pathology.
4. Radiologic technologists. I. Kowalczyk, Nina. II. Mace, James
D. Radiographic pathology for technologists. III. Title.
    [DNLM: 1. Pathology. 2. Radiography. QZ 4 M141r 1993]
RC78.M185 1993
616.07'57 — dc20
DNLM/DLC
for Library of Congress

NWST
1 AFK1333

93-23391
CIP

94 95 96 97 / 9 8 7 6 5 4 3 2 1

Preface

In the years that have passed since our first edition, medical imaging has continued its relentless pace of development. New ways of doing old things are rapidly moving to establish their own place. Digital radiography and fluoroscopy, for example, are beginning to emerge as tools useful in diagnosis. Radiologists benefit from these advances, as well as referring physicians who have access to laser printer–generated copies of films and images transmitted electronically through teleradiology applications.

MRI, CT, and sonography have also seen spectacular improvements in imaging capabilities. Changes in practice patterns are occurring as a result of the rise of these modalities. Myelography, for example, may be largely relegated to a limited role in diagnosis of back ailments as spine MRI studies prove their clinical efficacy while eliminating the obvious patient discomfort and complications. Ultra-thin slices and the development of volumetric analysis are opening new opportunities for CT. Further refinements and diagnostic capabilities of ultrasound are announced frequently, causing many to predict as much as 25% growth by the end of the decade.

This vast array of choices complicates the task of referring physicians in selecting exactly the right modality for imaging a particular pathology. Radiologists, too, are having to wrestle with the necessity to subspecialize as a result of the increasing demands placed on them by the sophistication of these modalities. Radiologic technologists are equally challenged in learning the nuances of the various modalities to provide the optimal diagnosis for referring and interpreting physicians. Never before has the first sentence in the preface of our first edition been truer: *The education of all health professionals becomes increasingly complex as knowledge expands exponentially.*

The goal of the second edition remains largely the same as the first. While many courses in the curriculum are devoted to the science of imaging, radiographers must also have an appreciation of the art involved in their profession. Although interpretation and diagnosis of images remains the purview of rigorously trained physicians, the radiographer who can enhance an image to provide an optimal diagnosis serves a critical role in medicine. This text provides a good basic understanding of diseases seen by diagnostic imaging and therefore helps the radiographer see their work in a different light, one which is focused on the importance of practicing the discipline as an art *and* science.

It is assumed that the didactic instruction of which this text is a part occurs in the latter part of a student radiographer's education. Brief reviews of anatomy and physiology begin each chapter primarily to reacquaint the reader with those aspects of the particular body system to be studied. Where appropriate, the effect of a given disease on technical factors employed in traditional diagnostic radiography is noted. Images chosen to illustrate diseases include conventional radiographs as in the first edition, although the reader should note significant improvement in their quality and captioning. Also, additional emphasis has been placed on the role of CT, MRI, and ultrasonography in depiction of certain pathologies.

Other enhancements to the first edition include a substantively bolstered text. Not only are disease processes included that were omitted in the first edition, but all discussions have been improved to include more information about symptoms and treatments. The glossary has expanded accordingly. The reader is cautioned, however, that it is not the authors' intent to provide an all-encompassing pathology textbook for all audiences. Rather, an overview of diseases seen radiographically with broad coverage of a given topic is the approach taken. The intended user is the radiographer, both student and practitioner. Readers interested in more information are provided several additional references at the conclusion of each chapter to guide them in their search for more in-depth knowledge.

Furthermore, other new items included in the second edition help the reader more fully appreciate radiographic pathology. Each chapter begins with a set of learning objectives, designed to help the reader focus on items of importance. In addition, each chapter concludes with a number of multiple choice questions to help assess learning. Answers are provided at the back of the book.

Our sincere hope is that this textbook enhances the radiographer's education and possibly appreciation of the importance of their work. We found that creating a second edition was, perhaps, even more work than producing the first. Deciding where to begin and end discussion of a particular topic was difficult. Recognizing that nothing can ever be "one size fits all," we believe our second edition offers significant improvements to our readers, the radiography community. Any role this book can play in improving the results of the science and art of our discipline is most gratifying.

James D. Mace
Nina Kowalczyk

Acknowledgments

As noted in the preface, creation of the first edition of this text was a lot of work! Little did we know that doing it again as a second edition was, arguably, even more. Support for the project was unequivocal from a variety of sources, perhaps most importantly our spouses, Cheryl and Doug. Their love, enthusiasm, and willingness to help out in whatever way possible provided an unending source of support for our efforts.

Much of the team that helped produce the first edition remained intact for this one. Again, our sincere gratitude is extended to our physician reviewers, Rebecca Gibbons, MD, and Greg Gibbons, MD. Their review of the textual content was invaluable in assuring accuracy, a characteristic most important to the users of this text. Help from other physicians was also forthcoming, and appreciated. In particular, much thanks to Phil Shaffer, MD; Bill Wiand, DO; Geof Wiot, MD; and Gordon Taylor, MD for their assistance in procuring images, as well as lending guidance to the text development.

A particular thanks goes to the American College of Radiology for their generous granting of rights for use of their radiographic teaching file (copyright 1988) for many of the illustrations in this text. Their images and supporting material have significantly improved the quality of illustrations in the second edition, and we are indebted to them. Appreciation is also extended to Riverside Methodist Hospitals, The Ohio State University Hospitals, and Children's Hospital, all of Columbus, Ohio, for use of images from their facilities. Much credit, too, goes to the Media Department of Riverside Methodist Hospitals for their superb photography of these images. Correct exposure of radiographs is not always an easy chore, but in this they excelled!

Our editorial research consultants were also invaluable in this project. Much thanks to Esther Bennett, RT; Cindy Burns, RT; Vic Krell, RT; Roberta Dials, RT; Lynn Joe-Morgan, RT; Lynn Shepherd, RT; Sheryl Najmulski, RT; Julie Gill, RT; and Michelle Crager. Running down the details and doing a lot of the ''legwork'' saved us innumerable hours in the preparation of this second edition. Their support and willingness to help in any way possible was a great source of stress relief. Many others contributed images, too, and we are most appreciative of their assistance.

Finally, we could identify hundreds of others who supported one or both editions, or simply inspired us. Some must be mentioned for their contributions to our careers. Phil Ballinger and Bill Finney of the School of Allied Medical Professions at The Ohio State University served as excellent role models for each of us. Many of the hundreds of students with whom they've interacted owe some of their success to these two fine representatives of academia and radiologic technology.

Although we are somewhat removed from mainstream radiologic technology education, our own students through the years have served, too, as a source of inspiration, both at The Ohio State University and Riverside Methodist Hospitals in Columbus, Ohio, and at Providence Hospital in Sandusky, Ohio. Teaching was never just a job; it was a conscious choice that we relished and approached with enthusiasm. Our experiences with our students have contributed to this book as well. For all those others who have also played a role, we are appreciative. Our gratitude and sincere thanks are extended to them and all of the above for their role in this textbook.

Reviewers

Robert Champa, MA, RT(R)
Clinical Instructor
Cooperative Radiography Program
Memorial Hospital of Burlington County
Mount Holly, NJ

Sharyn D. Gibson, MHS, RT(T)
Head, Radiologic Technologies Department
The School of Health Professions
Armstrong State College
Savannah, GA

Darrell McKay, PhD
Professor/Department Chair
Health Technology
St. Louis Community College
St. Louis, MO

Jordan B. Renner, MD
Associate Professor of Radiology
    and Medical Allied Health Professions
The University of North Carolina at Chapel Hill
Chapel Hill, NC

Bonnie Young, RT
Education Coordinator
Community School of Radiologic Technology
Springfield, OH

Contents

1   Introduction to Pathology, 1
Pathologic Terms, 1
Disease Classifications, 3

2   The Skeletal System, 10
Anatomy and Physiology Review, 10
Imaging Considerations, 13
Congenital/Hereditary Diseases, 14
Inflammatory Disease, 23
Metabolic Disease, 33
Traumatic Disease, 39
Visceral Cranial Fractures, 59
Vertebral Column, 68
Neoplastic Disease, 73

3   The Respiratory System, 86
Anatomy and Physiology Review, 86
Imaging Considerations, 88
Congenital/Hereditary Diseases, 111
Inflammatory Diseases, 113
Traumatic Diseases, 132
Neoplastic Diseases, 139

4   The Abdomen and Gastrointestinal System, 147
Anatomy and Physiology Review, 148
Imaging Considerations, 153

Congenital/Hereditary Anomalies, 165
Inflammatory Diseases, 173
Degenerative Diseases, 186
Bowel Obstructions, 188
Neurogenic Diseases, 197
Diverticular Disease, 199
Traumatic Disease, 205
Neoplastic Diseases, 209

5   The Hepatobiliary System, 219
Anatomy and Physiology Review, 219
Imaging Considerations, 222
Inflammatory Diseases, 228
Metabolic Diseases, 234
Neoplastic Diseases, 235

6   The Urinary System, 242
Anatomy and Physiology Review, 242
Imaging Considerations, 245
Congenital/Hereditary Diseases, 254
Inflammatory Diseases, 264
Degenerative/Metabolic Disease, 267

7   The Reproductive System, 286
The Female Reproductive System, 287
Anatomy and Physiology Review, 287
Imaging Considerations, 288
Congenital Abnormalities, 291
Inflammatory Disease, 291
Neoplastic Diseases, 292
Disorders during Pregnancy, 302
The Male Reproductive System, 303
Anatomy and Physiology Review, 303
Imaging Considerations, 304
Neoplastic Diseases, 305

8   The Cardiovascular System, 309
Anatomy and Physiology Review, 309
Imaging Considerations, 314
Congenital/Hereditary Diseases, 319

Valvular Disease, 323
Congestive Heart Disease, 324
Degenerative Diseases, 326
Aneurysms, 329
Venous Thrombosis, 331

9   The Hemopoietic System, 336
Anatomy and Physiology Review, 336
Imaging Considerations, 339
Acquired Immune Deficiency Syndrome, 342
Neoplastic Disease, 343

10   The Central Nervous System, 348
Anatomy and Physiology Review, 348
Imaging Considerations, 353
Congenital/Hereditary Diseases, 361
Inflammatory Disease, 366
Traumatic Disease, 372
Neoplastic Diseases, 381

Answer Key, 404

Glossary, 406

Bibliography, 424

Contents in Brief

1 Introduction to Pathology, 1

2 The Skeletal System, 10

3 The Respiratory System, 86

4 The Abdomen and Gastrointestinal System, 147

5 The Hepatobiliary System, 219

6 The Urinary System, 242

7 The Reproductive System, 286

8 The Cardiovascular System, 309

9 The Hemopoietic System, 336

10 The Central Nervous System, 348

1

Introduction to Pathology

▼
Upon completion of Chapter 1, the reader should be able to:
- Define common terminology associated with the study of disease.
- Differentiate between signs and symptoms.
- Distinguish between a disease diagnosis and its prognosis.
- Describe the different types of disease classifications.
- Cite characteristics that distinguish benign from malignant neoplasms.
- Identify the difference in origin for carcinoma vs. sarcoma.

Pathology is basically the study of disease. Many types of disease exist, and in general, many conditions can be readily demonstrated radiographically. For the radiography student to better understand specific pathologic conditions, one must first have a working knowledge of common pathologic terms. This chapter will serve as a brief introduction to terms associated with pathology.

PATHOLOGIC TERMS

Any abnormal disturbance of the function or structure of the human body as a result of some type of injury is called a *disease*. After injury, *pathogenesis* occurs. This refers to the sequence of events producing cellular changes that ultimately lead to observable changes known as *manifestations*. These manifestations can display in a variety of fash-

1

ions. A *symptom* refers to the patient's perception of the disease. Symptoms are subjective, and only the patient can identify these manifestations. For example, a headache is considered a symptom. A *sign* is an objective manifestation and can be detected by the physician during examination. A fever, swelling, and/or a skin rash are all considered signs. A group of signs and symptoms that characterizes a specific abnormal disturbance is a *syndrome*. However, some disease processes, especially in the early stages, do not produce symptoms and are termed *asymptomatic*.

Etiology is the study of the cause of a disease. In addition to the normal agents that can cause disease (e.g., viruses, bacteria, trauma, heat) a number of other causes are known. Proper infection control practices are important in a health care environment to prevent *nosocomial* disease. Staph infection following hip replacement surgery is an example of a nosocomial disease, i.e., one acquired from the environment. The etiology of the disease in this case could be poor infection control practices. *Iatrogenic* reactions are those adverse responses that occur from medical treatment itself (e.g., a collapsed lung that occurs in response to a complication that arises in arterial line placement). If no causative factor can be identified, the disease is termed *idiopathic*.

The length of time over which the disease is displayed may vary. Acute diseases usually have a quick onset and last a short period of time, whereas a *chronic* disease may present more slowly and last a very long time.

Two additional terms are encountered when referring to the identification and outcome of a disease. A *diagnosis* is the name of a disease an individual is believed to have, and the prediction of the course and outcome of the disease is called a *prognosis*.

Government agencies compile statistics annually regarding the incidence, or rate of occurrence, of disease (Table 1-1). *Epidemiology* is the investigation of disease in large

▼**Table 1-1**   Deaths, death rates, and percent of total deaths for the 10 leading causes of death, 1990

Rank	Cause of Death	Number	Death Rate per 100,000	Percent of Total
1	Heart disease	720,058	289.5	40.9
2	Malignant neoplasms	505,322	203.2	28.8
3	Cerebrovascular disease	144,088	57.9	8.2
4	Accidents	91,983	37.0	5.2
5	Chronic obstructive pulmonary disease	86,679	34.9	4.9
6	Pneumonia and influenza	79,513	32.0	4.5
7	Diabetes	47,664	19.2	2.7
8	Suicide	30,906	12.4	1.7
9	Chronic liver disease and cirrhosis	25,815	10.4	1.5
10	HIV infection	25,188	10.1	1.4

Modified from The U.S. Department of Health and Human Services, Monthly Vital Statistics Report, Volume 41, Number 17, January 7, 1993.

groups. The *prevalence* of a given disease refers to the number of cases found in a given population. The *incidence* of disease refers to the number of new cases found in a given time period. Diseases of high prevalence in an area where a given causative organism is commonly found are said to be *endemic* to that area. For example, histoplasmosis is a fungal disease of the respiratory system endemic to the Ohio and Mississippi River valleys. It is not uncommon to see a relatively high prevalence of it in these areas. Its appearance in great numbers in the far Western states, however, could represent an epidemic.

The *mortality rate* is the number of deaths caused by a particular disease averaged over a population. The incidence of sickness sufficient to interfere with an individual's normal daily routine is referred to as *morbidity rate*. It is fairly easy to obtain accurate data concerning the mortality rate of a specific population, but somewhat more difficult to obtain accurate data about the morbidity rate.

DISEASE CLASSIFICATIONS

Diseases can be grouped into several broad categories. Those in the same category may not necessarily be closely related, but groupings such as those discussed in the following tend to produce lesions that are similar in *morphology*, i.e., their form and structure. Pathologies discussed in this text are generally grouped into classifications of:

1. congenital/hereditary
2. inflammatory
3. degenerative
4. metabolic
5. traumatic
6. neoplastic.

Congenital and Hereditary Disease

Diseases that are present at birth and result from genetic or environmental factors are termed *congenital*. It is estimated that 2% to 3% of all live births show one or more congenital abnormalities, although some of these may not be visible until a year or so after birth. A major category of congenital diseases is due to abnormalities in the number and distribution of chromosomes. In *somatic cells* (those other than germ cells), chromosomes exist in the nucleus of each cell in pairs, with one member from the male parent and the other from the female parent. In humans, chromosomes are normally composed of 22 pairs of *autosomes* (those other than the sex chromosomes) and one pair of sex chromosomes. Down syndrome is a congenital condition caused by an autosomal mitosis error, leading to an extra twenty-first chromosome so that the affected individual has 47 chromosomes rather than the normal 46.

Hereditary diseases are caused by developmental disorders genetically transmitted from either parent to child through abnormalities of individual genes in chromosomes and are derived from ancestors. For example, hemophilia is a well-known hereditary disease in which proper blood clotting is absent. A genetic abnormality present on the sex chromosome is a sex-linked inheritance; those on one of the other 22 chromosomes is an autosomal inheritance. The inherited disease may be *dominant* (transmitted by a single gene from either parent) or *recessive* (transmitted by both parents to an offspring). Amniocentesis, typically guided by ultrasound, is a standard procedure used prenatally to assess the presence of certain hereditary disorders.

A congenital defect is not necessarily hereditary, however, since it may have been acquired in utero. Intrauterine injury during a critical point in development can occur from maternal infections, radiation, or drugs. Abnormalities of this type occur sporadically and cannot generally be recognized before birth. However, their likelihood is greatly lessened by following proper precautions against infection, avoiding radiation (particularly during early term of pregnancy), and avoiding of drugs or agents not specifically recognized by a physician as safe.

Inflammatory Disease

An *inflammatory* disease results from the body's reaction to a localized injurious agent. Types of inflammatory diseases include infective diseases, which result from invasion by microorganisms such as viruses, bacteria, or fungi; toxic diseases, which result from poisoning by biologic substances; and allergic diseases, which are an overreaction of the body's own defenses.

Some diseases in this classification are considered *autoimmune disorders*. Under normal conditions, antibodies are formed in response to foreign antigens. In certain diseases, however, they form against and injure the patient's own tissues. These are known as *autoantibodies,* and diseases associated with them are autoimmune disorders. Rheumatoid arthritis is an example of an autoimmune disorder.

An inflammatory reaction (i.e., *inflammation*) is a generalized pathologic process that is nonspecific to the agent causing the injury. The body's purpose in creating an inflammatory reaction is to localize the injurious agent and prepare for subsequent repair and healing of the injured tissues. Substances released from the damaged tissues can cause both local and systemic effects (Fig. 1-1). Those effects seen local to the injury include capillary dilatation to allow fluids and leukocytes, specifically, to infiltrate into the area of damage. Cellular *necrosis* (death) is common to acute inflammation, and the leukocytes serve to remove the dead material through phagocytosis. The characteristics of such acute inflammation include heat, redness of skin, swelling, pain, and some loss of function as the body tends to protect the injured part. If the inflammatory process is significant, system effects such as an elevation of body temperature become evident.

Chronic inflammation differs from that of the acute stage in that damage caused by an injurious agent may not necessarily result in tissue death. In fact, necrosis is relatively uncommon in cases of chronic inflammation. It differs also in the duration of the inflammation, with chronic conditions lasting for long periods of time. Certain conditions discussed in this text evidence chronic inflammation (e.g., pulmonary emphysema as described in Chapter 3).

The repair of tissues damaged from an inflammatory process attempts to return the body to normal. Tissue *regeneration* is the process in which damaged tissues are replaced by new tissues that are essentially identical to those replaced. While this is the most desirable type of repair, tissues vary in their ability to replace themselves. Damaged nerve cells, for example, are not likely to readily regenerate. Fibrous connective tissue repair is the alternative to regeneration, but it is less desirable because it leads to scarring and

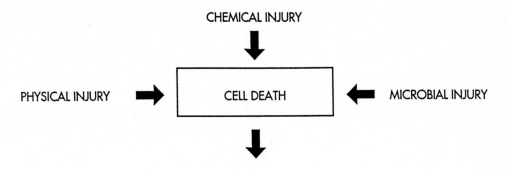

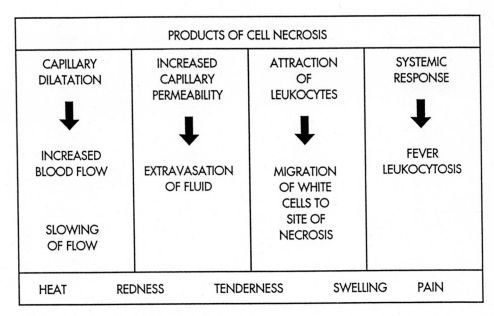

Fig. 1-1. Local and systemic effects of cell necrosis induced by various agents.   (From Crowley LV: *Introductory concepts in pathology,* Chicago, 1972, Year Book.)

fibrosis. Damaged tissues are replaced by a scar and lack the structure and function of the original tissue.

Infection refers to an inflammatory process caused by a disease-causing organism. Under favorable conditions, the invading pathogenic agent multiplies and causes injurious effects. Generally, localized infection is usually accompanied by inflammation, but inflammation can occur without infection. *Virulence* refers to the ease with which an organism can overcome body defenses. An organism with high virulence is likely to produce progressive disease in susceptible persons, while one of low virulence can produce disease only in highly susceptible persons under favorable conditions.

Degenerative Disease

Degenerative diseases are caused by a deterioration of the body. Although they are usually associated with the aging process, some degenerative conditions may exist in younger patients. For instance, an individual may develop a degenerative disease following a traumatic injury, regardless of age.

The process of aging results from the gradual maturation of physiologic processes that reach a peak, then gradually fade (i.e., degenerate) to a point where the body can no longer survive. Heredity, diet, and environmental factors are known to affect the rate of aging. Over time, the functional abilities of tissues decrease either because their cell numbers are reduced or the function of each individual cell declines, with both typically participating in pathologies resulting from aging. Atherosclerosis, osteoporosis, and osteoarthritis are three diseases commonly associated with the aging process. Each is discussed later in this text.

Metabolic Disease

Metabolism is the sum of all physical and chemical processes in the body. Diseases caused by a disturbance of the normal physiologic function of the body are classified as *metabolic* diseases. These include endocrine disorders (e.g., diabetes and hyperparathyroidism) and disturbances of fluid and electrolyte balance.

Endocrine glands secrete their products (hormones) into the bloodstream to regulate various metabolic functions. The major endocrine glands include the pituitary, thyroid, parathyroids, adrenal glands, pancreatic islets, ovaries, and testes. An endocrine disorder may consist of hypersecretion, causing an overactivity of the target organ, or insufficient secretion, resulting in underactivity. The clinical effects of endocrine disturbance depend on the degree of dysfunction and the age and sex of the individual.

Dehydration is the most common disturbance of fluid balance and is due to insufficient intake of water or excessive loss of it. Electrolytes are mineral salts (most commonly sodium and potassium) dissolved in the body's water. Depletion of them may occur because of vomiting, diarrhea, or use of diuretics (substances that promote the excretion of salt and water). Disturbance of either the fluid or electrolyte balances upset *homeostasis,* the body's normal internal resting state.

Traumatic Disease

Another general classification of diseases is *traumatic*. These diseases may result from mechanical forces such as crushing or twisting of a body part or from the effects of ionizing radiation on the human body. In addition, disorders resulting from extreme hot or cold temperatures, such as burns and frostbite, are also classified as traumatic.

Trauma may injure a bone, resulting in fractures. These are covered extensively in the Chapter 2. It may also injure soft tissues. A *wound* is an injury of soft parts associated with rupture of the skin. Traumatic injuries may injure soft tissues even if the skin is not broken. Bleeding into the tissue spaces as a result of capillary rupture is known as a *bruise* or *contusion*.

Neoplastic Disease

Neoplastic disease results in new, abnormal tissue growth. Normally, growing and maturing cells are subject to mechanisms that control their growth rate. When this control mechanism goes awry, an overgrowth of cells develop, resulting in a neoplasm. *Lesion* is a term used to describe the many types of cellular change that can occur in response to disease. Some lesions may be visible immediately (e.g., a burn) while others may be detectable initially only through diagnostic means such as laboratory testing.

An abnormal growth of cells leads to the formation of both benign and malignant tumors, or neoplasms. A *benign neoplasm* remains localized and is generally noninvasive, as opposed to a *malignant neoplasm,* which continues to grow, spread, and invade other tissues. *Cancer* is a general term often used to denote various types of malignant neoplasms. The spread of cancer cells is termed *metastasis*. Certain types of cancer appear more often as metastases from other areas rather than originating in a given organ. More discussion of this occurs in subsequent chapters.

It is important to note that the terms *cancer* and *carcinoma* are not synonymous. A *carcinoma* is one type of cancer and is derived from epithelial tissue. Another cancer is a *sarcoma*, which arises from connective tissue. Radiography plays a major role in the diagnosis of a variety of neoplastic diseases.

The treatment of cancer consumes enormous financial, emotional, and other resources in health care. While the state-of-the-art is continually advancing, the primary treatment modalities are surgery, chemotherapy, and radiation therapy. The choice of which modality or combination of modalities depends on many factors, including the type of cancer, its location and stage, and the treating oncologist. The goal of treatment may be *curative,* allowing the patient to remain free of disease for 5 years or more, or *palliative,* which is designed to relieve pain when curing isn't possible.

The Staging of Cancer. Decisions regarding the appropriate treatment of malignant tumors and in determining prognosis and end results are guided by classifications that "stage" the disease. Although several clinical classifications of cancer exist, the *TNM System* emerged in the 1950s and is now considered a recognized standard, as endorsed by the American Joint Committee on Cancer (AJCC). The AJCC is cosponsored by several prominent health organizations, including the American Cancer Society and the American College of Radiology.

The TNM system is based on the premise that cancers of similar histology or origin are similar in their patterns of growth or extension. "T" refers to the size of the untreated primary cancer or tumor. As the size increases, lymph node involvement (i.e. "N") occurs, eventually leading to distant metastases (i.e., "M"). The addition of numbers to these three letters indicates the extent of malignancy and the progressive increase in size or involvement of the tumor. T0, for example, indicates that no evidence of a primary tumor exists, while T1, T2, T3, and T4 indicate an increasing size or extension. N0 indicates lack of regional lymph node metastasis, while N1, N2, and N3 indicate increasing involvement of regional lymph nodes. Finally, M0 indicates no distant metastasis while M1 indicates the presence of distant metastasis.

In addition, other descriptors are used to categorize a given tumor further according to its primary site, histopathologic type and grade, lymphatic or venous invasion, and residual tumor classification. The combination of all of these allows the TNM system to serve as a shorthand notation for description of the clinical extent of a given malignant tumor. It facilitates treatment planning, provides an indication of prognosis, assists in evaluating treatment results, facilitates information exchange between treatment centers, and allows for unambiguous categorization of malignancies to aid in the continuing investigation of cancer.

CONCLUSION

There is no doubt that technological advances in the field of radiology have done much to relieve human suffering. But it is important to recognize that radiography alone cannot provide a definitive diagnosis. Radiography must be used in conjunction with other diagnostic and therapeutic modalities to provide the best treatment for each specific disease process. The following chapters will provide the student radiographer with a better understanding of disease processes of the various physiologic systems. This information should help students to analyze and critique each radiograph to ensure that they provide optimal information to assist physicians in their diagnosis.

▼ QUESTIONS

1. The prediction of the course and end of a disease and an outlook based on that prediction best defines its:
   - **a.** diagnosis
   - **b.** etiology
   - **c.** prognosis
   - **d.** syndrome

2. Disorders resulting from extreme heat or cold are classified as:
   - **a.** congenital
   - **b.** inflammatory
   - **c.** neoplastic
   - **d.** traumatic

3. A compression fracture of the lumbar spine that results from steroid treatments for pain reduction of arthritis would be an example of _____ disease.
   - **a.** degenerative
   - **b.** iatrogenic
   - **c.** idiopathic
   - **d.** traumatic

4. A disease such as Tay-Sachs syndrome that is transmitted genetically is termed:
   - **a.** congenital
   - **b.** hereditary
   - **c.** metabolic
   - **d.** neoplastic

5. Sickness sufficient to interfere with normal daily routines is termed:
   - **a.** etiology
   - **b.** morbidity
   - **c.** mortality
   - **d.** pathogenesis

6. Which of the following would be considered a symptom of a disease process?
   - **a.** bloody stool
   - **b.** nausea
   - **c.** skin rash
   - **d.** swelling

7. A disease that presents slowly and lasts over a long period of time is said to be:
   - **a.** acute
   - **b.** asymptomatic
   - **c.** chronic
   - **d.** congenital

8. Which of the following types of disease classifications is usually associated with the normal aging process?
   - **a.** congenital
   - **b.** degenerative
   - **c.** inflammatory
   - **d.** metabolic

9. Which of the following statements are true?
   1. The presence of neoplastic disease always results in patient death.
   2. Carcinomas and sarcomas derive from different types of tissues.
   3. The spread of cancerous tissue to other sites is referred to as metastasis.
   - **a.** 1 and 2
   - **b.** 2 and 3
   - **c.** 1 and 3
   - **d.** 1, 2, and 3

10. The leading cause of death in the American population for all groups is:
    - **a.** accidents
    - **b.** AIDS
    - **c.** cancer
    - **d.** heart disease

11. If 4,000 cases of a given disease are found in the inhabitants of a given population, its _____is defined.
    - **a.** incidence
    - **b.** morphology
    - **c.** metabolism
    - **d.** prevalence

12. Autoimmune disorders are a type of which disease classification?
    - **a.** congenital
    - **b.** degenerative
    - **c.** inflammatory
    - **d.** traumatic

13. The relative ease with which an organism can overcome normal bodily defenses against it refers to:
    - **a.** infection
    - **b.** necrosis
    - **c.** pestulence
    - **d.** virulence

14. Endocrine gland dysfunction will likely result in which type of disease?
    - **a.** degenerative
    - **b.** iatrogenic
    - **c.** metabolic
    - **d.** neoplastic

15. A general term to describe the many types of cellular changes that occur in response to disease is:
    - **a.** contusion
    - **b.** lesion
    - **c.** metastasis
    - **d.** morphology

2

The Skeletal System

▼

Upon completion of Chapter 2, the reader should be able to:

- Describe the anatomical components of the skeletal system on a macroscopic and basic microscopic level.
- Identify and explain the criteria for assessing technical adequacy of skeletal radiographs.
- Characterize a given condition as congenital, inflammatory, arthritic, metabolic, traumatic, or neoplastic.
- Specify the pathogenesis, signs and symptoms, and prognosis of the skeletal pathologies cited in this chapter.
- Discuss the healing process involved with fractures and identify complications associated with skeletal trauma.
- Describe and classify skeletal fractures according to the various classifications discussed in this chapter.
- Explain the role of various imaging modalities in the diagnosis and treatment of skeletal pathologies.

ANATOMY AND PHYSIOLOGY REVIEW

The skeletal system is comprised of 206 separate bones and is responsible for body support, protection, movement, and blood cell production. This system is commonly divided into the axial skeleton (Fig. 2-1), which contains 80 bones, and the appendicular skeleton (Fig. 2-2), which contains 126 bones. Bone is a type of connective tissue, but it differs from other connective tissue because of its matrix of calcium phosphate. The skeletal system shares

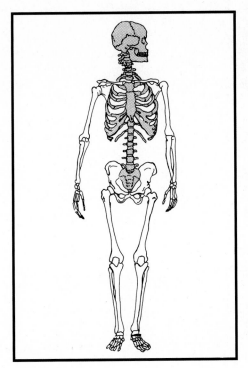 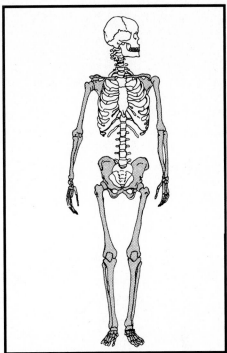

Fig. 2-1, left. Axial skeleton. (From Bontrager KL: *Textbook of Radiographic Positioning and Related Anatomy,* ed 3, St Louis 1993, Mosby.)

Fig. 2-2, right. Appendicular skeleton. (From Bontrager KL: *Textbook of Radiographic graphic Positioning and Related Anatomy,* ed 3, St Louis, 1993, Mosby.)

the majority of the body's calcium and phosphorus. The construction of this matrix further classifies bone tissue as either *compact* (dense) or *cancellous* (spongy) (Fig. 2-3).

The outer portion of bone is composed of compact bone and the inner portion, termed the *medullary canal,* is made up of cancellous bone. Bone marrow is located within the medullary canal and is interspersed between the *trabeculae.* This intricate, weblike bony structure is visible on a properly exposed radiograph of the skeletal system and is often referred to as the trabecular pattern. The term *diploe* is specific to the cancellous bone located within the skull. The red bone marrow is responsible for the production of both erythrocytes and leukocytes. At the approximate age of 20 years, the majority of the red bone marrow is replaced by yellow bone marrow composed mainly of fat.

Osteoblasts are the bone-forming cells that line the medullary canal and are interspersed throughout the periosteum. They are responsible for bone growth and thickening, ossification, and regeneration. *Osteoclasts* are specialized cells that break down bone to enlarge the medullary canal and allow for bone growth. This production and breakdown of bone plays an important role in serum calcium and phosphorus equilibrium. Approx-

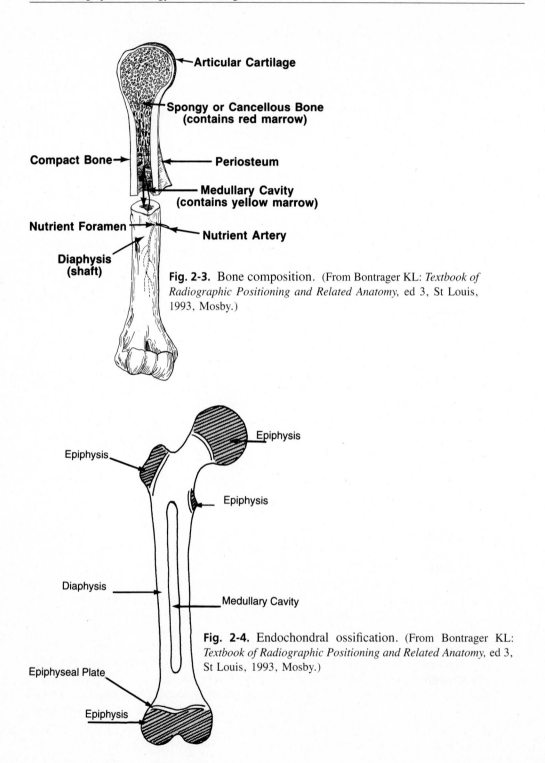

Fig. 2-3. Bone composition. (From Bontrager KL: *Textbook of Radiographic Positioning and Related Anatomy,* ed 3, St Louis, 1993, Mosby.)

Fig. 2-4. Endochondral ossification. (From Bontrager KL: *Textbook of Radiographic Positioning and Related Anatomy,* ed 3, St Louis, 1993, Mosby.)

imately 99% of the body's calcium is found within the skeletal system and certain metabolic disease processes may alter this percentage, resulting in either hypocalcemia or hypercalcemia.

The bones of the skeletal system may also be classified according to their shape to include long, short, flat, and irregular bones. The diaphysis of a long bone refers to the shaft portion, whereas the epiphysis refers to the end portion (Fig. 2-4). The metaphysis refers to the growth zone between the epiphysis and diaphysis. A cartilaginous growth plate is located between these two areas in the bone of a growing child. Radiographically, these growth areas appear radiolucent. As the body matures, this cartilage calcifies and is no longer radiographically visible in the adult.

The periosteum is a fibrous membrane that encloses all of the bone except the joint surfaces and is crucial to supplying blood to the underlying bone. Osteoblasts located within the periosteum increase bone thickness relative to individual activities. The more physical stress a bone is under, the thicker the compact portion develops; therefore it is common medical practice to allow patients with healing fractures of the hip or femur to bear weight on the injured bone, thus helping to reduce the healing period. Disuse atrophy occurs when a bone is not allowed to bear weight and results in significant decalcification and thinning of the bone.

The 206 bones of the body are connected to each other by one of three types of joints. Fibrous (synarthrodial) joints form firm, immovable joints such as the sutures of the skull. Cartilaginous (amphiarthrodial) joints such as those found between the vertebral bodies, are slightly movable. Synovial (diarthrodial) joints are freely movable joints. The ends of the bones composing a synovial joint are lined with articular cartilage and are held together by ligaments. The joint capsules are lined by a synovial membrane responsible for the secretion of synovia, a lubricating fluid containing mucin, albumin, fat, and mineral salts.

IMAGING CONSIDERATIONS

When one examines a skeletal radiograph, it is important to begin by properly orienting the film and recognizing the radiographic projection. The radiographic exposure technique selected can be very important in achieving a proper diagnosis. Proper technique is achieved when the soft tissues and bony structures of interest are both visible. Any motion of the part in question impairs the visibility of detail present.

Soft tissue areas often hold clues to the diagnosis and should be examined. Any signs of muscle wasting, soft tissue swelling, calcifications, opaque foreign bodies, or the presence of gas may indicate disease. Any analysis of the configuration of the bone and its relationship to other bones serves to detect or exclude fractures, dislocations, congenital anomalies, or acquired deformities.

The interface between cortical (compact) bone and soft tissue is also important. Any periosteal new bone formation seen may be a response to trauma, tumors, or infection. Juxtaarticular erosions are often seen in cases of arthritis. Cortical reabsorption can be demonstrated as smudgy, irregular loss of the cortical margin. In addition, the internal bone structure is important and should be examined for abnormally altered texture, alterations in the amount of mineralization, or foci of destruction. Careful consideration of all areas mentioned assists the physician in achieving the correct diagnosis.

CONGENITAL/HEREDITARY DISEASES
Osteogenesis Imperfecta

Osteogenesis imperfecta is a serious, autosomal dominant, congenital disease affecting the newborn skeletal system. Because of the abnormal fragility of their bones, infants afflicted with this disease are born with multiple fractures that heal but only lead to new fractures (Fig. 2-5). This results in limb deformities and may lead to dwarfism. This rare condition tends to improve after childhood. In some cases, however, a hearing disorder persists because of abnormal connective tissue around the auditory ossicles.

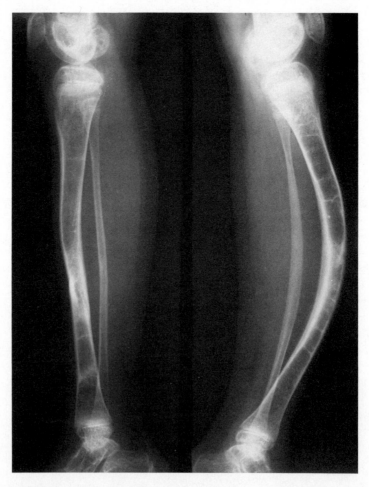

Fig. 2-5. Tibia/fibula radiograph demonstrating bowed lower extremities resulting from osteogenesis imperfecta tarda. This condition was recognized shortly after the child began to walk. (Courtesy of The American College of Radiology, Reston, Virginia.)

Achondroplasia

The most common inherited disorder affecting the skeletal system resulting in bone malformation and dwarfism is *achondroplasia*. The cartilage located in the epiphyses of the long bones does not convert to bone in the normal manner, thus patients with this type of osteochondrodysplasia present with a normal trunk size and shortened extremities (Fig. 2-6). Additional clinical manifestations of this disorder include extreme lumbar spine lordosis, bow legs, and a bulky forehead. Occasionally, orthopedic surgery may be necessary in management of complications associated with achondroplasia. In addition, these patients may receive genetic and social counseling.

Osteopetrosis

Osteopetrosis and ''marble bone'' are terms used to characterize a variety of disorders involving an increase in bone density and defective bone contour, often referred to as

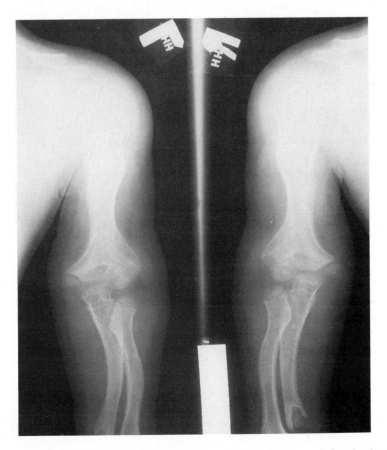

Fig. 2-6. Radiographs of shortened upper extremities caused by a defect in the endochondral bone formation associated with achondroplasia. (Courtesy of The American College of Radiology, Reston, Virginia.)

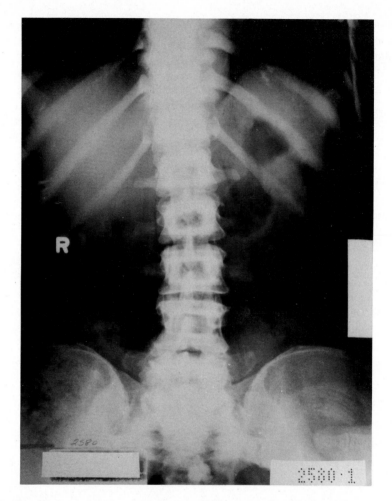

Fig. 2-7. An AP lumbar spine radiograph demonstrating uniform sclerosis of the bone associated with osteopetrosis. (Courtesy of The American College of Radiology, Reston, Virginia)

skeletal modeling. These disorders include osteoscleroses, craniotubular (affecting the cranium and tubular long bones) dysplasias, and craniotubular hyperostoses. It is important for the technologist to be aware that both the osteosclerotic and craniotubular hyperostotic disorders require an increase in exposure factors to adequately penetrate the bony anatomy because of abnormal bone density (Fig. 2-7). In some cases, adequate radiographic density may never be achieved.

Albers-Schönberg disease is a fairly common form of osteosclerotic osteopetrosis. This benign skeletal anomaly involves increased bone density in conjunction with fairly normal bone contour. In fact, many patients afflicted with Albers-Schönberg disease are asymptomatic and it is often discovered after radiographing the patient for an unrelated problem. Although this is a hereditary disorder, the bone sclerosis is not radiographically visible at birth. As the individual ages, radiographic manifestations of the osteopetrosis become visible, especially in the region of the cranium and spine, however general health is unimpaired.

Craniotubular dysplasias are a group of hereditary diseases mainly resulting in abnormal or defective bone contour of the cranium and long bones. Radiographs are useful in demonstrating this alteration in contour, scleroses, and changes within the cortical bone. Craniotubular hyperostoses include a variety of fairly rare hereditary diseases causing both an increase in bone density and abnormal bone modeling. Both of these craniotubular anomalies present in childhood. Although these disorders do not normally impair the individual's general health, bony overgrowth may entrap cranial nerves, resulting in some dysfunction such as facial palsy and/or deafness.

Hand and Foot Malformations

A variety of abnormalities of the fingers and toes may occur during fetal development but can be surgically corrected at birth. Failure of the fingers or toes to separate is called *syndactyly* and gives the physical appearance of webbed digits. *Polydactyly* (Fig. 2-8, p. 18) refers to the presence of extra digits.

Clubfoot (talipes) is a congenital malformation of the foot that prevents normal weight-bearing. The foot is most commonly turned inward at the ankle. This congenital malformation is more common in males than in females and may occur bilaterally. It is generally corrected by casting or splinting the foot in correct anatomical position.

Congenital Dislocation of the Hip

A malformation of the acetabulum often results in *congenital hip dislocations*. Since the acetabulum does not completely form, the head of the femur is displaced superiorly and posteriorly (Fig. 2-9, p. 18). Many times, the ligaments and tendons responsible for proper placement of the femoral head are also affected. Congenital dislocations of the hip occur more frequently in females than in males. This anomaly is most commonly treated with immobilization through casting or splinting the affected hip.

Vertebral Anomalies

Scoliosis refers to an abnormal lateral curvature of the spine (Fig. 2-10, p. 19), and although this is a hereditary disorder, it does not generally become visually apparent until adolescence. Scoliosis tends to affect females more frequently than males, and radiography is important in the diagnosis and treatment of this disorder. The lateral curves are usually convex to the right in the thoracic region and to the left in the lumbar region of the spine. Radiographic evaluation requires initial anteroposterior (AP) or posteroanterior (PA) and lateral standing radiographs with follow-up radiographs on a fairly routine basis. Good radiation protection techniques are vital because of the large size of the exposure field, the young age of the patient, and the frequency of the examinations. Special attention is necessary in shielding the breasts of young, female patients during radiographic examination throughout the treatment process. Scoliosis may be corrected surgi-

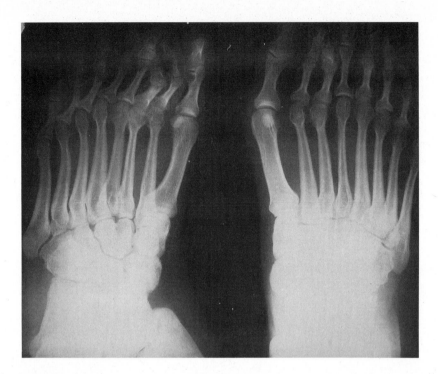

Fig. 2-8. A foot radiograph demonstrating additional digits associated with familial poly-dactyly. (Courtesy of The American College of Radiology, Reston, Virginia.)

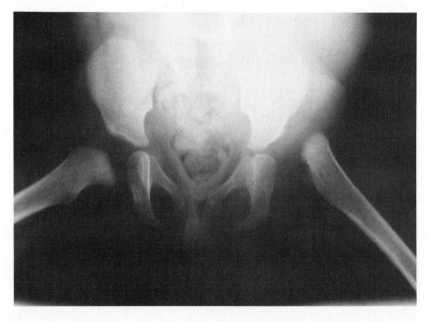

Fig. 2-9. A frog leg lateral projection of the pelvis on an infant demonstrating congenital dislocation of the left hip. (Courtesy of The American College of Radiology, Reston, Virginia.)

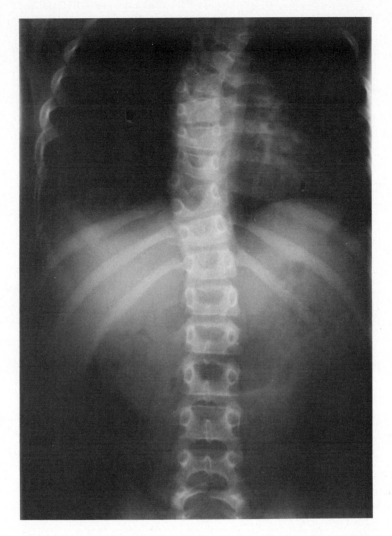

Fig. 2-10. An AP spine radiograph of a child with congenital scoliosis. (Courtesy of The American College of Radiology, Reston, Virginia.)

cally or by placing the individual in a brace or body cast. Treatment depends on the site of the deformity and the severity of the curvature.

A *transitional vertebra* is one that takes on the characteristics of both vertebrae on each side of a major division of the spine. Most frequently, such vertebrae occur at the junction between the thoracic and lumbar spine, or the junction between the lumbar spine and sacrum. The first lumbar vertebra may have rudimentary ribs articulating with the transverse processes (Fig. 2-11), as may the seventh cervical vertebra. A cervical rib may

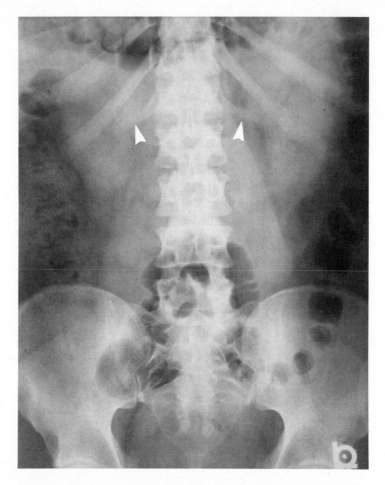

Fig. 2-11. An AP lumbar spine radiograph demonstrating bilateral lumbar ribs. (Courtesy of Riverside Methodist Hospitals, Columbus, Ohio.)

exert pressure on the brachial nerve plexus or the subclavian artery, requiring surgical removal of the rib.

Spina bifida is an incomplete closure of the vertebral canal, which is particularly common in the lumbosacral area (Fig. 2-12). Frequently, such patients have no visible abnormality or neurologic deficit, but failure of bony fusion of the two laminae is visible radiographically (spina bifida occulta). In more severe cases, the spinal cord or nerve root may be involved, which results in varying degrees of paralysis. Treatment of spina bifida is determined based on the extent of the anomaly and requires the services of a variety of physicians.

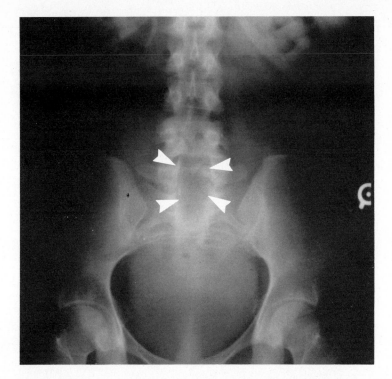

Fig. 2-12. An abdominal radiograph of a patient with spina bifida occulta of the lower lumbar vertebrae. (Courtesy of Riverside Methodist Hospitals, Columbus, Ohio.)

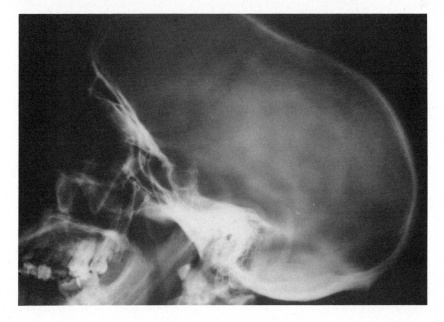

Fig. 2-13. A lateral skull radiograph demonstrating premature closure of the sagittal suture. This results in dolichocephaly and prominent convolutional markings caused by the increased intracranial pressure. (Courtesy of The American College of Radiology, Reston, Virginia.)

Cranial Anomalies

The premature or early closure of any of the cranial stutures is called *craniosynostoses*. This congenital anomaly causes an overgrowth of the unfused sutures to allow the brain to grow, thus altering the shape of the head (Fig. 2-13, p. 21). Although this defect may be corrected with surgery, brain damage may occur.

Anencephaly is a congenital abnormality in which the brain and cranial vault do not form (Fig. 2-14). In most cases only the facial bones are formed. This abnormality results in death shortly after birth and may be diagnosed before birth by both diagnostic medical sonography and radiography.

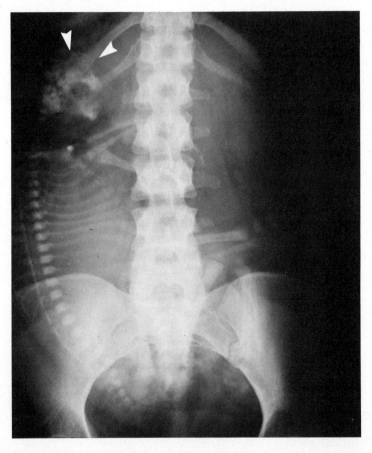

Fig. 2-14. An abdominal radiograph of a pregnant female carrying a fetus with anencephaly. Notice the lack of the cerebral cranial bones. (Courtesy of Riverside Methodist Hospitals, Columbus, Ohio.)

INFLAMMATORY DISEASE
Osteomyelitis

Osteomyelitis is an infection of the bone and bone marrow, most often caused by staphylococcus delivered via the bloodstream. It may, however, result from direct infection such as might occur with an open fracture. In the former case, infants and children are generally affected because of their lowered resistance in combination with the virulence of the organism. Generally, the osteomyelitis develops at the ends of the long bones of the lower limbs in adults and the metaphysis in children.

The acute stage of osteomyelitis is characterized by the formation of an abscess leading to an inflammatory reaction within the bone that causes a rise in internal bone pressure. Because of the constriction of periosteum, blood vessels compress and thrombose, leading to bone necrosis within 24 to 48 hours. Unfortunately, it is not until about 14 days that new periosteal bone repair is evident radiographically to indicate the presence of the disease. Therefore it is imperative that the condition is recognized clinically and treated with antibiotics and local drainage.

Initially, radiographs may demonstrate soft tissue swelling in the area around the affected bone (Fig. 2-15, p. 24). Follow-up radiographs may be performed 10 to 14 days after medical treatment to aid in the diagnosis.

With the effective use of antibiotics, osteomyelitis seldom passes the acute stage. Chronic osteomyelitis is characterized by extensive bone destruction with irregular, sclerotic reaction throughout the bone. A *sequestrum* is the essentially dead, devascularized bone that appears very dense. An *involucrum* is a shell of new supporting bone laid down by the periosteum around the sequestrum. An accurate diagnosis is extremely important in helping to distinguish osteomyelitis from a neoplastic bone disease.

Radiography is not a very sensitive means of diagnosing the condition because a fair amount of destruction must occur before the changes of osteomyelitis are visible radiographically. Nuclear medicine bone-scan studies are much more sensitive and will demonstrate the bone destruction as a "hot spot" on the final image. In addition, magnetic resonance imaging (MRI) now has a significant role in detection of osteomyelitis.

Tuberculosis

Tuberculosis of the bone is a chronic inflammatory disease that affects the ends of long bones or the spine. Radiographically the ends of the long bones display a "worm-eaten" appearance, with the disease slowly destroying the epiphyses, spreading to the articular cartilage, and in some cases infecting the joint space (Fig. 2-16, p. 25). Tuberculosis of the spine is also called Pott's disease. It destroys the spine, causing softening and eventual collapse of the vertebrae, which results in paravertebral abscess formation and exerts abnormal pressure on the spinal cord.

Arthritis

Joint inflammation is known as *arthritis* and may be caused by a variety of etiologic factors. An accurate clinical history is of extreme importance because different types of arthritis are characterized by specific features. It is important to identify the number of joints involved, the location of the joints involved, and the presence of another disease

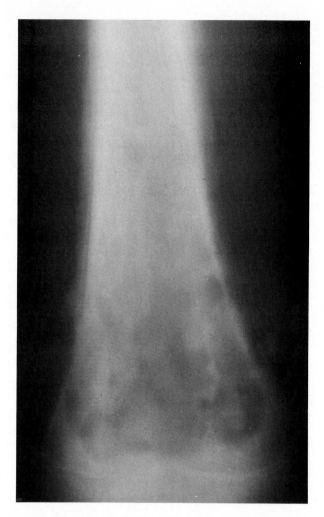

Fig. 2-15. A tomogram of a right knee demonstrating acute osteomyelitis of the femur. The 12-year-old female complained of swelling and pain. (Courtesy of The American College of Radiology, Reston, Virginia.)

process. Some types of arthritis involve several joints, but others involve only one joint. In addition, certain types of arthritis have a predilection for specific joints while sparing others. Finally, some types of arthritis are associated with specific disease processes caused by a host of factors such as bacteria or autoimmune response. Arthritis may be further classified as acute or chronic; the most common forms are chronic and disabling.

   Acute Arthritis. Acute arthritis is commonly called *pyogenic arthritis* and it is caused by a variety of factors including staphylococci, streptococci, and gonococci. Common clinical symptoms of acute arthritis are pain, redness, and swelling of the

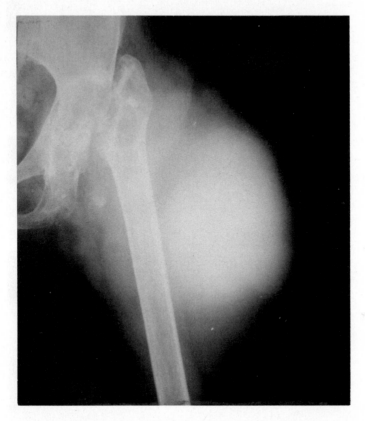

Fig. 2-16. A hip radiograph of a 47-year-old male with extensive destruction of the femoral head and neck caused by tuberculosis of the hip with a cold abscess. (Courtesy of The American College of Radiology, Reston, Virginia.)

affected joint, often accompanied by a fever. Generally the pyogenic or pus-forming organisms enter the body via a wound, as in the case of an open fracture, or the organisms may spread to the joint from a bone infected with osteomyelitis. Pyogenic arthritis usually responds rapidly to antibiotic therapy. The early radiographic changes demonstrate an increase in joint space, bony destruction, and joint dislocation. Radiographs obtained during the healing stage demonstrate recalcification and sclerosis, often resulting in joint ankylosis.

Rheumatoid Arthritis. *Rheumatoid arthritis* may fluctuate in severity and is thought to be an autoimmune disease. It usually occurs between the ages of 30 to 40 years and is three times more common in females than in males. Symptoms include pain, swelling, and stiffness of the affected joint with periods of activity or exacerbations and remissions of the disease process. Rheumatoid arthritis is a systemic disease of connective tissue characterized by chronic inflammation and overgrowth of the synovial tissues. As

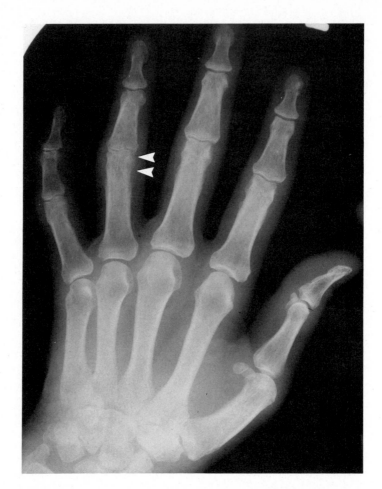

Fig. 2-17. A hand radiograph demonstrating soft tissue joint swelling associated with early rheumatoid arthritis. (Courtesy of The American College of Radiology, Reston, Virginia.)

the synovial tissues proliferate, they progressively destroy the cartilage, bone, and the supporting structures. In addition, blood chemistry analysis will identify the presence of an autoantibody against gamma globulin, also known as the serologic rheumatoid factor.

While any joint may be involved, rheumatoid arthritis typically begins in the peripheral joints, particularly in the small bones of the hands and feet. The radiographic changes seen early in this disease are soft tissue swelling and osteoporosis of the affected bones (Fig. 2-17). As the disease progresses, cortical erosion with joint space narrowing occurs because of the overgrowth of synovial tissue into the articular spaces. This severe damage makes the joint unstable and leads to deformity caused by displacement of the bones. The late changes of this condition can be quite severe, resulting in bone and cartilage de-

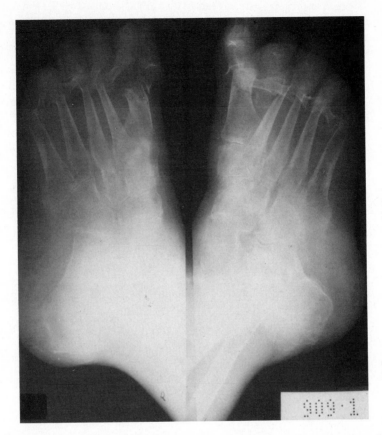

Fig. 2-18. Radiographs of a foot demonstrating subluxations at the metatarsophalangeal joints resulting from late rheumatoid arthritis. (Courtesy of The American College of Radiology, Reston, Virginia.)

struction and subluxation or dislocation of the involved joint (Fig. 2-18). Eventually the joints become ankylosed (fused), which requires surgical intervention. Surgical procedures such as synovium excision, dislocation corrections, joint reconstructions, and prosthetic joint replacements may be performed to improve joint function (Fig. 2-19, p. 28).

Ankylosing Spondylitis. *Ankylosing spondylitis* is a progressive form of arthritis mainly involving the spine. It tends to affect males between the ages of 10 to 30 years. Early radiographic changes demonstrate bilateral narrowing and fuzziness of the sacroiliac joints. Eventually the sacroiliac joints become obliterated and the condition progresses up the spine. Later radiographic changes show calcification of the bones of the spine with ossification of the vertebral ligaments. The articular cartilage is destroyed and fibrous adhesions develop. These adhesions lead to bone fusion and calcification of the annulus fibrosis of the intervertebral disks and the anterior and lateral spinal ligaments. The spine becomes a rigid block of bone, giving the condition its characteristic nickname of ''bamboo spine'' (Figs. 2-20 and 2-21, pp. 29 and 30).

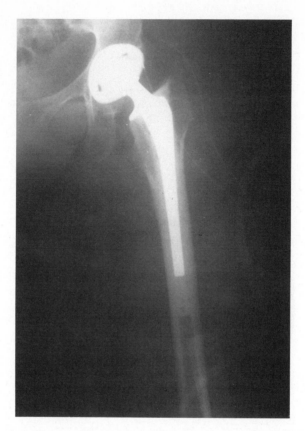

Fig. 2-19. A portable radiograph of a left hip demonstrating proper placement of a prosthetic hip replacement. (Courtesy of The Ohio State University Hospitals, Columbus, Ohio.)

Osteoarthritis. The most common type of arthritis is *osteoarthritis,* also known as degenerative joint disease. It affects males and females equally and results from a non-inflammatory deterioration of the joint cartilage that occurs with the normal ''wear and tear'' of aging. It may also be secondary to bone stress associated with trauma. Osteoarthritis generally affects the large, weight-bearing joints of the body (Fig. 2-22, p. 31) or the interphalangeal joints of the fingers. In joints afflicted with this disease, the articular cartilage degenerates and is gradually worn away, exposing the underlying bone. Radiographically this loss of articular cartilage appears as a narrowing of the joint space. An overgrowth of articular cartilage occurs on the peripheral surfaces of the joint and often calcifies, which results in *osteophytes* or bone spurs that are visible radiographically (Fig. 2-23, p. 31). In terms of radiographic diagnosis, the formation of osteophytes helps to distinguish osteoarthritis from other types of arthritis.

Clinically, an individual with osteoarthritis presents with pain and progressive stiffening of the affected joint. Treatment consists of surgical prosthetic joint replacement, which greatly relieves the pain and allows a return of joint mobility.

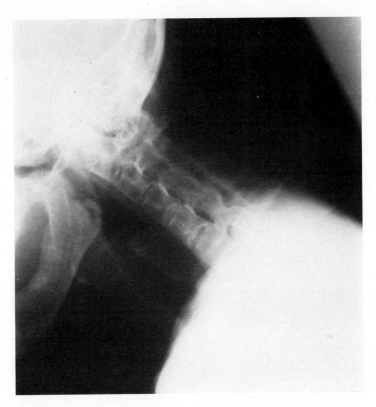

Fig. 2-20. A lateral cervical spine radiograph depicting ankylosing spondylitis with granulation tissue beneath the anterior longitudinal ligament destroying the corners of the contiguous vertebra. (Courtesy of The American College of Radiology, Reston, Virginia.)

Inflammation of Associated Joint Structures. The specialized connective tissues that attach muscle to bone are called *tendons*. They are enclosed in a sheath that is susceptible to inflammation. Inflammation of the tendon sheath is called *tenosynovitis* and it may spread to the associated tendon, resulting in *tendinitis*. *Bursae* are sacs lined with a synovial membrane and they are found in locations where tendons pass over bony prominences. If the bursa becomes inflamed, it is called *bursitis*. Inflammation of these associated structures may be caused by acute or chronic trauma, acute or chronic infection, inflammatory arthritis, gout, and rarely by pyogenic or tuberculous organisms. These inflammatory conditions are characterized by pain, localized tenderness, and limited motion of the involved joint. In cases of chronic bursitis, the walls of the bursa become thickened and calcium deposits may be visible radiographically within the bursa (Fig. 2-24, p. 32). Chronic tendinitis may also cause the formation of calcium deposits in either the affected tendon or associated sheath. These calcium deposits that form in the shoulder joint as a result of chronic trauma often cause rotator cuff tears, which can be detected on shoulder arthrogram and magnetic resonance examinations of the shoulder.

Text continued on page 32.

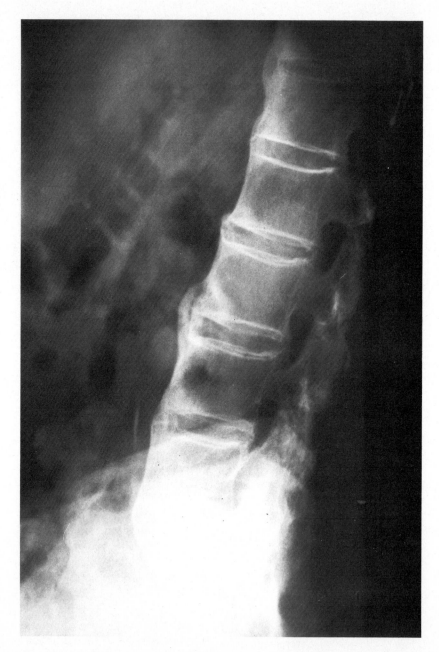

Fig. 2-21. A lateral lumbar spine radiograph on a 64-year-old male with ankylosing spondylitis. Notice the fusion of the vertebrae into a solid block of bone. (Courtesy of The Ohio State University Hospitals, Columbus, Ohio.)

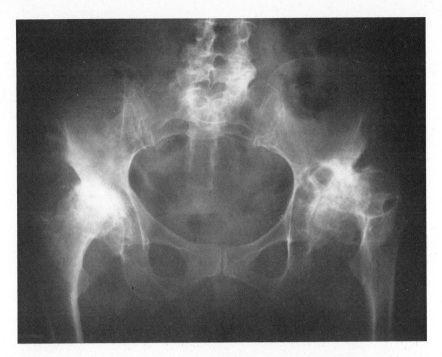

Fig. 2-22. A radiograph of the pelvis demonstrating osteoarthritis of the hip secondary to congenital subluxation. This 68-year-old female had a history of painful hips and limping. (Courtesy of The American College of Radiology, Reston, Virginia.)

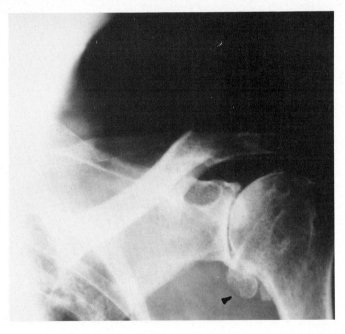

Fig. 2-23. A shoulder radiograph demonstrating the formation of an osteophyte at the inferior lip of the glenoid labrum due to primary osteoarthritis. (Courtesy of The American College of Radiology, Reston, Virginia.)

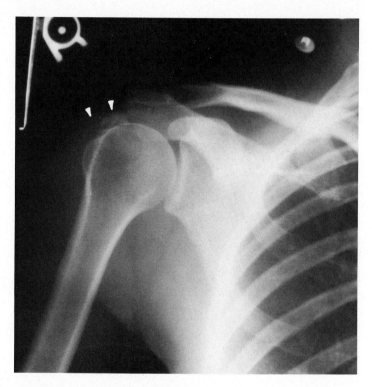

Fig. 2-24. A shoulder radiograph demonstrating radiopaque calcium deposits within the bursa caused by chronic bursitis. (Courtesy of Riverside Methodist Hospitals, Columbus, Ohio.)

Common medical treatment of bursitis and tendinitis include nonsteroidal antiinflammatory agents in combination with analgesics. In severe cases, corticosteroid injections may be used. In cases in which the tendons or bursae ossify, surgical intervention is necessary, especially in conjunction with rotator cuff tears.

Gouty Arthritis. *Gouty arthritis* is an inherited metabolic disorder in which excess amounts of uric acid are produced and deposited in the joint and adjacent bone. The condition occurs more frequently in males and most commonly affects the metatarsophalangeal joint of the great toe. It is characterized by acute attacks with intervals of remission.

The crystallization of uric acid within the joint causes an acute inflammatory reaction. Large masses of these sodium urate crystalline deposits are called *tophi*. Bony changes include erosion (Fig. 2-25) with overhanging edges. One long-term complication of gout is the formation of radiolucent kidney stones caused by increased excretion of uric acid by the kidneys. Treatment of gout consists of medications to either promote excretion of uric acid by the kidneys or to inhibit the production of uric acid within the body.

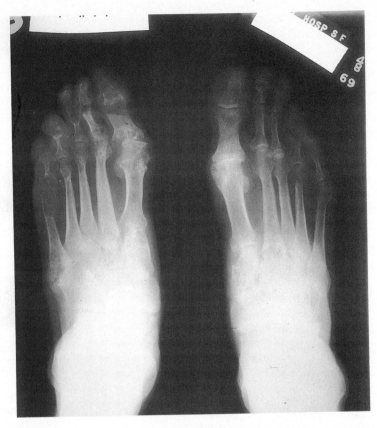

Fig. 2-25. Bilateral feet demonstrate multiple erosions of the bone, some associated with soft-tissue tophi, as consistent with gout. Asymetry of these lesions helps distinguish them from rheumatoid arthritis. (Courtesy of The American College of Radiology, Reston, Virginia.)

METABOLIC DISEASE
Osteoporosis

A prime determinant of radiographic film density is the amount of calcium present in the bone structure. *Osteoporosis* is an increasingly known metabolic bone disorder common in women past menopause. The disease is characterized by an abnormal decrease in bone density caused by failure of osteoblasts to lay down bony protein matrix. The normal equilibrium associated with osteoid production and withdrawal is quite complicated and depends on a combination of dietary intake and absorption, hormonal interplay, and normal stress or muscular activity. In postmenopausal women, for example, the lack of hormone estrogen creates a weakened bony matrix, contributing to the development of "porous" bones. As this condition becomes more severe, these bones are subject to compression fractures as they can literally "cave in" from the weakness. The bony changes caused by osteoporosis are best demonstrated in the spine (Fig. 2-26), where decreased bone density stands out clearly against the bony cortex. This condition requires a decrease in exposure technique.

Osteoporosis is by far the most common form of metabolic bone disease and can be differentiated from osteomalacia by examining serum enzyme levels. Patients with osteoporosis have normal serum enzyme levels whereas patients with osteomalacia present with a decrease in serum phosphorus. Treatment generally includes an increase in dietary intake of calcium, vitamin D, and sex hormone supplements.

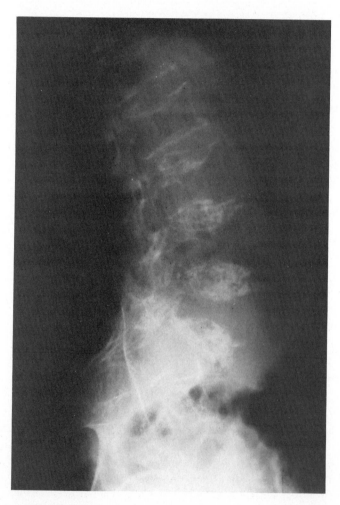

Fig. 2-26. A lateral lumbar spine radiograph of an elderly female who complained of back pain. The radiograph revealed severe osteoporosis with compression fractures of the vertebrae. (Courtesy of Riverside Methodist Hospitals, Columbus, Ohio.)

Osteomalacia

Osteomalacia is a condition caused by a lack of calcium in the tissues and a failure of bone tissue to calcify. This normally results from an inadequate intake or absorption of calcium, phosphorus, or vitamin D. With this condition, the bones remain spongelike, resembling osteoporosis in radiographic appearance. Laboratory analysis and other testing is necessary to differentiate the diagnosis. If osteomalacia occurs before growth plate closure, it is known as *rickets* (Fig. 2-27). Proper nutritional education is vital to populations susceptible to osteomalacia because adequate calcium, phosphorus, and vitamin D intake can prevent or frequently cure this disorder.

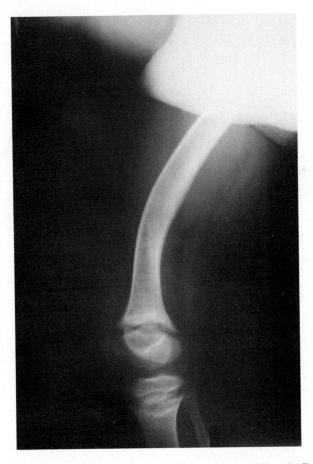

Fig. 2-27. A radiograph of a femur of a child diagnosed with Vitamin-D resistant rickets. Notice the bowing of the extremity. (Courtesy of The American College of Radiology, Reston, Virginia.)

Paget's Disease (Osteitis deformans)

Paget's disease is a metabolic disorder of unknown etiology that is fairly common in the elderly population, affecting males twice as frequently as females. This disease process may affect one or more bones, most commonly involving the pelvis, spine, skull (Fig. 2-28) and the long bones (Fig. 2-29). Paget's disease is characterized by two stages in which the bone undergoes continuous destruction, called the *osteolytic stage* and simultaneous replacement by abnormally soft and poorly mineralized material, called the *osteoblastic stage*. The osteoid material that replaces the normal bone tissue is very bulky and porous with exceptional vascularity. Although this osteoid matrix is thicker than the normal bone, its softness often leads to weight-bearing, stress-induced deformities and fractures. As the skull enlarges, additional complications may occur because of impingement of the cranial nerves. These complications include hearing and vision disturbances. In addition, individuals with Paget's disease have an increased risk of developing osteogenic sarcoma, a malignant neoplastic disease of the skeletal system. Radionuclide bone

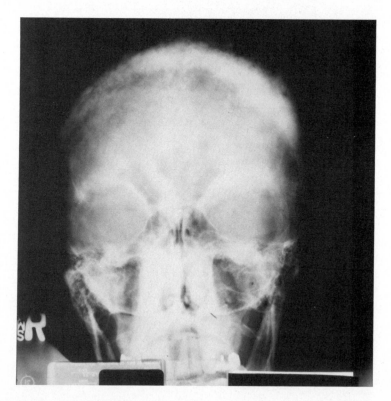

Fig. 2-28. A PA skull radiograph depicting an advanced proliferative phase of Paget's disease. Notice the changes within the inner and outer tables of the skull. (Courtesy of The American College of Radiology, Reston, Virginia.)

scans readily detect Paget's disease, even in its very early stages. Radiographically, the affected bones typically demonstrate cortical thickening with a coarse, thickened trabecular pattern. Mixed areas of radiolucent osteolysis and radiopaque osteosclerosis may be seen. Blood chemistry results indicate very high alkaline phosphatase levels with normal serum calcium and phosphorus. There is no known cure for this disease. If the bone lesions are asymptomatic, no treatment is necessary. In symptomatic cases medications are administered to decrease bone resorption.

Hyperparathyroidism

Hyperparathyroidism is a fairly common disease of the endocrine system, but it will be discussed in this chapter because of its affect on the skeletal system. This disease is often very mild and may go undetected for a long period of time. Remember that the skeletal system is involved in the balance of serum calcium and phosphorus levels and that the body strives to keep this ratio constant. Hyperparathyroidism applies to any disorder that

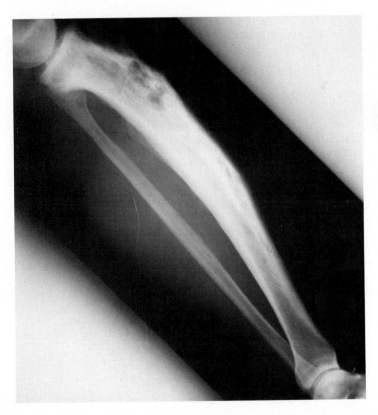

Fig. 2-29. A radiograph of the tibia on the same patient as in Fig. 2.28 demonstrating the effect of advanced proliferative Paget's disease on the tibia. (Courtesy of The American College of Radiology, Reston, Virginia.)

disrupts the calcium-phosphate ratio and results in an elevated level of parathyroid hormone (PTH). Excess PTH secretion overstimulates the osteoclasts that are responsible for
bone removal, thus leading to bone destruction. This osteoclastic activity results in a
decreased bone density, so a decrease in radiographic exposure is necessary to produce a
quality radiographic image.

There are basically three types of hyperparathyroidism: primary hyperparathyroidism, secondary hyperparathyroidism, and a third type caused by ectopic production of
a parathyroid-like hormone. Treatment varies with each specific cause of hyperparathyroidism and is very complex.

Primary hyperparathyroidism arises from an adenoma, carcinoma, or hyperplasia of
the parathyroid gland and may be treated surgically. The excess production of PTH causes

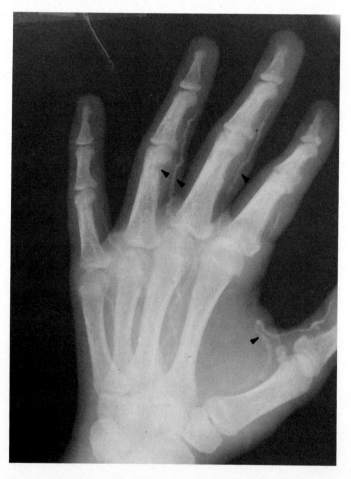

Fig. 2-30. A hand radiograph of an individual with secondary hyperparathyroidism. Notice the subperiosteal resorption of bone and calcification of the arteries of the hand.
(Courtesy of The American College of Radiology, Reston, Virginia.)

bone destruction, an increased absorption of calcium by the intestines and kidneys, and an increase in urine calcium, which predisposes the individual to renal stones. The net effect of these reactions to the high level of PTH is an increase in serum calcium with a decrease in serum phosphate. Individuals affected with primary hyperparathyroidism may first present with symptoms of renal colic, but radiographic investigation demonstrates sub-periosteal bone resorption, especially in the diaphyses of the phalanges and clavicles. Bone resorption is also radiographically evident in the teeth.

Secondary hyperparathyroidism (Fig. 2-30) represents a response to hypocalcemia, hyperphosphatemia, or hypomagnesemia. It is caused by a very complex metabolic dis-order that is beyond the scope of this text and is most commonly seen in individuals with chronic renal disease. Decreased renal function leads to a loss of the kidney's ability to produce vitamin D and compromises their ability to excrete phosphate.

Acromegaly

Although *acromegaly* is an endocrine disorder caused by a disturbance of the pituitary gland, it is also briefly mentioned in this chapter because of its effect on the skeletal system. This disorder is caused by excessive secretion of growth hormones in the adult, which is often due to a pituitary adenoma. Acromegaly is a slowly progressive disease that may be diagnosed years after the individual is symptomatic. An increase in growth hormone in the adult produces a thickening and coarsening of the bones because the epiphyses have closed and the bone cannot grow in length. Radiographic studies dem-onstrate an enlarged sella turcica and changes in the skull, often obliterating the diploe found between the inner and outer tables of the cortical bone. Individuals with acromegaly present with a prominent forehead and jaw, widened teeth, abnormally large, spade-like hands (Fig. 2-31, p. 40), and a coarsening of facial features (Fig. 2-32, p. 41). This disorder is frequently treated with a combination of surgery and radiation therapy used to eradicate the adenoma.

TRAUMATIC DISEASE
Fractures

General radiography is extremely important in the evaluation of skeletal trauma and serves several purposes. The most obvious of these is to diagnose the presence of a fracture or dislocation. If a fracture is present, for example, a determination can be made as to whether the underlying bone is normal or whether the fracture is pathologic in nature. Before the fracture is stabilized, radiographs are taken to show the position of the bone ends. Post-reduction films indicate the success of the fracture reduction. Finally, subsequent radio-graphs are taken to assess healing and any possible complications of fractures.

In any case of trauma it is essential to have at least two projections of the part, preferably taken at right angles to one another. A minimum of two projections is also necessary to adequately determine fracture alignment. These radiographs should demon-strate the joint above and below the area of trauma because there may be dislocation, and because the injury may transfer force to a point distal or proximal to the point of injury. An example of this would be a fracture or dislocation of the fibular head concurrent with an ankle or distal tibial fracture.

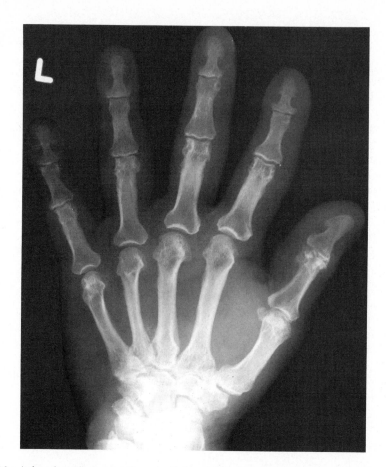

Fig. 2-31. A hand radiograph of an individual diagnosed with acromegaly. Notice the spade-like appearance of the hand. (Courtesy of The American College of Radiology, Reston, Virginia.)

Frequently, fractures are obvious by clinical examination, but radiographic changes in appearance may be subtle. Fractures usually appear as a radiolucent line, but they may be thin and easily overlooked. Occasionally a fracture appears as a radiopaque line if the fragments overlap. A step in the cortex, as indicated by a break in the normal bony contour, is a second radiographic indication. Other signs include interruption of the bony trabeculae, bulging or buckling of the cortex, soft tissue swelling, and/or joint effusion.

Skeletal trauma usually causes significant soft tissue injuries, including neurovascular damage, capsular and ligamentous tears, cartilage injury, and hemoarthroses. Such injury may be assessed in several ways. Stress radiographs on a joint determine ligamentous stability. Radiographs of both extremities are often used to compare epiphyseal appearance. Arteriography may also be used to assess any vascular damage occurring as a result of skeletal trauma.

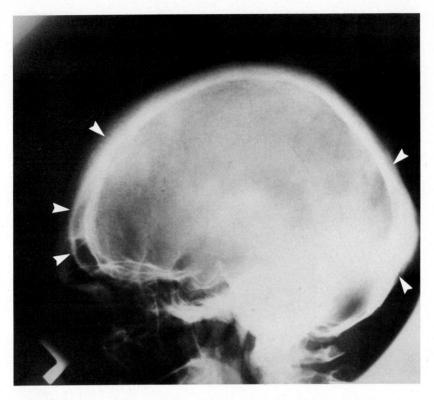

Fig. 2-32. A skull radiograph depicting the changes caused by acromegaly. (Courtesy of The American College of Radiology, Reston, Virginia.)

When performing radiography of the skeletal system, it is critical for the technologist to choose the appropriate exposure factors and film/screen combination to produce a radiograph demonstrating good soft tissue definition in addition to achieving good penetration of the bony anatomy. If the soft tissue is too dark or the associated bony anatomy too light (i.e., no trabecular pattern), then the radiograph is of compromised diagnostic quality.

A *fracture* is a discontinuity of bone caused by mechanical forces either applied to the bone or transmitted directly along the line of a bone. When a fracture occurs, blood vessels are broken as a result of the break in the endosteum and periosteum. As blood, and lymph and tissue fluids infiltrate this area, swelling and pain result.

Initially the break in the bone is filled by a large clot that temporarily bridges the fracture. Within 2 to 3 days osteoblasts begin to slowly appear around the injured bone. Immobilization of the injured site is critical because any unnatural movement interferes with the deposition of the calcified matrix necessary for permanent union of the fracture. *Provisional callus* is mainly composed of cartilage and begins to form approximately 1

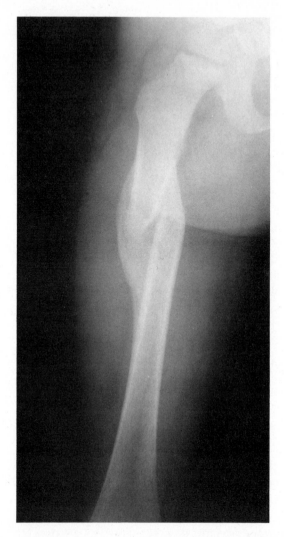

Fig. 2-33. A femoral radiograph demonstrating advanced callus formation following a transverse fracture of the femur. (Courtesy of The American College of Radiology, Reston, Virginia.)

week after the fracture. As calcium continues to be deposited within the provisional callus, it is replaced by *bony callus* (Fig. 2-33), which is responsible for rigidly uniting the fracture site. Although the break is rigidly united within 4 to 6 weeks, excess bone still encircles the external fracture site and excess bone is still found within the marrow space at this time. Remodeling of the bone and total healing requires months. Weight-bearing force on the fracture site tends to guide the modeling process, so in many cases the patient may be instructed to begin using the affected limb in a limited fashion at this point in the healing process. If everything goes well during the healing process, the bone may repair to the point that the fracture site is no longer visible on subsequent radiographs. Proper healing greatly depends on the initial immobilization (casting, splinting, pinning, or plating), proper alignment or reduction of the fracture, and proper metabolic activity, which includes good vascularity and blood supply, proper nutrition, and normal hormone levels. Bacterial infections of the fracture site may inhibit callus formation, thus complicating the healing process.

Delayed union is a term referring to a fracture that does not heal within the usual amount of time. If a fracture is not reduced properly or is not properly immobilized, malunion may occur. *Malunion* refers to a fracture that heals in a faulty position, thus impairing the normal function or cosmetic appearance of the affected body part. The most serious complication is nonunion. *Nonunion* refers to a fracture in which healing does not occur and the fragments do not join. This is often due to lack of vascularization. Injuries to other soft tissue structures or organs can be associated with skeletal fractures, such as a rib fracture that penetrates the lung and results in a pneumothorax. Additional complications of skeletal fractures include muscular ossification and fat emboli occurring in bones containing yellow bone marrow.

Fracture Classifications. Several means of classifying fractures exist. One distinction is whether the fracture is open or closed. An *open* fracture is one in which the bone has penetrated the skin. This type of fracture leaves an open route for bacteria to enter from outside the body, which may lead to possible infection. As described earlier, the intrusion of bacteria can alter the healing process and precautions must be taken to prevent infection from setting into the bone or surrounding soft tissue structures. A *closed* fracture is one in which the skin is not penetrated, thus reducing the chance of infection.

Fractures may be classified according to the mechanics of stress that produce the break or the appearance of the fracture line. This includes torsion (twisting), transverse, linear, and spiral fractures. When one of the fractured bone ends is jammed into the cancellous tissue of another fragment, it is called an *impacted* fracture (Fig. 2-34, p. 44).

Fractures may also be classified according to their location such as intertrochanteric (transcervical), supracondylar, or transcondylar fractures. Often they may not fit into a specific classification because they may demonstrate mixed features. The following pages discuss the appearance of common types of fractures.

Comminuted Fractures. Sometimes one or more fragments separate along the edges of the major fragment, in addition to the major line of the fracture. Such fractures are said to be *comminuted* (Fig. 2-35, p. 45). Comminuted fractures differ from multiple fractures as follows. In the case of a multiple fracture, each fracture is complete, leaving a fragment of intact shaft between them. Comminuted fractures do not represent a complete thickness of bone as do multiple fractures. Occasionally, the bone involved in a comminuted fracture may be extensively shattered, as might occur from a gunshot wound. Such fractures are also particularly apt to be compound.

A *butterfly fracture* is a comminuted fracture in which there are one or two butterfly wing or wedge-shaped fragments split off from the main fragments. A *splintered fracture* is a comminuted fracture with long, sharp-pointed fragments.

Complete, Noncomminuted Fractures. *Complete, noncomminuted fractures* are those in which the bone has separated into two fragments. The fractures may be recognized according to the direction of the fracture line. A *spiral* or *oblique fracture* is an

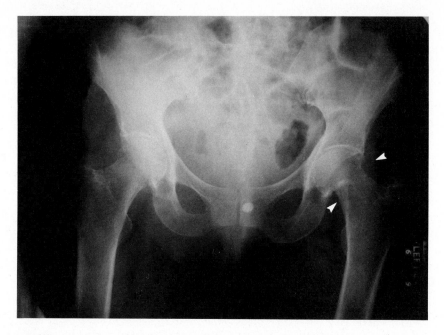

Fig. 2-34. A pelvis radiograph on an elderly female with trauma to her left hip. The radiograph demonstrates an impacted fracture of the left hip. (Courtesy of The American College of Radiology, Reston, Virginia.)

example of this type. Such a fracture usually results from a rotary-type injury that twists the bone apart and is particularly common in the shafts of long bones (Fig. 2-36, p. 46). A *transverse fracture* (Fig. 2-37, p. 47) is another type of complete, noncomminuted fracture. Demonstrated radiographically, such a fracture through normal bone is invariably ragged along the fracture line. A *pathologic fracture* is commonly a transverse fracture occurring in abnormal bone that is weakened by various diseases (Fig. 2-38, p. 48). It may result from the disease process itself or from a relatively minor trauma. Often, pathologic fractures may be the first indication of the presence of pathology. *Multiple fractures* are another type of complete, noncomminuted fracture in which two or more complete fractures occur involving the shaft of a single bone (Fig. 2-39, p. 49).

Avulsion Fractures. *Avulsion fractures* occur when a fragment of bone is pulled away from the shaft. These usually occur around joints because of ligament, tendon, and muscle tearing, as associated with a sprain or dislocation (Fig. 2-40, p. 49). A *chip fracture* is an avulsion fracture of a small fragment or chip of bone from the corner of a phalynx or other long bone. These are very common in the fingers and are often very tiny.

Incomplete Fractures. *Incomplete fractures* are those in which only part of the bony structure gives way, with little or no displacement. A common example of this is the *greenstick fracture,* in which the cortex breaks on one side without separation or breaking of the opposing cortex (Fig. 2-41, p. 50). The effect is similar to that of trying to break

Text continued on page 51.

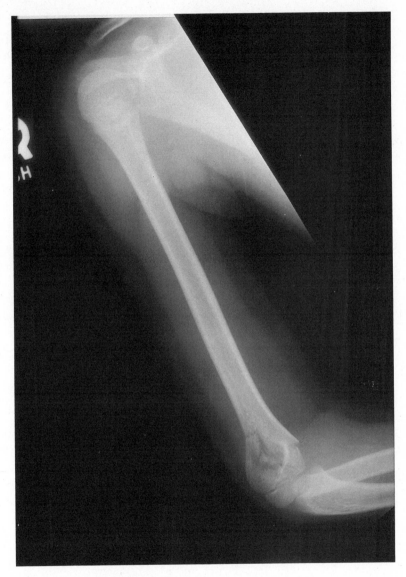

Fig. 2-35. A humerus radiograph on an individual in a motor vehicle accident. The radiograph revealed a comminuted fracture of the humerus. (Courtesy of Riverside Methodist Hospitals, Columbus, Ohio.)

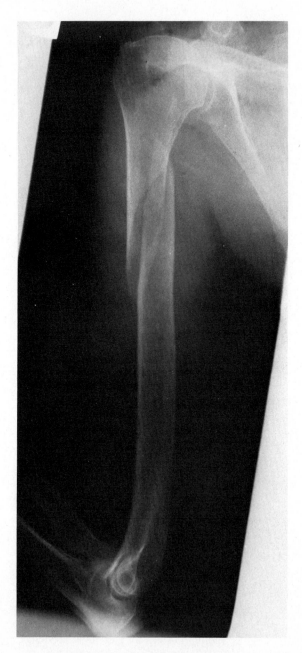

Fig. 2-36. A humerus radiograph of an individual who sustained a twisting injury of the humerus. The radiograph demonstrates a spiral fracture of the humerus. (Courtesy of Riverside Methodist Hospitals, Columbus, Ohio.)

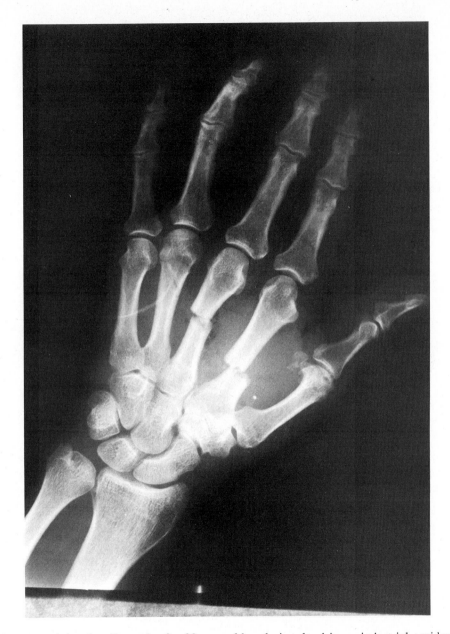

Fig. 2-37. A hand radiograph of a 32-year-old male involved in an industrial accident, demonstrating transverse fractures of the second and third metacarpals. (Courtesy of Riverside Methodist Hospitals, Columbus, Ohio.)

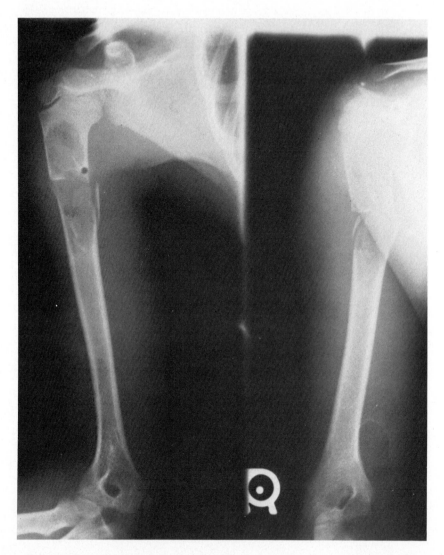

Fig. 2-38. A humerus radiograph demonstrating a pathologic fracture through a bone cyst. The patient had complained of pain and denied a history of trauma associated with this fracture. (Courtesy of Riverside Methodist Hospitals, Columbus, Ohio.)

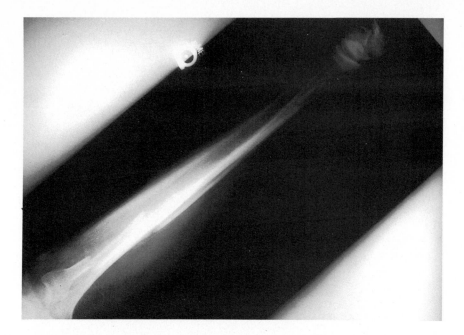

Fig. 2-39. A forearm radiograph of an individual involved in a motor vehicle accident. The radiograph revaled multiple fractures of the forearm. (Courtesy of Riverside Methodist Hospitals, Columbus, Ohio.)

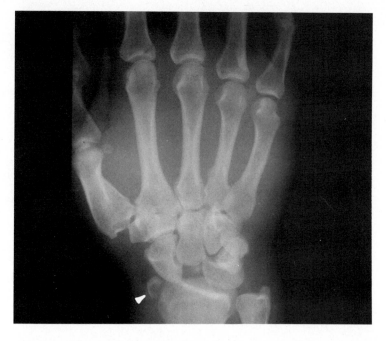

Fig. 2-40. A wrist radiograph obtained following trauma to the wrist resulting in perilunate dislocation with an associated avulsion fracture of the distal radius. (Courtesy of The American College of Radiology, Reston, Virginia.)

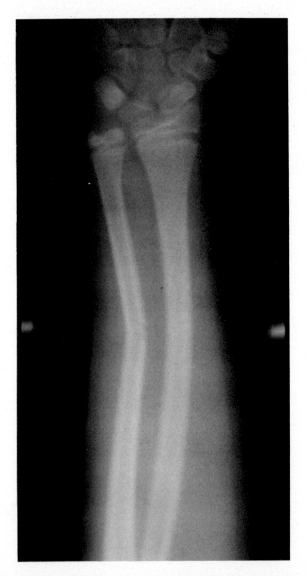

Fig. 2-41. A forearm radiograph of a child who sustained a fall demonstrating a greenstick fracture of the middle portion of the ulna. Notice the incomplete break of the cortex of the ulna. (Courtesy of Riverside Methodist Hospitals, Columbus, Ohio.)

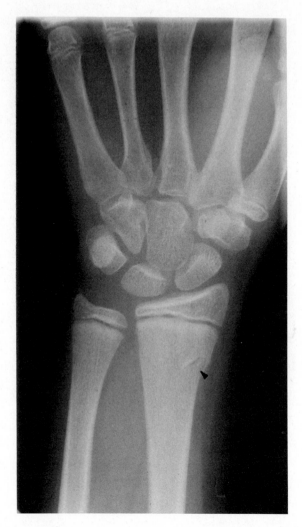

Fig. 2-42. A forearm radiograph of a 14-year-old female who fell on her hand, resulting in a torus fracture of the distal radius. (Courtesy of The American College of Radiology, Reston, Virginia.)

a green twig, hence its name. Greenstick fractures are found almost exclusively in infants and children because of the softness of the cancellous bone. A *torus fracture* is a greenstick fracture in which the cortex folds back upon itself, producing only a slight irregularity (Fig. 2-42).

Incomplete fractures may also occur in demineralized bone, such as occurs with osteoporosis. The bone in question breaks only partway through, resulting in a sharp angular deformity without displacement.

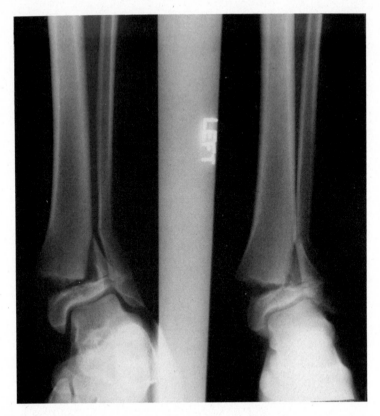

Fig. 2-43. A lower leg radiograph demonstrating an epiphyseal-metaphyseal fracture of the tibia with a transverse diaphysieal fracture of the distal fibula. (Courtesy of The American College of Radiology, Reston, Virginia.)

Penetrating fractures are a type of incomplete fracture resulting from penetration by a sharp object such as a bullet or a knife. Frequently there is a comminution at the site of the injury.

Growth Plate Fractures. *Growth plate fractures* are those that involve the end of a long bone of a child (Fig. 2-43). The fracture may be limited to growth plate cartilage, and is thus not directly visible unless displacement occurs, or it may extend into the metaphysis, epiphysis, or both. Crush injuries of the growth plate can also occur. Comparison projections are often used with such fractures to compare growth plate appearances. Healed injuries of this type may result in an alteration of the length of the involved bone.

Stress and Fatigue Fractures. *Stress fractures* are fractures that usually occur as a result of a strong, violent force. They are generally found at the point of muscular attachments such as in the fibula of a runner. Stress fractures may not be clearly visible on plain radiographs but may be diagnosed with radionuclide bone scans of the affected area. *Fatigue fractures* occur at sites of maximal strain on a bone, usually in connection

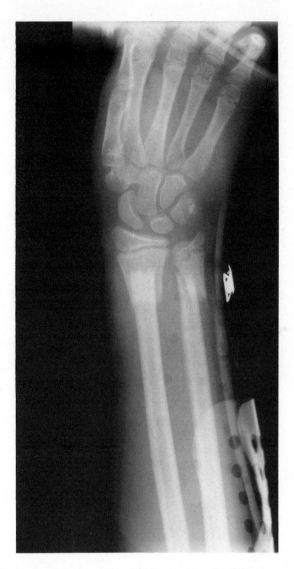

Fig. 2-44. A radiograph of a wrist on an elderly woman who fell on an outstretched hand. The radiograph demonstrates a classic Colle's fracture. (Courtesy of Riverside Methodist Hospitals, Columbus, Ohio.)

with unaccustomed activity. Most frequently fatigue fractures are found in the metatarsals, particularly the second metatarsal. Other common names for fatigue fractures include march, stretch, or insufficiency fractures.

Fractures Classified According to Location. Some fractures occur in selected areas and are usually easily recognized. One of these is the *Colle's fracture* (Fig. 2-44), which is a fracture through the distal one-inch of the radius. The distal fragment is usually

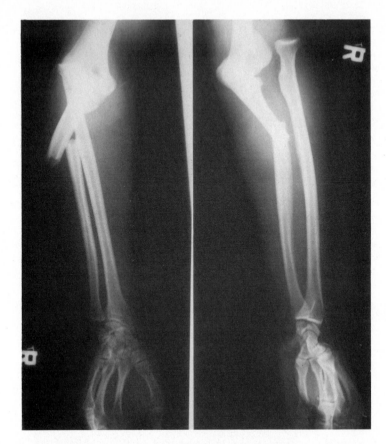

Fig. 2-45. A forearm radiograph of an individual who fell off a cliff, landing on an outstretched hand with the elbow partially flexed. The radiograph demonstrates a Monteggia fracture of the forearm. (Courtesy of The American College of Radiology, Reston, Virginia.)

angled backward on the shaft with impaction along the dorsal aspect. An avulsion fracture of the ulnar styloid process is also a frequent occurrence. This is the most common wrist fracture, and it usually results from falling on an outstretched hand. A *Smith's fracture* is a reverse Colle's fracture with displacement toward the palmar aspect of the hand.

A *Boxer's fracture* occurs when the fifth metacarpal fractures as a result of a blow to or with the hand. A *Monteggia fracture* is one of the proximal third of the ulnar shaft, with anterior dislocation of the radial head (Fig. 2-45). A *Pott's fracture* involves both malleoli, with dislocation of the ankle joint (Fig. 2-46).

As mentioned earlier, radiographic signs of some fractures are subtle at best. Such is sometimes the case with the elbow. The elbow "*fat pad sign*" (Fig. 2-47, p. 56) can be an indicator of a nonvisualized, underlying fracture of the bones of the elbow. In the

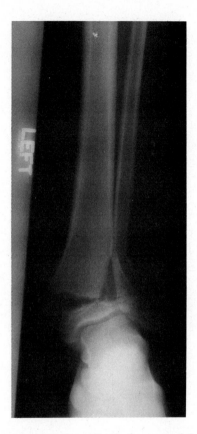

Fig. 2-46. An ankle radiograph depicting a Pott's fracture of the ankle demonstrated by a dislocation of the joint with a fracture of both malleoli. (Courtesy of Riverside Methodist Hospitals, Columbus, Ohio.)

elbow, there is normally a small accumulation of fat adjacent to the anterior surface of the distal humerus. This radiolucency is normally visible radiographically. A similar pad is found along the posterior surface but is normally not visualized radiographically. If the joint capsule is distended by fluid as a result of a fracture, the posterior fat pad becomes displaced from the bone and is visible on the lateral projection of the elbow. Visualization of a posterior fat pad is considered to be a sign of a possible underlying fracture. The anterior fat pad may also be displaced, giving a sail-shaped appearance. This is a prime example of how soft tissue demonstration can assist in making a diagnosis.

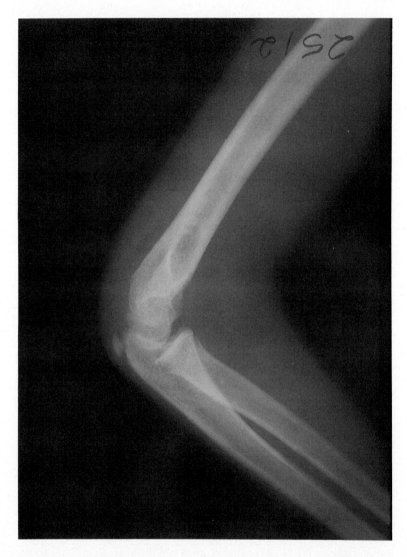

Fig. 2-47. Lateral elbow radiograph demonstrates the fat pad sign associated with a radial head fracture.   (Courtesy of Riverside Methodist Hospitals, Columbus, Ohio.)

Cerebral Cranial Fractures. Vascular markings in the skull, either venous or arterial, are routinely demonstrated as linear translucencies and can occasionally be mistaken for fractures (Fig. 2-48). In most cases a fracture will appear more translucent than a vascular marking because a fracture will traverse the full thickness of the skull. Although the edges of the fractures may branch abruptly, they can be seen to fit together, whereas venous channels have irregular edges that cannot be fitted together. The sutures between the individual cranial bones remain visible radiographically, even after they become fused. To an untrained eye, these sutures may also resemble a fracture.

In most cases the location of the skull fracture is more important than the extent of the fracture. If the fracture crosses an artery, an arterial bleed may occur, resulting in an epidural hematoma. A fracture that enters the mastoid air cells or a sinus communicates with a potentially infected space, which would allow the contamination to spread throughout the cranium, possibly resulting in encephalitis or meningitis.

Fractures visible after skull trauma are generally classified as either linear, depressed, or basilar skull fractures. *Linear fractures* appear as straight, sharply defined, nonbranch-

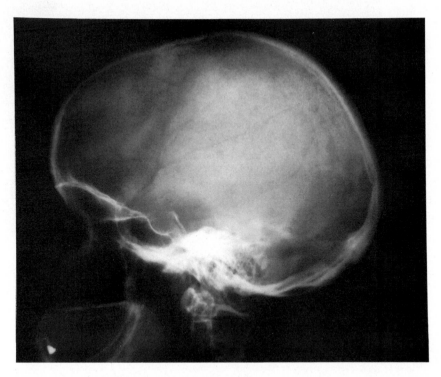

Fig. 2-48. A lateral skull radiograph demonstrating normal vascular markings within the cerebral cranium. (Courtesy of The American College of Radiology, Reston, Virginia.)

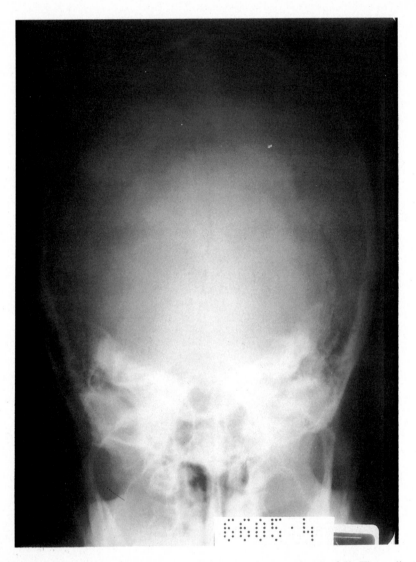

Fig. 2-49. A Towne skull radiograph of a small child who sustained a fall. The radiograph reveals a linear skull fracture of the parietal bone. (Courtesy of Riverside Methodist Hospitals, Columbus, Ohio.)

ing lines and are intensely radiolucent (Fig. 2-49). A *depressed fracture* appears as a curvilinear density because the fracture edges are overlapped (Fig. 2-50). This type of fracture may cause injury to the cerebral cortex and bleeding into the subarachnoid space. A depressed fracture is best demonstrated when the X-ray beam is directed tangential to the fracture.

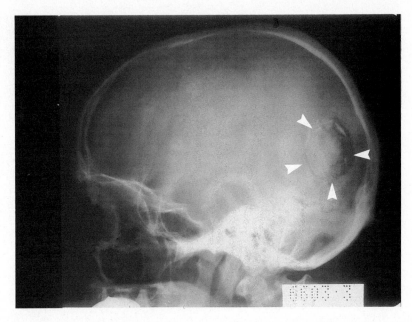

Fig. 2-50. A lateral skull radiograph of a child who was struck in the head with a baseball bat. The radiograph demonstrates a depressed fracture of the frontal bone. (Courtesy of Riverside Methodist Hospitals, Columbus, Ohio.)

Basilar skull fractures are very difficult to demonstrate radiographically. Air-fluid levels in the sphenoid sinus and/or clouding of the mastoid air cells are often the only radiographic finding suggesting a fracture. Therefore it is important to include a cross-table lateral skull radiograph with the trauma skull radiographic series.

Visceral Cranial Fractures. Injury to the soft tissues of the eyes, nose, and mandible is often accompanied by bony fractures. Facial bone fractures generally result from a blow to the face. In addition, facial and/or head trauma may indicate a possible cervical spine fracture.

A zygomatic arch fracture may be difficult to recognize initially because of the edema. However, a fracture may be indicated by clinical signs, which include black eyes, flattening of the cheek, and/or a restriction of the movement of the mandible.

Careful examination by palpation is performed by the physician because a fracture of the zygomatic arch may be present without accompanying facial fractures. A depressed fracture of the zygomatic arch may also be difficult to demonstrate radiographically (Fig. 2-51, p. 60). An oblique submentovertical projection may be used to best demonstrate the extent of the fracture.

A parieto-acanthial (Water's method) is also of value in examining the fractures of the zygomatic arch.

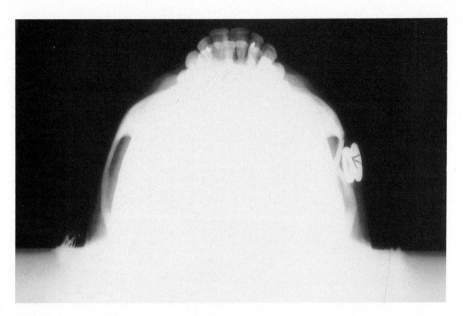

Fig. 2-51. A submentovertical projection of the zygomatic arch demonstrating a depressed fracture of the zygomatic arch resulting from a direct blow to the left cheek. (Courtesy of The Ohio State University Hospitals, Columbus, Ohio.)

The mandible is very prone to fracture because of the prominence of the chin, therefore any patient suffering a head or face injury should be clinically examined for a mandibular fracture. Anatomically the mandible is strongest at the center and weakest at the ends with the most common site for fracture at the angle (31%) followed by the condyles (18%). Mandibular fractures (Fig. 2-52), are generally detected by the patient's inability to open the mouth and pain when moving the mandible. These fractures also cause a misalignment of the patient's teeth. Care must be taken to demonstrate all areas of the mandible (body, ramus, and symphysis) when ruling out mandibular fractures.

Fractures of the maxilla are serious because of the adjacent nasal cavity, paranasal sinuses, orbit, and close proximity of the brain. The maxilla also transmits cranial nerves and major blood vessels. Maxillary fractures may be divided into three major classifications: horizontal, pyramidal, and transverse. A *horizontal* fracture of the maxilla (LeFort I) refers to a separation of the body of the maxilla from the base of the skull above the palate and below the zygomatic process. This type of fracture results in a freely movable jaw. A *pyramidal* fracture (LeFort II) involves vertical fractures through the maxilla at the malar and nasal bones forming a triangular shaped separation of the maxilla. A *transverse* fracture (LeFort III) is the most extensive and serious type of maxillary fracture; it extends across the orbits and results in separation of the visceral and cerebral cranium.

A *blow-out fracture* results from a direct blow to the front of the orbit, thus transferring the force to the orbital walls and floor. This fracture occurs in the thinnest, weakest

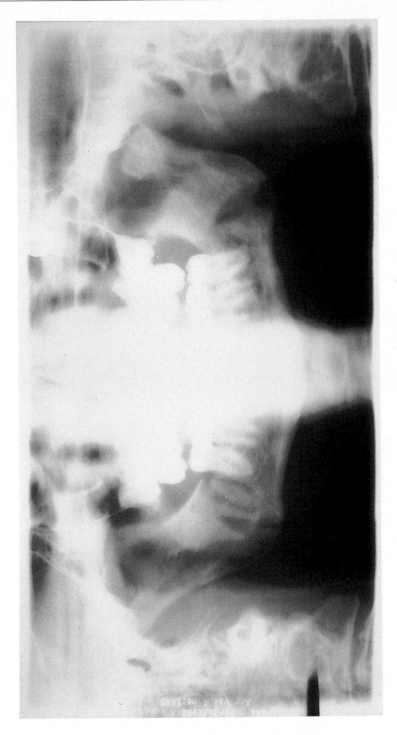

Fig. 2-52. A panoramic projection of the mandible demonstrating a fracture. (Courtesy of The Ohio State University Hospitals, Columbus, Ohio.)

portion of the orbit, i.e., the orbital floor just above the maxillary sinuses. If this condition is not diagnosed and treated, impairment of extraocular movements will develop. A parieto-acanthial projection (modified Water's method) provides the most information in the radiographic diagnosis of blow-out fractures (Fig. 2-53).

A *tripod fracture* occurs when the zygomatic or malar bone is fractured at all three sutures: frontal, temporal, and maxillary (Fig. 2-54). This fracture results in a free-floating zygoma and may cause facial disfigurement if not diagnosed and properly treated.

The most frequently fractured facial bone is the nasal bone. A nasal bone fracture may be accompanied by a fracture of the ascending process of the maxillae and/or the nasal septum, which is composed of the vomer and the perpendicular plate of the ethmoid bone. A nose bleed, or epistaxis, is usually present with a nasal bone fracture. Radiographs of nasal bone fractures are obtained in addition to a clinical examination to confirm a fracture. Lateral projections demonstrate anterior/posterior displacement, whereas a parieto-acanthial or intraoral projection demonstrates lateral/medial displacement of the bone fragments (Fig. 2-55).

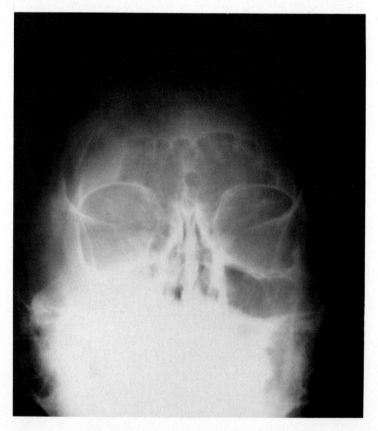

Fig. 2-53. A parieto-acanthial projection of the facial bones on an individual who sustained a direct blow to the left orbit from a racquetball. The radiograph demonstrates a blow-out fracture of the left orbit. (Courtesy of The Ohio State University Hospitals, Columbus, Ohio.)

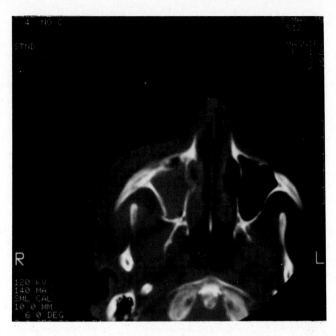

Fig. 2-54. A CT image demonstrating a tripod fracture of the right zygomatic bone. (Courtesy of Riverside Methodist Hospitals, Columbus, Ohio.)

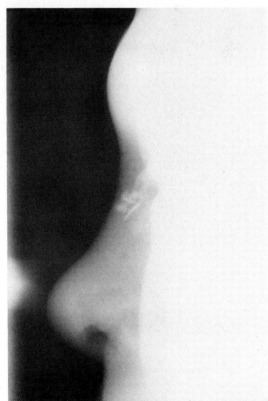

Fig. 2-55. A lateral nasal bone radiograph of a 20-year-old male who was struck in the face. The radiograph demonstrates a nasal bone fracture.(Courtesy of The Ohio State University Hospitals, Columbus, Ohio.)

Dislocations

Often a dislocation and a subluxation are considered synonymous. This is incorrect. A *dislocation* implies that a bone is out of its joint and not in contact with its normal articulation. A *subluxation* is a partial dislocation, often occurring with a fracture. The common sites of dislocations are the shoulder, hip, and acromioclavicular joint.

Shoulder joints most commonly dislocate anteriorly (Fig. 2-56). Such dislocations are readily detectable radiographically since the humeral head usually locates below the glenoid fossa and coracoid process. Posterior dislocations of the shoulder (Fig. 2-57) are more difficult to diagnose, as they may appear normal on an AP radiograph. A trans-scapular ("Y") projection is useful in locating the humeral head in this case.

With traumatic dislocation of the hip, the femoral head is most commonly displaced posteriorly to lie against the sciatic notch (Fig. 2-58). It may also displace anteriorly and lie adjacent to the pubis or obturator foramen. Congenital hip dislocations are usually unilateral and are recognized by a shortening of the extremity. If the condition is not recognized until the child begins to walk, conservative therapies may be replaced by surgical intervention.

Acromioclavicular joint separations (Fig. 2-59, p. 66) are more common with children than adults. The typical film sequence for this diagnosis involves radiographs taken with and without weights. A joint separation is assessed by determining the alignment between the acromial end of the clavicle and the acromion process of the scapula.

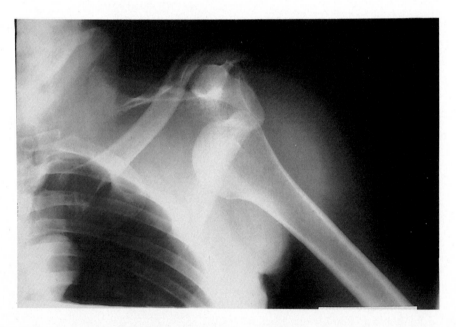

Fig. 2-56. A shoulder radiograph demonstrating an anterior dislocation of the humeral head. Note the location of the humeral head below the glenoid fossa and coracoid process. (Courtesy of Riverside Methodist Hospitals, Columbus, Ohio.)

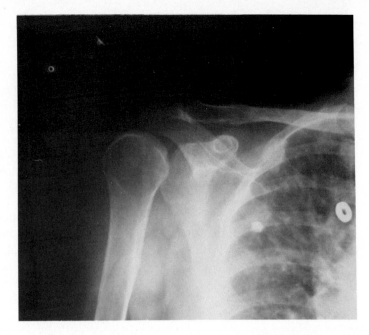

Fig. 2-57. A shoulder radiograph demonstrating a posterior dislocation of the humerus with the humeral head overlapping the rim of the glenoid fossa. The humeral head is also displaced slightly superolaterally. (Courtesy of The American College of Radiology, Reston, Virginia)

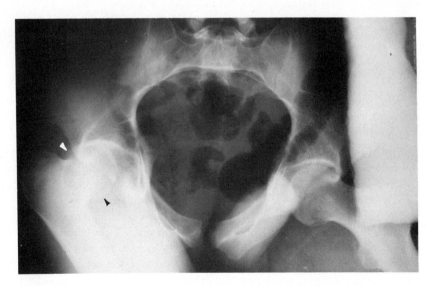

Fig. 2-58. A pelvis radiograph of a 25-year-old male whose right knee struck the dashboard in a motor vehicle accident resulting in a posterior dislocation of the right femoral head. (Courtesy of The American College of Radiology, Reston, Virginia.)

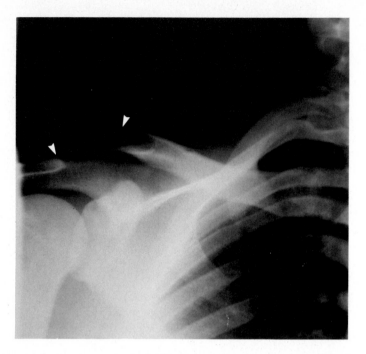

Fig. 2-59. A weight-bearing acromioclavicular radiograph demonstrating a dislocation as evidenced by uneven alignment of the acromial end of the clavicle and the acromion process of the scapula. (Courtesy of The Ohio State University Hospitals, Columbus, Ohio.)

Battered Child Syndrome

Battered child syndrome is a term associated with a physical form of child abuse. Physical child abuse often co-exists with both emotional and sexual abuse. This syndrome affects males and females equally; approximately 25% of cases involve children under the age of 2 years. In addition, about 20% of the children who survive physical abuse suffer permanent injuries. An accurate incidence of child abuse is difficult to ascertain, but statistics indicate that approximately 2000 deaths per year result from child abuse.

Physical signs of battered child syndrome include bruises, burns, abrasions, and fractures in various stages of healing. In most cases the explanation for the injury is inconsistent with the actual injury. Radiographic signs of child abuse include hematomas and single or multiple fractures of varying ages, especially in areas where it is difficult for the child to self-inflict the injury (Fig. 2-60). Often, fractures may indicate that an extremity has been twisted or turned until it breaks and/or multiple rib fractures indicating repeated traumatic injuries generally inflicted by a parent or guardian. All emergency room personnel should be familiar with signs of child abuse and are ethically required to report suspected cases of child abuse to the proper authorities.

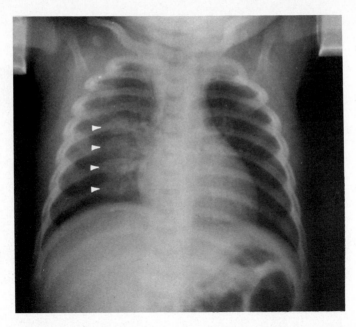

Fig. 2-60. A pediatric chest radiograph revealing numerous rib fractures with adjacent soft tissue masses resulting from hemorrhage surrounding the fracture sites. (Courtesy of The American College of Radiology, Reston, Virginia.)

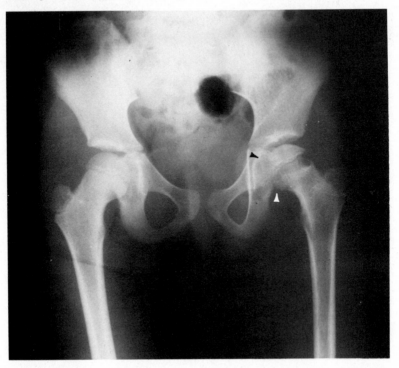

Fig. 2-61. An AP pelvis radiograph of a young male demonstrating Legg-Perthes disease of the left femoral head. Notice the asymmetry of the femoral heads. (Courtesy of The American College of Radiology, Reston, Virginia.)

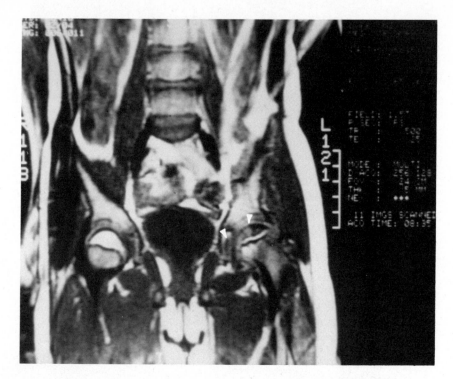

Fig. 2-62. An MRI of the same patient as depicted in Fig. 2-53. The image demonstrates a low signal intensity in the left femoral epiphysis consistent with Legg-Perthes disease. (Courtesy of The American College of Radiology, Reston, Virginia.)

Legg-Perthes Disease

Legg-Perthes disease is a term associated with ischemic necrosis of bone. Ischemia results from poor blood supply to the bone that leads to hypoxia. Ischemic necrosis of the bone affects the epiphyses and may be easily mistaken for tuberculosis of the skeletal system. The etiology of this disorder is unknown and the disease process is fairly quiet. Perthes refers specifically to ischemic necrosis of the head of the femur. It tends to occur in males between the ages of 5 to 10 years and often follows injury or trauma to the affected hip. Clinically these patients present with a limp that is accompanied by little or no pain. Radiographically the bone in the center of the epiphysis is fragmented and the head of the femur is flattened (Fig. 2-61). Magnetic resonance images normally demonstrate a low signal intensity from the affected hip in Legg-Perthes disease (Fig. 2-62).

VERTEBRAL COLUMN

The causes of vertebral column injuries include direct trauma, hyperextension-flexion injuries (whiplash), osteoporosis, or metastatic destruction. Radiographic indications of spinal column injuries include the interruption of smooth, continuous lines formed by the vertebrae stacking on each other (Fig. 2-63). Also, the vertebral bodies may lose some

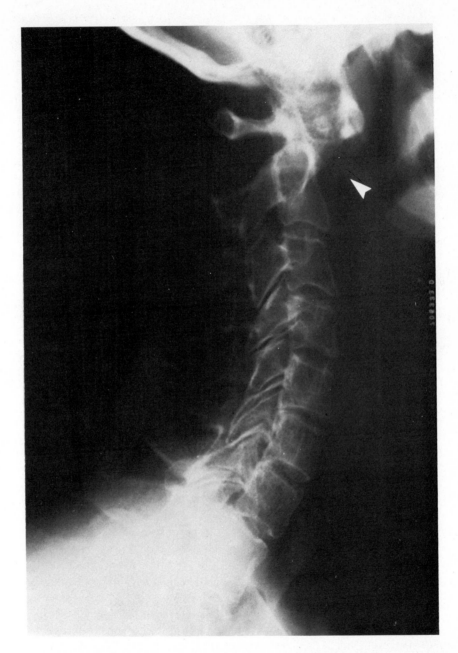

Fig. 2-63. A lateral cervical spine radiograph of an individual involved in a motor vehicle accident, demonstrating subluxation of the first and second cervical vertebrae as evidenced by the uneven alignment of the vertebral bodies. (Courtesy of The American College of Radiology, Reston, Virginia.)

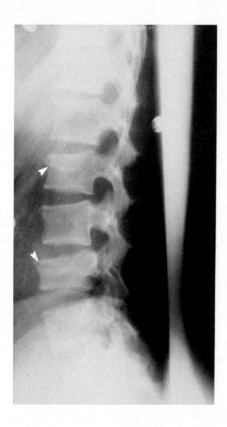

Fig. 2-64. A lateral lumbar radiograph demonstrating compression fractures of the second and fourth lumbar vertebral bodies with no apparent fracture of the posterior elements of the spine. (Courtesy of The American College of Radiology, Reston, Virginia.)

height, or the interspace may narrow. Muscle spasm as a result of trauma may cause a reversal or straightening of the normal spinal curvatures.

Perhaps the most common condition of the vertebral column is generalized back pain, typically in the lumbar area. Such back pain may not always result from bony involvement. Disk disease can cause muscle spasm with pain referral throughout the back. Finally, back pain may be secondary to referred pain from the hip.

Compression fractures are the most frequent type of injury involving a vertebral body. Usually the damage is limited to the upper portion of the vertebral body, particularly to the anterior margin. Such fractures generally occur in the thoracic and lumbar vertebrae (Fig. 2-64). Cervical spine injuries may involve the odontoid process, usually at the junction of the odontoid and the body of the second cervical vertebra. A *Hangman's fracture* is a fracture of the arch of the second cervical vertebra and is usually accompanied by anterior subluxation of the second cervical vertebra on the third cervical vertebra. A Hangman's fracture results from acute hyperextension of the head.

Spondylolysis exists when there is a cleft, or breaking down, of the body of a vertebra between the superior and inferior articular processes (pars interarticularis). Typically, this occurs in the arch of the fifth lumbar vertebra and appears radiographically as a "collar" or "broken neck" on the "Scotty dog" appearance and is demonstrated on an oblique projection of the lumbar spine (Fig. 2-65). When forward slippage of the vertebral column off a vertebra

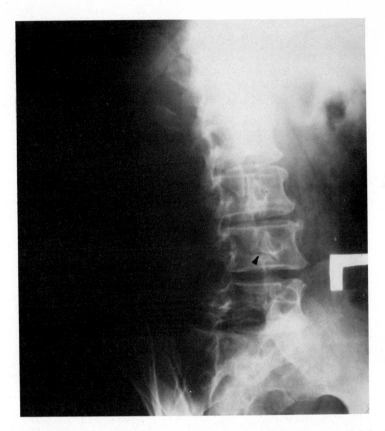

Fig. 2-65. An oblique radiograph of the lumbar spine demonstrating spondylolysis of the fourth and fifth lumbar spine on the left side. Notice the ''break in the scotty dog's neck.'' (Courtesy of The American College of Radiology, Reston, Virginia.)

occurs because of spondylolysis, it is known as *spondylolisthesis*. The patient with this condition may present symptoms identical to those of a herniated disk. Such slippage commonly occurs at the L5/S1 junction and is best detected on a lateral projection (Fig. 2-66, p. 72).

Radiography of the trauma patient with vertebral trauma is critical. Fractures and/or dislocations of the spine are classified as stable or unstable. The spine may be visualized as two columns, with the anterior column being composed of the vertebral bodies and intervertebral disks and the posterior column being composed of the posterior elements (e.g., spinous processes, lamina). If either the anterior column or the posterior column of the spine are fractured or dislocated, the injury is classified as stable. However, in cases in which both columns are involved in the injury, it is classified as unstable. In all cases, the patient should be immobilized until cross-table lateral radiographs have been obtained and cleared by a physician. To rule out possible fractures and/or dislocations, the lateral cervical spine radiograph must include all seven vertebrae in their entirety, including spinous processes and intervertebral disk spaces. At times this may require assistance in depressing the patient's shoulders or the use of the twining (swimmer's method) projection to clearly demonstrate the entire seventh cervical vertebra. A twining projection may also be necessary to demonstrate the upper thoracic vertebra in a lateral projection. Additional trauma projections of the cervical spine such as the pillar projection or trauma oblique projections may be requested to better demonstrate the complex anatomy of the spine.

Fractures and/or dislocations of the vertebrae may impinge on the spinal cord and cause significant damage. The responsibility of the technologist in terms of proper patient handling and obtainment of diagnostic quality images cannot be overemphasized. Often, tomography of the vertebral column may be used to better demonstrate vertebral anatomy. Computed tomography (CT) also plays a vital role in the diagnosis and treatment of vertebral fractures/dislocations and associated problems. CT of the spine may be used preoperatively to serve as a "road map" to the surgeon because this imaging modality clearly demonstrates the size, number, and location of various fracture fragments. CT may

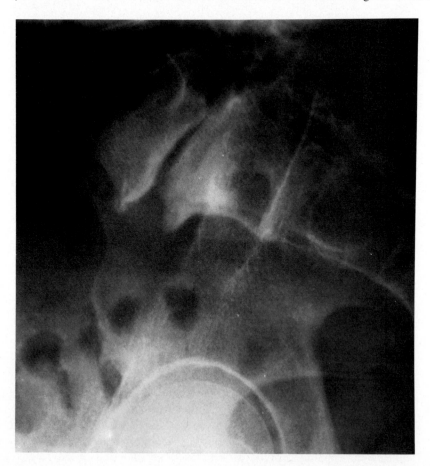

Fig. 2-66. An L5/S1 spot radiograph of a female complaining of low back pain, demonstrating spondylolisthesis of this joint. (Courtesy of Riverside Methodist Hospitals, Columbus, Ohio.)

also be used postoperatively to demonstrate the outcome of the surgery. There is still a role for conventional tomography in spinal fractures, especially with horizontal fractures. In certain situations, MRI may be used to evaluate the extent of ligamentatous and soft tissue injury and/or injury to the spinal cord.

NEOPLASTIC DISEASE

Many varieties of bone tumors exist and are seen in patients of all ages. The diagnosis of a bony abnormality is often made radiographically on the basis of the patient's age, pattern of bone destruction, the location of the tumor, and its position within the bone. For example, benign lesions often expand the bone and demonstrate sharp, sclerotic margins. Malignant neoplasms often infiltrate, permeate, and destroy anatomic margins.

Radiographic studies contribute greatly to the diagnosis and management of bone tumor patients. Plain films are used to disclose the lesions and show the growth characteristics that assist in determining their benign or malignant nature. In conjunction with conventional tomography and CT, plain radiographs identify malignant growth patterns and the proper site for biopsy. Sometimes, seemingly unrelated examinations, such as a barium enema or chest radiograph, are ordered by the physician to rule out distant metastases.

Osteochondroma (Exostosis)

The most common benign bone tumor is the *osteochondroma* (Fig. 2-67), which arises from the growth zone between the epiphysis and diaphysis of long bones, also called the meta-

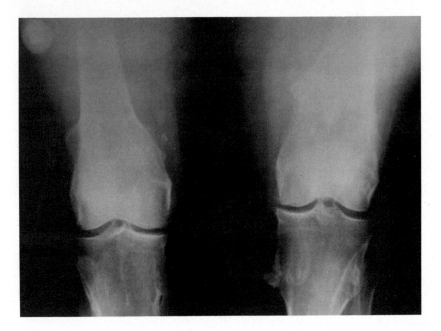

Fig. 2-67. Bilateral AP knee radiographs demonstrating osteochondroma with exostoses within the knee joint. (Courtesy of The American College of Radiology, Reston, Virginia.)

physis. Most commonly it involves the lower femur or upper tibia and is capped by growing cartilage. The cortex of an osteochondroma blends with the normal bone and the growth tends to protrude up and away from the nearest joint, most commonly the knee. Exostoses or excessive bone growth may appear as singular or multiple lesions and are normally diagnosed in childhood or adolescence. Multiple exostoses is believed to be a hereditary disorder and usually appears at an earlier age than does the single lesion osteochondroma. In addition, multiple exostoses may transform to malignant neoplasms such as chondrosarcoma. Many times osteochondromas are asymptomatic unless the affected long bone is traumatized, which results in a pathologic fracture of the diseased bone.

Osteoma

An *osteoma* is a fairly rare benign growth most commonly located in the skull. These lesions are composed of very dense, well-circumscribed, normal bone tissue that usually

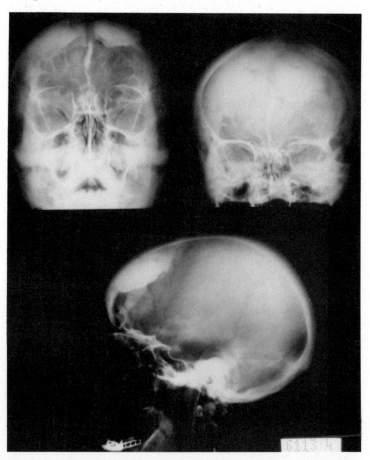

Fig. 2-68. Various skull projections demonstrating hyperostosis frontalis interna. (Courtesy of The American College of Radiology, Reston, Virginia.)

projects into the orbits or paranasal sinuses. Another term associated with osteoma of the skull is *hyperostosis frontalis interna* (Fig. 2-68).

Endochondroma

An *endochondroma* is a slow-growing benign tumor composed of cartilage. It grows in the marrow space and most commonly affects the small bones of the hands and feet in individuals between the ages of 10 and 30 years. These benign tumors do not invade the surrounding tissue as they grow; however, they do expand the cortical bone, causing thinning. Radiographically endochondromas appear as radiolucent lesions containing small, stippled calcifications (Fig. 2-69). The erosion of the cortex may cause pain and swelling and increase the incidence of pathologic fractures. Multiple growths, termed *endochondromatosis,* may also occur in childhood and, like multiple osteochondromas, may undergo malignant transformation.

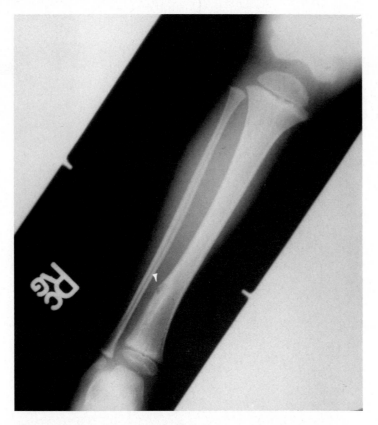

Fig. 2-69. An AP tibia/fibula radiograph demonstrating an endochondroma of the distal tibia as evidenced by small, scattered, well-defined, oval lucent defects. (Courtesy of The American College of Radiology, Reston, Virginia.)

Simple Bone Cyst

A *simple bone cyst* is a wall of fibrous tissue filled with fluid. These frequently occur in the long bones of children, most commonly in the humerus (Fig. 2-70) and knee. The cyst is usually first noticed when the patient presents with pain caused by the increased tumor growth or as a result of a pathologic fracture.

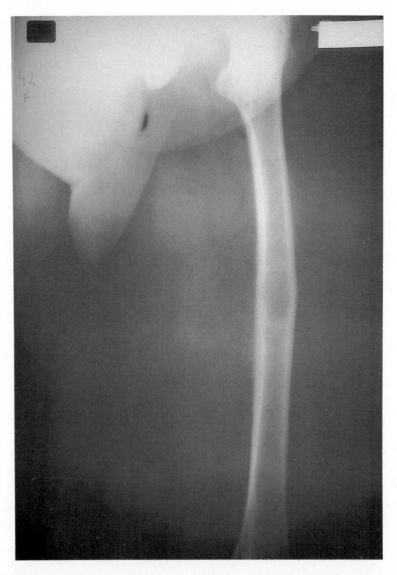

Fig. 2-70. An AP radiograph demonstrating a well-circumscribed radiolucency consistent with a simple bone cyst. (Courtesy of Riverside Methodist Hospitals, Columbus, Ohio.)

Radiographically, simple bone cysts appear radiolucent with well-defined margins from the normal bone surrounding the lesion. Occasionally, the cyst may be surrounded by a thin rim of sclerotic bone. Small cysts tend to heal and obliterate themselves; larger cysts require surgical intervention. The benign bone cyst is treated by surgical excision and packing with bone chips to obtain complete healing.

Osteoid Osteoma

Another common benign tumor of the skeletal system is the *osteoid osteoma*. These fibrous tumors occur twice as often in males compared with females and almost always develop before the age of 30 years. Osteoid osteomas are most commonly found in the femur, tibia, or spine of the young adult. They arise within the cortical bone and erode the underlying bone tissue, resulting in a lytic lesion called a *nidus*. The area of erosion is surrounded by a zone of dense, sclerotic bone, making the radiographic appearance of osteoid osteomas very distinctive (Fig. 2-71). In some cases, however, the rim of hyper-

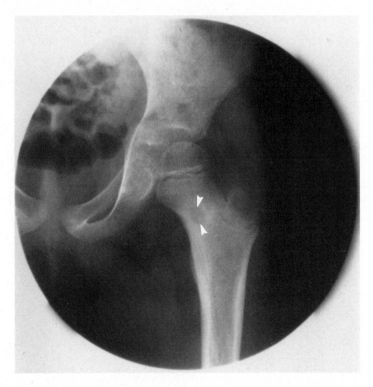

Fig. 2-71. An AP hip radiograph of a 7-year-old female who complained of a 2-month history of aching pain. The radiograph demonstrates an osteoid osteoma as evidenced by the well-defined defect in the cortical area of the femoral neck. (Courtesy of The American College of Radiology.)

trophied bone may obscure the lytic center, requiring the use of tomography to better visualize the nidus. Radionuclide bone scans are also of value in identifying and localizing osteoid osteomas. The erosion of the surrounding tissue causes extreme pain, often occurring at night, which is relieved by aspirin. Treatment of an osteoid osteoma requires surgical removal of the nidus.

Osteoclastoma (Giant Cell Tumor)

Osteoclastoma refers to a group of tumors characterized by the presence of numerous, multinucleated, osteoclastic giant cells. Unlike the previously mentioned neoplastic diseases, giant cell tumors may be either benign or malignant. Approximately 50% of osteoclastoma are benign, 35% recur after surgical excision, and 15% are aggressively malignant from the beginning. This neoplasm affects the sexes equally and is found in individuals between the ages of 20 to 30 years. Anatomically this disease tends to affect the ends or epiphyses of long bones, especially the lower femur, upper tibia, and lower radius. It begins in the medullary canal and expands outward, producing a clublike deformity of the end of the long bone. In addition, soft tissue extensions may be present, but giant cell tumor does not involve the joint space.

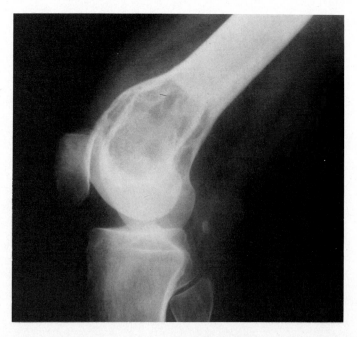

Fig. 2-72. A lateral knee radiograph of a 30-year-old male who complained of a painful knee for approximately 2 months. The radiograph demonstrates a benign osteoclastoma of the knee. (Courtesy of The American College of Radiology.)

Clinical signs and symptoms of an osteoclastoma are nonspecific and include pain, tenderness, an occasional palpable mass, or an occasional pathologic fracture. Because this is an osteoclastic disease process, bone and cartilage formation generally do not occur in these lesions, therefore the technologist must decrease exposure factors to avoid over-penetration of the affected bone. Radiographically, a giant cell tumor presents as a mass of osteolytic or cystic areas surrounded by a thin shell of bone giving it the classic "soap bubble" appearance (Fig. 2-72). Treatment of an osteoclastoma consists of surgical excision and bone grafting.

Osteosarcoma (Osteogenic Sarcoma)

Except for myeloma, the most common primary malignancy of the skeleton is the *osteosarcoma,* which arises from osteoblasts. This neoplasm is most frequently found in the metaphyses of long bones, with approximately 50% affecting the knee. Osteosarcoma can occur at any age but predominatly affects young males between the ages of 10 to 20 years and is rarely seen after the age of 50 years. It is occasionally seen in older individuals with Paget's disease or following high-level radiation exposure to the bone. Clinically, the patient may present with pain and swelling.

Osteosarcoma is a highly malignant disease with a poor prognosis because lung metastasis almost always occurs via the blood stream. This metastatic lung disease may appear as multiple, rounded, calcified shadows within the lung fields on a conventional chest radiograph. If the chest radiograph is clear, CT of the chest often demonstrates micrometastases, as they are commonly present in the lungs before the primary osteosarcoma is discovered. Secondary growths or spread to other bones is very rare with osteosarcoma. Although treatment of osteosarcoma includes amputation of the limb followed by chemotherapy, the 5-year survival rate is 5% to 20% with most patients dying within 12-18 months following diagnosis.

As the tumor grows from the metaphysis, it lifts the periosteum from the cortical bone and lays down spicules of new bone radiating out from the origin, which gives the radiographic appearance of a sun-ray or sunburst. This appearance is due to the radiopaque and radiolucent changes within the newly created space between the cortex of the metaphysis and the displaced periosteum. However, radiographic findings (Figs. 2-73 and 2-74, pp. 80 and 81) vary greatly in appearance because some osteosarcoma tumors produce very little osteoid tissue and contain no calcifications, while others are densely opaque. In both cases, the radiograph would not display the characteristic sun-ray appearance. Accurate diagnosis must be made through biopsy of the questionable lesion.

Ewing's Sarcoma

Another primary malignant bone tumor is a *Ewing's sarcoma.* This neoplasm occurs at a younger age than any other primary malignant bone neoplasm, usually between the ages of 5 to 15 years and rarely occurs after the age of 30 years. It is also more common in males than females.

Unlike osteosarcoma, Ewing's sarcoma arises from the medullary canal and involves

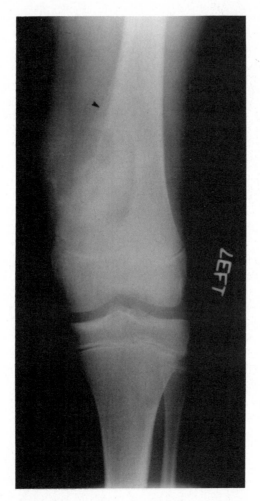

Fig. 2-73. A PA projection of the knee on a 14-year-old male with painful swelling above the left knee. The radiograph demonstrated cortical destruction along the posteromedial margin of the distal femur consistent with an osteosarcoma of the left femur. (Courtesy of The American College of Radiology, Reston, Virginia)

the bone more diffusely, giving rise to uniform thickening of the bone. These lesions tend to be very extensive, often involving the entire shaft of a long bone. Also unlike osteogenic sarcoma, Ewing's sarcoma does not begin at the end of a long bone. It does, however, tend to affect the extremities and pelvis. Although Ewing's sarcoma is a fairly rare disease, it is extremely malignant and carries a very poor prognosis, with a 5-year survival rate of 0% to 12%. Clinical symptoms are nonspecific and include pain and

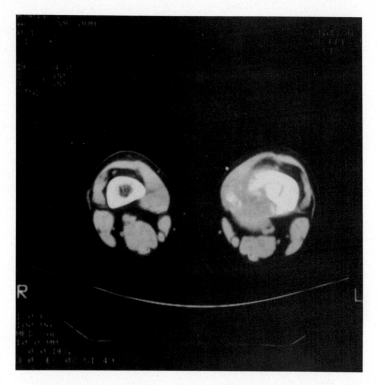

Fig. 2-74. An MRI of the left femur on the same patient described in Fig. 2-73. MRI is helpful in determining the medullary extension of the osteosarcoma. (Courtesy of The American College of Radiology, Reston, Virginia.)

tenderness of the affected area. The lesions undergo a combination of bone formation in the early stages and destruction in the later stages with new bone being formed on the surface (Fig. 2-75, p. 82). This process often gives a classic "onion skin" or laminated appearance radiographically. Ewing's sarcoma is responsive to radiation therapy; however, it often returns following therapy, thus accounting for the poor prognosis.

Chondrosarcoma

A *chondrosarcoma* is a malignant tumor of cartilaginous origin and is composed of atypical cartilage. It is only about half as common as osteosarcoma and comprises approximately 10% of all malignant tumors of the skeletal system. Males are three times as likely as females to develop chondrosarcoma and it is more common in older adults. As mentioned earlier in this chapter, benign exostoses and multiple endochondromas may be

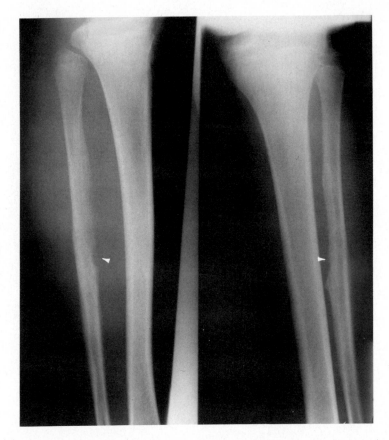

Fig. 2-75. Lower leg radiographs on a 12-year-old male complaining of left leg pain demonstrating a Ewing's sarcoma of the tibia as indicated by the lytic defect in the proximal diaphysis of the fibula. (Courtesy of The American College of Radiology, Reston, Virginia.)

transformed into chondrosarcomas. However, this accounts for only about 10% of the cases, with approximately 90% of chondrosarcomas arising afresh without prior cartilaginous lesions. Chondrosarcomas may be bulky and they tend to destroy the bone as they extend through the cortex into the surrounding soft tissue. These lesions have the ability to implant or "seed" into the surrounding soft tissue, so careful excision is a necessity. While neither radiation therapy nor chemotherapy are effective in the treatment of chondrosarcomas, adequate excision leads to a good prognosis with a 5-year survival rate of 25% to 50%.

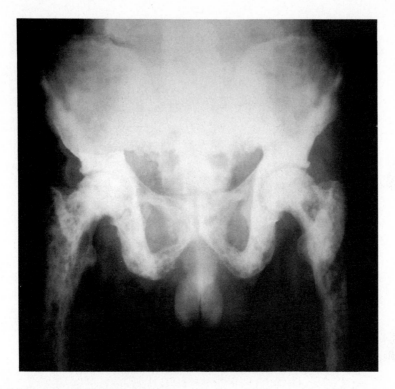

Fig. 2-76. An AP pelvis radiograph on an elderly male diagnosed with carcinoma of the prostate. There is diffuse metastatic disease to the pelvis from the prostatic primary. (Courtesy of The American College of Radiology, Reston, Virginia.)

Metastases From Other Sites

Any type of cancer can metastasize to bone, but metastatic disease from carcinomas are the most common malignant tumors of the skeleton, with secondary bone tumors of any origin far outnumbering primary bone tumors. The bones of the skeletal system that contain red bone marrow are the major bones affected by metastatic disease because of their good vascularization (Fig. 2-76). These include flat bones (such as the ribs, sternum, pelvis, and skull), the vertebrae, and the upper ends of the femora and humeri. Skeletal surveys and radionuclide bone scans are indicated on all known cancer patients who present with skeletal complaints. Many times a pathologic fracture is the first presenting symptom of such disease.

The most common primary sites for metastatic bone cancer are the breast, lung, prostate, kidney, and thyroid gland with the tumor spreading via proximity, the blood stream, or the lymphatic system. Treatment of metastatic disease is dependent on the primary disease, but radiation therapy in combination with either chemotherapy or hormone therapy is commonly used to manage such patients.

▼   QUESTIONS

1. Specialized cells responsible for the formation of bone are termed:
   a. chondroblasts   c. osteoclasts
   b. osteoblasts   d. both b and c

2. A freely movable joint is classified as:
   a. amphiarthrodial   c. synarthrodial
   b. diarthrodial   d. triarthrodial

3. Bone marrow is located anatomically within the:
   a. cortex   c. periosteum
   b. medullary canal   d. trabeculae

4. The end portion of a long bone is referred to as the:
   a. epiphysis   c. diploe
   b. diaphysis   d. metaphysis

5. The human body normally contains_____ bones.
   a. 156   c. 197
   b. 175   d. 206

6. The most common inherited disorder that results in dwarfism is:
   a. achondroplasia   c. osteogenesis imperfecta
   b. Alber-Schönberg disease   d. spina bifida

7. The term *marble bone* is often associated with which skeletal disorder?
   a. achondroplasia   c. osteopetrosis
   b. osteomalacia   d. osteoporosis

8. The formation of extra digits is termed:
   a. adactyly   c. syndactyly
   b. polydactyly   d. talipes

9. An abnormal lateral curvature of the spine is referred to as:
   a. ankylosing spondylitis   c. spondylolisthesis
   b. scoliosis   d. spondylolysis

10. Osteomyelitis is a(n)_____disease of the skeletal system.
    a. arthritic   c. inflammatory
    b. congenital   d. neoplastic

11. The most common type of arthritis affecting both sexes equally is:
    a. ankylosing spondylitis   c. osteoarthritis
    b. gout   d. rheumatoid arthritis

12. Which type of arthritis is believed to be an autoimmune disease?
    a. bursitis   c. osteoarthritis
    b. gout   d. rheumatoid arthritis

13. Rickets is a type of_____ affecting children.
    a. hyperparathyroidism   c. osteopetrosis
    b. osteomalacia   d. osteoporosis

14. A fracture of the skeletal system in which the bone has penetrated the skin is termed:
    - **a.** closed
    - **b.** comminuted
    - **c.** compound
    - **d.** noncomminuted

15. Fractures that occur at sites of maximal strain on a bone, usually in connection with unaccustomed activity are classified as _____ fractures.
    - **a.** avulsion
    - **b.** fatigue
    - **c.** growth plate
    - **d.** stress

16. The most common anatomical site for a mandibular fracture is (are) the:
    - **a.** angle
    - **b.** body
    - **c.** condyle
    - **d.** symphysis

17. A fracture that heals in a faulty position is termed:
    - **a.** callus
    - **b.** delayed union
    - **c.** malunion
    - **d.** nonunion

18. Shoulder dislocations are most commonly displaced:
    - **a.** anteriorly
    - **b.** posteriorly

19. The most common benign bone tumor is the:
    - **a.** endochondroma
    - **b.** osteoid osteoma
    - **c.** osteoma
    - **d.** osteochondroma

20. All of the following are malignant neoplasms of the skeletal system EXCEPT:
    - **a.** chondrosarcoma
    - **b.** Ewing's sarcoma
    - **c.** osteosarcoma
    - **d.** osteoma

3

The Respiratory System

▼

Upon completion of Chapter 3, the reader should be able to:

- Describe the anatomical components of the respiratory system.
- Distinguish between the results obtained and uses for the various projections of the chest.
- Describe the various types of tubes, lines, and catheters used in relation to the respiratory system.
- Characterize a given condition as congenital, inflammatory, traumatic, or neoplastic.
- Identify the pathogenesis of the chest pathologies cited and the typical treatments for them.
- Describe, in general, the radiographic appearance of each of the given pathologies.

ANATOMY AND PHYSIOLOGY REVIEW

The respiratory system serves to distribute air for the gas exchange with the circulatory system. This system is usually subdivided into the upper respiratory tract, which is comprised of the nose, mouth, pharynx, and larynx, and the lower respiratory tract, which consists of the trachea, bronchi, alveoli, and lungs (Fig. 3-1). The thoracic cavity comprises the right and left pleural cavities and the mediastinum. The parietal pleura lines the thoracic cavity, while the visceral pleura adheres directly to the lung tissue.

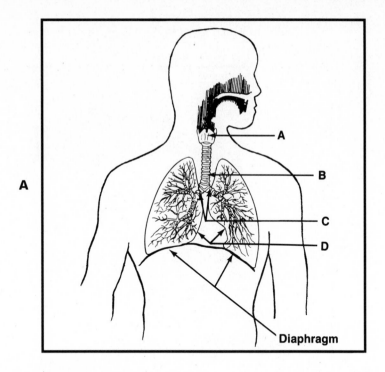

A

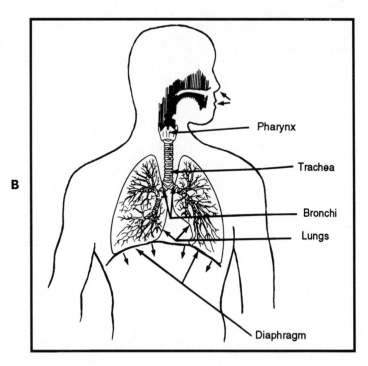

B

Fig. 3-1, *A.* The respiratory system. *B.* The trachea and its bifurcation at the carina. (From Bontrager KL: *Textbook of Radiographic Positioning and Related Anatomy,* ed 3, St Louis, 1993, Mosby.)

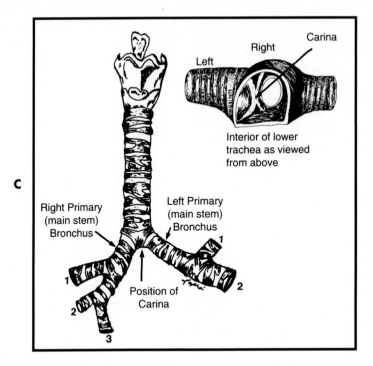

C

Carina

Right

Left

Interior of lower
trachea as viewed
from above

Right Primary
(main stem)
Bronchus

Left Primary
(main stem)
Bronchus

1

1

2

2

Position of
Carina

3

Fig. 3-1, *C.* The secondary bronchi and alveoli (From Bontrager KL: *Textbook of Radiographic Positioning and Related Anatomy,* ed 3, St Louis, 1993, Mosby.)

Anatomically, the mediastinum is divided into anterior, middle, and posterior portions. The anterior mediastinum contains the thyroid and thymus glands. The middle mediastinum contains the heart and great vessels, esophagus, and trachea. The posterior mediastinum contains the descending aorta and spine.

The anatomic bony structures of the thorax assist in both inspiration and expiration. These bony structures include the ribs, sternum, and thoracic vertebrae.

The paranasal sinuses are lined with respiratory epithelium and communicate with the nasal cavities, hence their inclusion in this chapter. The maxillary and ethmoid sinuses are the only paranasal sinuses present at birth. The frontal sinuses generally develop shortly after birth and are fully developed by the age of 10 years. The sphenoid sinus begins to develop around the ages of 2 or 3 years and is fully developed by late adolescence.

IMAGING CONSIDERATIONS

The examination most frequently performed in any radiology department is the chest radiograph. Although this examination may seem "routine," chest radiography provides important information concerning the soft tissues, bone, pleura, and mediastinum, in addition to the lung tissue.

Exposure Factor Conditions

Correct exposure-factor selection is critical, because this may hide and/or appear to create pathologic findings. This is particularly true for serial portable radiographs, since the interpreting physician relies heavily on consistent exposure conditions in analyzing the change in pathology following treatment. Institutions use various means of manually recording techniques for portables so that different technologists can use similar exposure conditions. Mobile phototiming devices are also available for portable situations and offer the advantage of exposure consistency associated with phototiming. Their use is a bit trickier in portable conditions, however, given the reduced number of sensors. Finally, the emergence of digital radiography (as described later) offers the potential to eliminate exposure repeats caused by inadequacy or inconsistency of technical factors.

Some sources describe pathologies, including those in the chest, as *additive* (harder than normal to penetrate) or *subtractive* (easier than normal to penetrate). In the respiratory system, any condition that adds fluid or tissue to the normally aerated chest (e.g., pneumonia) requires an increase in exposure to afford proper penetration. Similarly, any condition that increases the aeration of the chest (e.g., emphysema) reduces the amount of exposure required for proper densities to be achieved. Most experts agree that manipulation of the milliampere seconds (mAs) is the best approach for exposure adjustments since kilovoltage peak (kVp) changes affect image contrast, making it more difficult for the clinician to compare one film with another.

Phototiming of the exposure (i.e., automatic exposure control) facilitates the attainment of consistent exposures but requires careful analysis of the clinical history and conscious thought about the type of disease present and its location to ensure truly optimal radiographs. Activation of the photodetector, for example, over an area of significant aeration or *consolidation* (tissue or fluid accumulation), can result in an excessive or insufficient exposure, respectively, necessitating a repeat exposure. Again, experience with phototiming combined with careful thought when setting the phototimer can eliminate these mistakes.

Position and Projection

Patient position and projection are also critical exposure conditions that may distort the final image. *Position* refers to the arrangement of the patient's body (e.g., erect, supine, recumbent) while *projection* refers to the path of the X-ray beam (e.g., anteroposterior [AP] meaning entering through the body's anterior surface and exiting the posterior surface.) The standard projections for chest radiography are the posteroanterior (PA) and left lateral (Fig. 3-2, pp. 90 and 91). Each of these serves to place the heart closest to the film, since it lies in the anterior part of the chest and mostly to the left side. When combined with a standard 72-inch source-to-image distance (SID), magnification of the heart is minimized.

The Standard Chest Radiograph

On a normal erect PA chest film the costophrenic and cardiophrenic angles are demonstrated with the right hemidiaphragm appearing 1 to 2 cm higher than the left because of the liver. When a patient is radiographed in a recumbent position, the lower lung fields may be obscured because of abdominal pressure raising the level of the diaphragm (Fig. 3-3, p. 92).

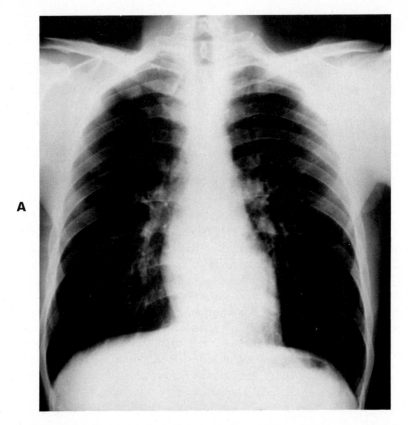

A

Fig. 3-2, A. Normal erect PA chest taken on a 24-year-old male. Straight inferior margin near diaphragm results from normal, physiologic accumulation of fat. (Courtesy of the American College of Radiology, Reston, Virginia.)

Other projections of the respiratory system are used less frequently than the PA and left lateral. The AP projection is the method of choice for portable radiography when the patient is often too ill to tolerate a visit to the department and assume an erect position. As much as possible, it is important that this view be taken in an erect position to demonstrate any air-fluid levels present. Maintenance of the beam perpendicular to the plane of the film is most important to avoid any foreshortening of the heart. Further, use of the 72-inch SID is most important for portable radiography to minimize magnification created by the heart, which is located further from the film in the AP projection.

AP or PA projections of the patient lying in a lateral decubitus position are also useful under specific conditions, such as free pleural fluid. The patient usually lies on the affected side; for example, the patient lies on his or her right side for a right lateral decubitus. In this position, any fluid present tends to layer out along the edge of the lung field, enhancing its visibility.

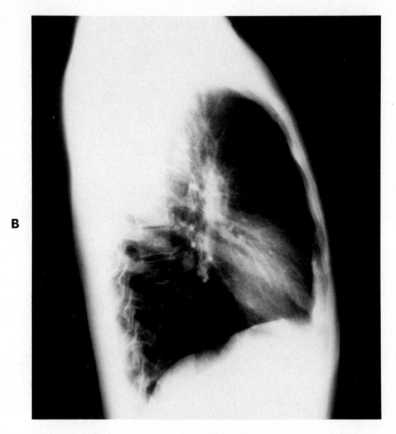

Fig. 3-2, *B.* Normal erect lateral chest of a 24-year-old male. Seen immediately behind the sternum is the internal thoracic muscle, arising from the sternum to insert on the second to sixth costal cartilages. (Courtesy of the American College of Radiology, Reston, Virginia.)

When evaluating the standard PA chest radiograph, the size and radiolucency of both lungs should be compared. Criteria for adequate inspiration and penetration of chest radiographs varies from institution to institution; however, a rule of thumb is that adequate inspiration should provide visualization of 10 posterior ribs within the lung field. Additionally, all thoracic vertebrae and intervertebral disk spaces should be faintly visible through the mediastinum on an adequately penetrated chest radiograph. The average movement of the lungs and diaphragm between inspiration and expiration is approximately 3 cm (Fig. 3-4, pp. 92 and 93).

Other Chest Studies

Oblique projections are useful in separating superimposed structures such as the sternum, esophagus, and thoracic spine. A lordotic chest radiograph is useful in demonstrating the apical regions of the lung, which are normally obscured by bony structures on the standard

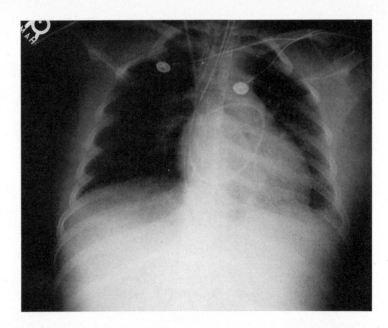

Fig. 3-3. Recumbant AP chest demonstrating obscuring of the lower lung fields. (Courtesy of Riverside Methodist Hospitals, Columbus, Ohio.)

A

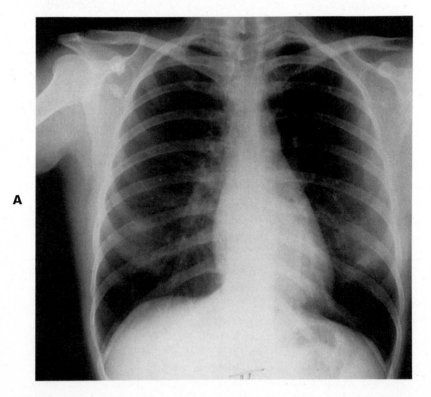

Fig. 3-4, *A.* Normal chest appearance on inspiration. (Courtesy of Riverside Methodist Hospitals, Columbus, Ohio.)

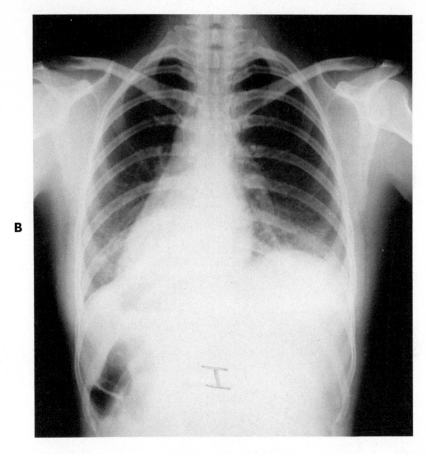

Fig. 3-4, *B.* Expiration film on the same patient demonstrates elevation of the diaphragm and a heart that is more transverse and appears larger. (Courtesy of Riverside Methodist Hospitals, Columbus, Ohio.)

PA projection (Fig. 3-5, p. 94). Certain diseases (e.g., tuberculosis) have a predilection for the apices. Fluoroscopy of the chest may be used to appraise the movements of the diaphragm, but it is generally performed to assist the physician in biopsy procedures. It is also useful in evaluation of a lung nodule vs. a pseudonodule, and in evaluation of cardiac, especially valvular calcification. Tomography of the chest is useful in the diagnosis of cavities and calcifications in the chest, but has been largely supplanted by computed tomography.

Computed tomography (CT) is becoming the method of choice for evaluation of pulmonary adenopathy (Fig. 3-6, p. 95). Standard radiographs are only about 50% sensitive to chest disease, typically displaying conditions farther advanced. In many cases, they are becoming a screening technique for CT analysis of questionable chest pathology. However, the excellent specificity of CT can be a problem because most people have

Text continued on p. 96.

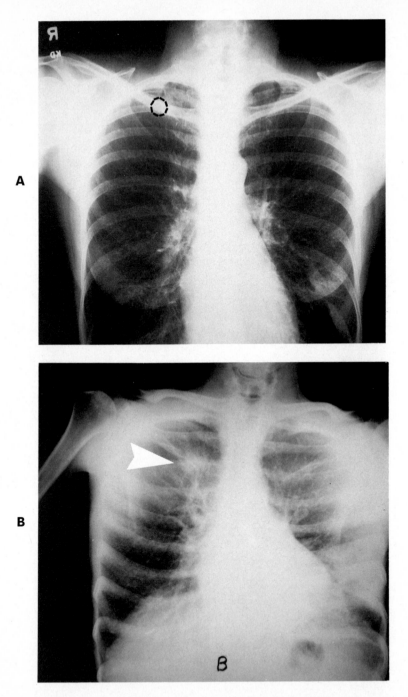

Fig. 3-5, *A.* PA chest radiograph reveals a suspicious density behind the right clavicle. *B.* Lordotic chest radiograph more clearly reveals coin lesion previously obscured by the right clavicle, later revealed to be cancer. (Courtesy of the American College of Radiology, Reston, Virginia.)

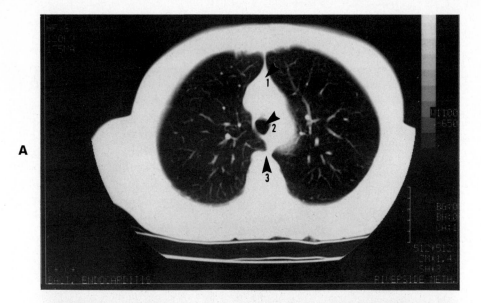

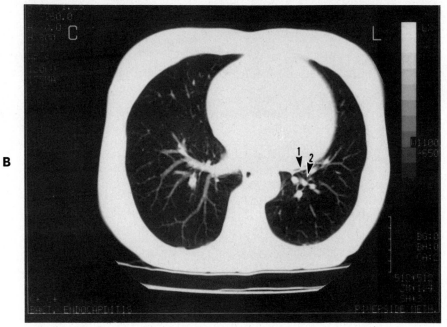

Fig. 3-6, *A.* Normal CT of the chest in the upper lungs with "lung windows", demonstrating *1,* the anterior junction line (sometimes seen on chest radiographs), *2,* the trachea, and *3,* the esophageal recess. *B.* CT view of the chest in the mid lungs, demonstrating *1,* a pulmonary vein (distinguished from an artery because of its oval shape), *2,* bronchi, and *3,* an artery (with characteristic rounded shape). (Courtesy of Riverside Methodist Hospitals, Columbus, Ohio.)

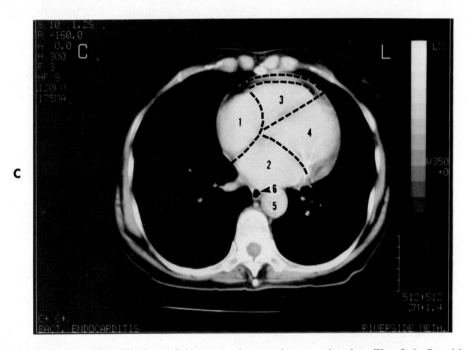

Fig. 3-6, *C.* A third CT view of the same chest at the same level as Fig. 3.6, *B,* with a window level adjusted to demonstrate the heart and surrounding structures. Seen are the heart's chambers, *1,* right atrium, *2,* left atrium, *3,* right ventricle, *4,* left ventricle, as well as other structures, including *5,* the aorta, and *6,* the esophagus (fitting in the esophageal recess). The azygos vein is the small rounded density immediately inferior to the esophagus. Also seen are a small pericardial effusion immediately above the right ventricle. The star-shaped calcification in the left atrium is a mitral annulus calcification. (Courtesy of Riverside Methodist Hospitals, Columbus, Ohio.)

granulomatous disease, which is often benign. A rule of thumb used in evaluating the character of a visualized nodule relates to its size: those less than 1 cm in size are usually benign and those greater than 1 cm are suspicious of malignancy. Also, the presence of calcium within a nodule is a reasonable indication of benignancy, particularly if in the middle of the lesion or diffusely present within the nodule. On the other hand, eccentric calcification may indicate malignancy.

The emergence of thin-cut CT, in which slice thicknesses range from 1.0 to 1.5 mm, holds great promise in evaluation of interstitial lung disease. Although typically a role of conventional radiography, this may become supplanted in time by the developing CT techniques, much like the role of traditional tomography has greatly declined in pulmonary evaluations. Magnetic resonance imaging (MRI) is not currently useful in evaluation of pulmonary lesions because of the associated motion. It does have use in mediastinal evaluation to separate adenopathy from vasculature, although this is usually done first by CT.

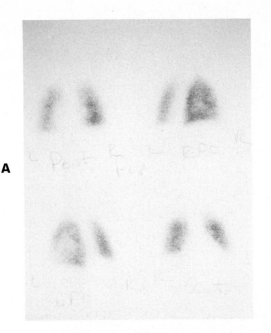 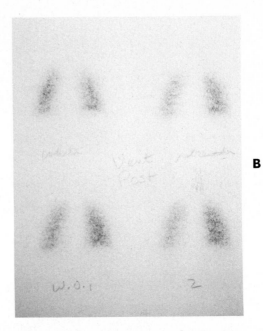

A   B

Fig. 3-7, *A.* Normal perfusion scan as evidenced by the sharply defined pleural margins and lung apices. *B.* A ventilation scan with radioactive xenon where the gas ''washout'' is not entirely normal in the right lung, as seen on the lower right image where the lungs are not of uniform density. This is suggestive of a partial obstruction of the right mainstream bronchus. (Courtesy of Riverside Methodist Hospitals, Columbus, Ohio.)

Perfusion and ventilation scans as performed in nuclear medicine are also useful in evaluating chest disease, particularly in the case of obstructive disease and pulmonary emboli. Injection of a radionuclide into the venous system for a perfusion causes it to become trapped in the pulmonary circulation, allowing for gamma camera visualization of its distribution. In a ventilation scan, the patient inhales a radioactive gas (such as xenon) and holds his or her breath while an image is taken of the gas distribution throughout the lungs (Fig. 3-7).

Digital (computed) radiography is beginning to emerge as an imaging modality important in chest radiography (Fig. 3-8), particularly in portable situations such as found in the intensive care unit. Most current applications feature photostimulable phosphor plate technology as replacements for the typical film-screen combination, with trade-offs of significant improvements in film latitude and reduced patient dosages, but somewhat less resolving capability than a conventional film-screen image. Sites using the technology report satisfaction of the referring physician with the image quality.

The improvement in exposure latitude possible with digital radiography, however,

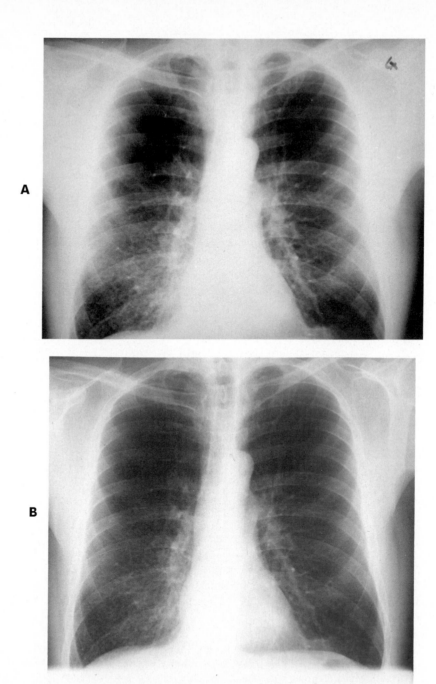

Fig. 3-8, *A.* PA chest radiograph taken on a patient, demonstrating proper exposure conditions for comparison to a chest radiograph taken with computed radiography. *B.* Digital radiograph on same patient produced with photo-stimulable phosphor plate technology, demonstrating nearly 33% dose reduction with increased scale of contrast. (Courtesy of Fuji Medical Systems, Stamford, Connecticut.)

allows for the virtual elimination of repeat radiographs for poor technique—a common complaint of radiologists reading these critical films. When combined with teleradiology and electronic image review capabilities, significant advantages emerge. These include the ability to maintain several days of on-line storage at the patient care site, elimination of lost films, and increased availability of the images. Digital radiography is rapidly emerging as a technique important in chest radiography and may gradually see larger adoption as the method of choice for digitizing much of the remaining analog imaging found in modern radiography.

Soft Tissues of the Chest

Various soft tissue densities are present on chest radiographs. These may vary with patient age, sex, and pathologic conditions. The pectoral muscles are normally demonstrated overlying and extending beyond the lung fields. Radiographs of both males and females demonstrate breast shadows in the midchest region (Fig. 3-9). These shadows are normally homogeneous in appearance, and female breasts may obscure the costophrenic

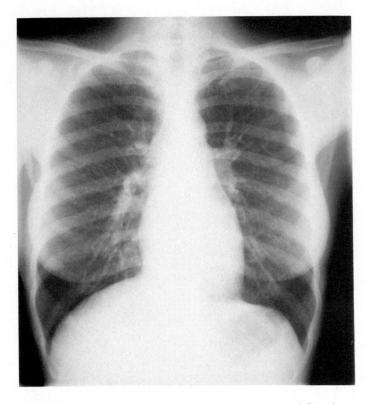

Fig. 3-9. Breast shadows are readily recognizable on the normal PA chest radiograph. (Courtesy of Riverside Methodist Hospitals, Columbus, Ohio.)

angles. Elevation of the breasts may be necessary to better demonstrate the bases of the lungs. Surgical removal of one or both breasts is also evident on a chest radiograph; breast prostheses, which appear as well-defined, circular radiopaque densities are also evident. Nipple shadows may be visible at the level of the fourth or fifth anterior rib spaces and may occasionally mimic nodules or masses in the chest. Differentiation of these soft tissue structures may be accomplished with the use of nipple markers, oblique projections of the chest, or chest fluoroscopy.

Bony Structures of the Chest

The ribs, sternum, and thoracic spine enclose the thoracic cavity. These structures assist the technologist in the assessment of the technical adequacy of chest radiographs. Congenital anomalies of the ribs may be demonstrated (Fig. 3-10) as well as calcified costal cartilages. This calcification generally occurs in patients in their late twenties and beyond.

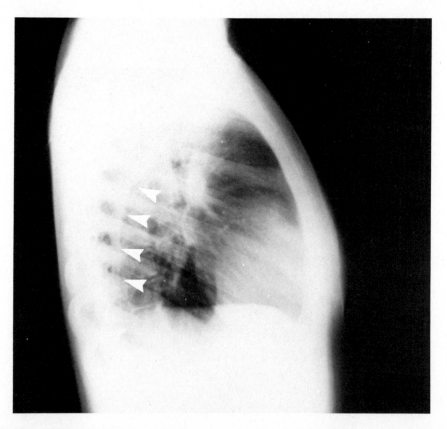

Fig. 3-10. Congenital intrathoracic rib seen as curving, tubular density in the posterior thorax. Usually, these are attached at one or both ends of a posterior rib and lie extrapleurally inside the thoracic cage. (Courtesy of the American College of Radiology, Reston, Virginia.)

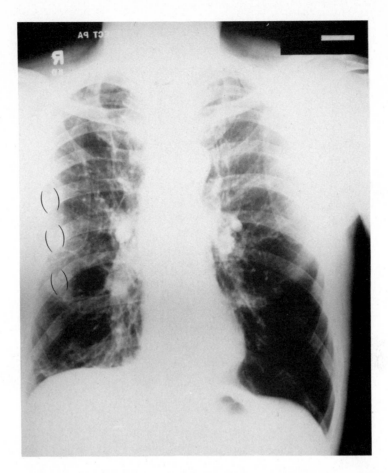

Fig. 3-11. Rib fractures of the fourth through ninth ribs. (Courtesy of the American College of Radiology, Reston, Virginia.)

Rib fractures may be seen (Fig. 3-11), sometimes with an accompanying pneumothorax. A depressed sternum (*pectus excavatum*) may also be demonstrated, possibly displacing the heart (Fig. 3-12, pp. 102 and 103). The thoracic spine may be assessed for scoliosis, which can affect the chest cavity, and kyphosis or compression fractures of the vertebrae.

The Mediastinum

The mediastinum contains all thoracic organs except the lungs. The heart occupies a large portion of the mediastinum, and its shape varies with age, degree of respiration, and patient position. Other organs contained within the mediastinum include the thyroid and thymus glands, and nervous and lymphatic tissues.

Radiographically, the mediastinum is divided into three sections. Anterior mediastinal masses generally arise from the thyroid gland, thymus gland, or lymphatic tissue.

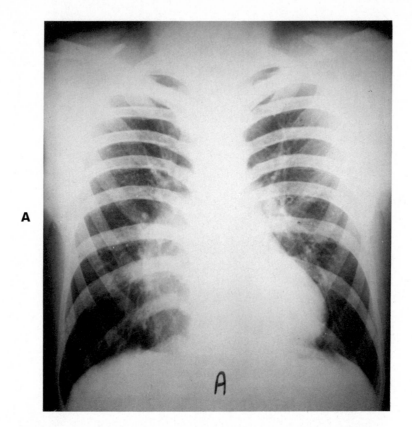

Fig. 3-12, *A.* Pectus excavatum on a 23-year-old male, indicated by vague density in medical portion of right lower lung field and obscuring of right heart margin. (Courtesy of the American College of Radiology, Reston, Virginia.)

Middle mediastinal masses are commonly lymphatic tissue, and posterior mediastinal masses usually arise from nervous or bony tissue.

In infants the mediastinum appears wide because the thymus is normally large in a healthy infant. On frontal projections, it may extend beyond the heart borders and caudally to the diaphragm, while on a lateral projection it may fill the anterior portion of the mediastinum, which is normally radiolucent later in life. This radiographic appearance is readily visible on both PA and lateral views and is referred to as the "sail sign" because of its characteristic appearance ((Fig. 3-13, p. 104). Diagnosis is difficult because the width of the upper mediastinum varies greatly with the phase of respiration. A crying child may present an opportune moment for the technologist to make an exposure by holding his or her breath, but the resultant Valsalva maneuver adds to the distortion of the thymus. True mediastinal masses are rare in infants and generally represent congenital malformations or neoplasms. In the elderly mediastinum, the aorta dilates and the aortic knob becomes much more visible.

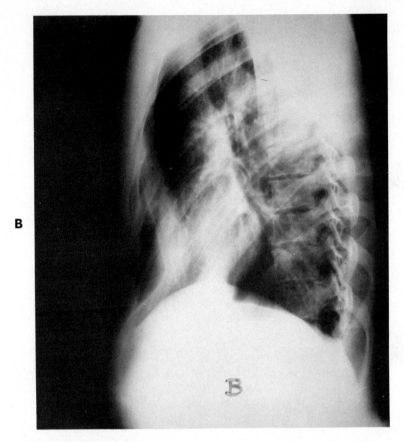

Fig. 3-12, *B.* Lateral projection demonstrating pectus excavatum, including compression of heart toward spine. (Courtesy of the American College of Radiology, Reston, Virginia.)

Mediastinal emphysema (pneumomediastinum) occurs when there has been a disruption in the esophagus or airway and air is trapped in the mediastinum (Fig. 3-14, p. 104). This may result from chest trauma, endoscopy, or violent vomiting. When unaccompanied by a pneumothorax, spontaneous mediastinal emphysema is usually self-limited, subsiding in a few days without complication. Air in the mediastinum from rupture of the esophagus (usually from vomiting) or a major bronchus (usually from trauma) is more serious and requires prompt diagnosis and surgical intervention. An esophogram may be performed to verify that a leak has not occurred.

When the pneumomediastinum is extensive, air may pass from the mediastinum into the subcutaneous tissues of the chest or neck, resulting in *subcutaneous emphysema* (Fig. 3-15, p. 105). Diagnosis of this may be made by feeling air bubbles in the skin of the chest or the neck.

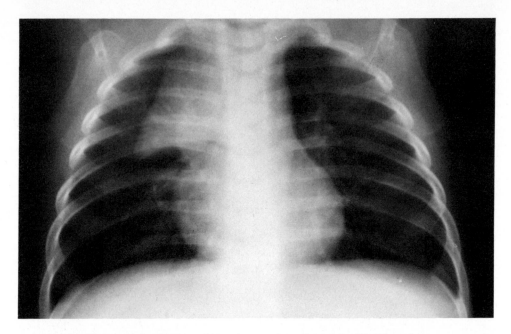

Fig. 3-13. Normal enlargement of the thymus in a 3-month-old infant demonstrates the "sail sign," evidenced by the uniform density increase in the right upper lung area.(Courtesy of the American College of Radiology, Reston, Virginia.)

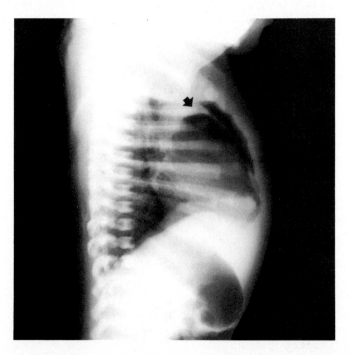

Fig. 3-14. Pneumomediastinum in a lateral chest projection of a full-term newborn, evidenced by air in the normally dense retrosternal space, with sharp outlining of the heart's anterior border. (Courtesy of the American College of Radiology, Reston, Virginia.)

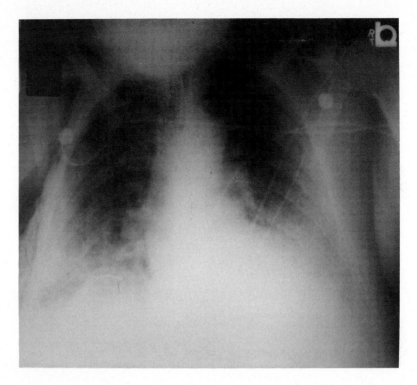

Fig. 3-15. Significant subcutaneous emphysema seen extending along entire right chest wall of this 70-year-old male. (Courtesy of Riverside Methodist Hospitals, Columbus, Ohio.)

Glandular enlargements of the thyroid gland are demonstrated by a displacement or narrowing of the trachea. The thyroid gland is usually located superior to the lung apices, but an ectopic thyroid gland may also displace the trachea.

Clinical manifestations of an ectopic thyroid gland are often absent, and the mass may be discovered accidentally when chest radiography is performed for some other purpose. Nuclear medicine studies are the modality of choice for detecting thyroid dysfunction and location.

Chest Tubes, Lines, and Catheters

A variety of tubes, lines, and catheters can be placed in relation to particular parts of the respiratory system. It is important for the technologist to be familiar with each of these and exercise great caution in attempting patient movement with any of these in place. It is best to have assistance from another technologist or nursing personnel to ensure the lines are free of any obstructions before patient movement occurs. Further, the technologist should always ask the patient's nurse if unsure if the patient is allowed to sit erect. The tube, film, and exposure technique should be established before the patient is moved. Patients in critical care units often can only be erect for a short period because of the instability of their blood pressure. Finally, it is best to cover cassettes with a pillowcase

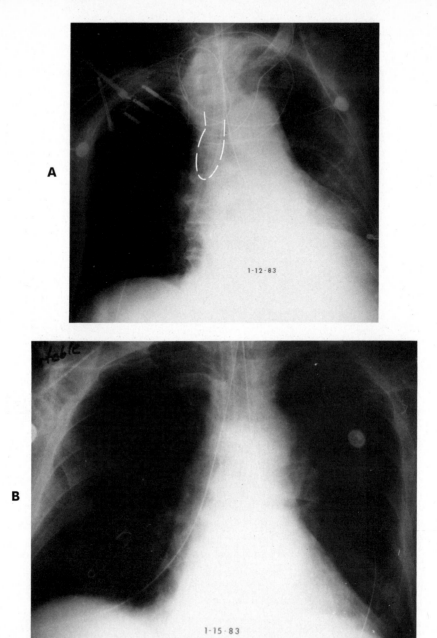

Fig. 3-16, A. Incorrect endotracheal (ET) tube placement creates shift of heart and mediastinum to the left with loss of air volume in the left lung. The ET tube tip lies in the proximal right main stem bronchus inferior to the carina. *B.* Correction of the endotracheal tube placement by withdrawal into the trachea following chest radiography demonstrates restoration of balanced lung ventilation. (Courtesy of the American College of Radiology, Reston, Virginia.)

or plastic bag to limit infection transfer and keep the cold cassette surface from touching the patient's back.

An *endotracheal* (ET) *tube* is a large, plastic tube inserted through the patient's nose or mouth into the trachea. It serves to help manage the patient's airway, allow for frequent suctioning, and/or allow for mechanical ventilation. Its proper position is below the vocal cords and above the *carina*, the bifurcation of the trachea (Fig. 3-16). Movement of the patient with an endotracheal tube should be done with great caution because inadvertent displacement or extubation may leave the patient without a patent airway.

A *chest tube* is also a large plastic tube inserted through the chest wall between the ribs. Its purpose is to allow for drainage of air (e.g., pneumothorax) and/or fluid (e.g., pleural effusion or hemothorax) from the thoracic cavity (Fig. 3-17). Those placed lower on the chest wall are usually for fluid drainage; those placed higher are usually for air removal. After open-heart surgery, a chest tube may be placed in the mediastinum for proper fluid drainage. Its location is midline, just below the sternum. It is important that bottles attached to the chest tube are kept below the level of the chest to allow for proper drainage.

Central venous pressure (CVP) *lines* are usually inserted via the subclavian vein, but they can also be placed through the jugular vein, antecubital vein, or the femoral vein. Proper insertion places the tip of the CVP catheter in the distal superior vena cava (SVC)

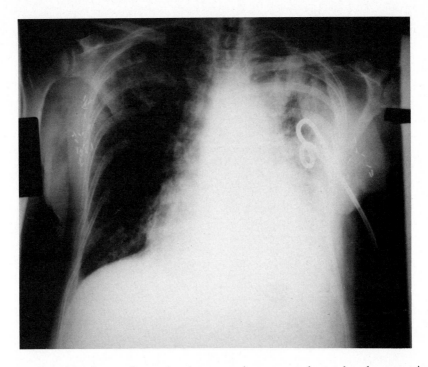

Fig. 3-17. Portable chest radiography demonstrating proper chest tube placement in the left lung, with a pleural reaction and fluid loculation in the lateral aspects of the left lung. (Courtesy of Riverside Methodist Hospitals, Columbus, Ohio.)

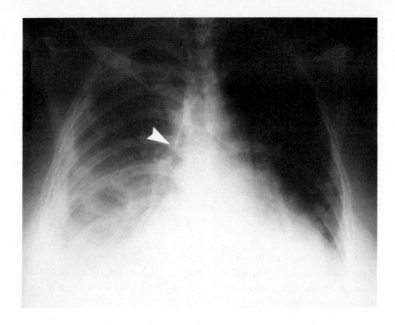

Fig. 3-18. Proper CVP line placement is demonstrated with the tip in the superior vena cava. Bilateral pleural effusions and cardiomegaly are also noted in this 71-year-old man. (Courtesy of Riverside Methodist Hospitals, Columbus, Ohio.)

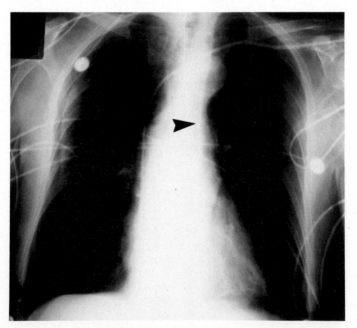

Fig. 3-19. Swan-Ganz catheter placement in the pulmonary artery, with the tip demonstrated by the arrow on this portable chest radiograph of this 69-year-old female. Occasionally, the catheter tip will enter a smaller pulmonary vessel. (Courtesy of Riverside Methodist Hospitals, Columbus, Ohio.)

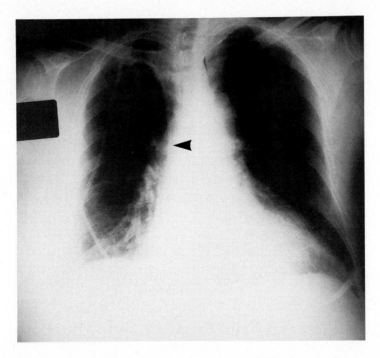

Fig. 3-20. Correct placement of a Hickman catheter within the superior vena cava as demonstrated on this portable chest radiograph of a 73-year-old female. (Courtesy of Riverside Methodist Hospitals, Columbus, Ohio.)

(Fig. 3-18). This catheter provides an alternative injection site to compensate for loss of peripheral infusion sites or to allow for infusion of massive volumes of fluids. In addition, it allows for measurement of central venous pressure, which indicates the patient's fluid status and provides function information about the heart's right side. A Swan-Ganz catheter has, however, largely supplanted a CVP for these purposes because it provides even greater accuracy in measurements.

A *Swan-Ganz* (pulmonary artery) *catheter* is usually inserted via the subclavian vein, but other injection sites include the antecubital vein, jugular vein, or femoral vein. It is a multilumen catheter that serves to evaluate cardiac function. The Swan-Ganz catheter measures pulmonary wedge pressure, reflecting left atrial pressure. It does not enter the heart's left side but is positioned in the pulmonary artery (Fig. 3-19). Inflation of the balloon at the tip of the catheter allows the tube to float into a smaller, pulmonary artery capillary. Diagnosis and management of heart failure resulting from myocardial infarction and cardiogenic shock represent the most common use of the catheter.

A *Hickman catheter* is usually inserted via subclavian vein. The tip of the catheter lies in the superior vena cava (Fig. 3-20). Its purpose is to allow for multiple tapping for injection of various agents, typically chemotherapeutics. Patients on whom these catheters are used typically have poor peripheral venous access because of the toxic effects of

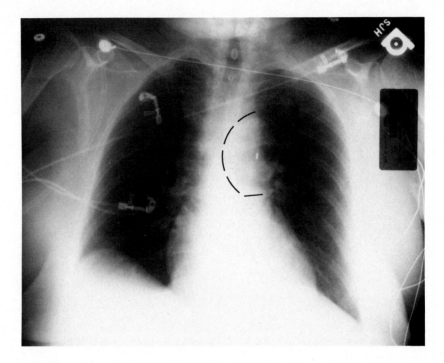

Fig. 3-21. Status postmyocardial infarction portable chest demonstrates proper placement of an intraaortic balloon pump in the descending thoracic aorta of this 76-year-old female. (Courtesy of Riverside Methodist Hospitals, Columbus, Ohio.)

chemotherapeutic drugs. Location in the subclavian vein provides ready access to the venous circulation and its blood flow return to the heart and relatively clean site.

An *intra-aortic balloon pump* (IABP) *catheter* is a specialized device inserted typically in surgery or at the bedside in critical care units. A 40-cc balloon at the distal end of the catheter allows for inflation and deflation by a pump to provide mechanical support of the left ventricle and thus the systemic circulation. Proper placement of the catheter is below the subclavian artery and above the renal arteries (Fig. 3-21). Particular caution should be used in moving these patients because movement may cause the balloon to float downward, possibly blocking the lower circulation.

Ventricular pacing electrodes may be placed for temporary or permanent purposes. Temporary pacing electrodes are inserted via the antecubital vein into the right ventricle. They provide electrical pacing of the heart in patients experiencing a very slow heart rate (i.e., *bradycardia*) as a substitute for misfiring of the heart's normal electrical system. Also, patients who have had open heart surgery may have these electrodes placed directly on the heart's surface and brought externally beneath the sternum at midline as a temporary precaution against heart arrhythmia problems. Permanent electrodes are used for permanent heart pacing needs. The pacemaker generator is inserted under the skin below the right clavicle, with the electrodes placed into the right ventricle (Fig. 3-22).

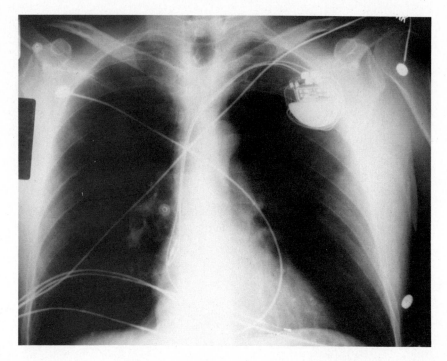

Fig. 3-22. Portable chest radiograph taken after pacemaker insertion demonstrates one pacemaker lead wire in the superior vena cava with the other near the apex of the right ventricle in this 52-year-old male. (Courtesy of Riverside Methodist Hospitals, Columbus, Ohio.)

CONGENITAL/HEREDITARY DISEASES
Cystic Fibrosis

A generalized disorder that affects the function of exocrine glands, *cystic fibrosis* involves many organs and not just the respiratory system. Other organs that can be affected include the salivary glands, small bowel, pancreas, biliary tract, female cervix, and male genital system. Although the basic cause of the disorder remains unknown, its complications are well-defined. In the respiratory system, gradually increasing secretions from hypertrophy of bronchial glands lead to obstruction of the bronchial system. The resultant plugging promotes infection followed by more tissue damage. Once the cycle is in motion, it is difficult to stop.

The disease remains the most common lethal genetic disease for Caucasian children, despite increasing life spans of 20 years of age or older because of improved treatments. Its diagnosis rests largely on certain clinical and laboratory findings, most notably elevated sodium and chloride levels in sweat. Radiographs taken over a period of years demonstrate gradually worsening structural abnormalities. Early changes of bronchial

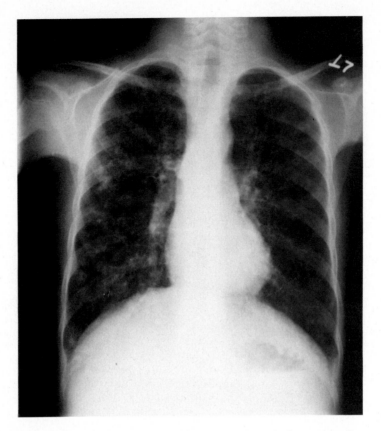

Fig. 3-23. Increased lung volume resulting from generalized obstructive disease and air trapping, which is characteristic of cystic fibrosis, as seen in this 9-year-old male. Also seen are areas of irregular aeration with cystic and nodular densities. (Courtesy of the American College of Radiology, Reston, Virginia.)

thickening and hyperinflation (Fig. 3-23) progress to extensive bronchiectasis, cyst formation, scarring, and overinflation of the lung and chest wall. Chest films are useful in revealing the origin and extent of the many respiratory complications (e.g., pneumonia) that plague cystic fibrosis patients. Treatment methods include antimicrobial drugs to combat infection, bronchodilators administered through inhalers, and respiratory physical therapy. Expert psychological guidance is also important in helping affected patients adjust to limitations to their quality of life.

Hyaline Membrane Disease

Also known as *respiratory distress syndrome*, hyaline membrane disease affects infants and is a disorder of prematurity. Incomplete maturation of the surfactant-producing system causes unstable alveoli, the structures in which gas exchanges occur in the lungs. Infants

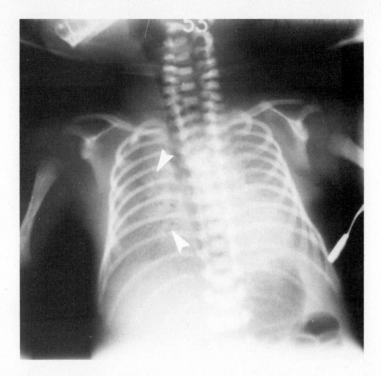

Fig. 3-24. Hyaline membrane disease in a pre-term infant as shown by the uniform opacity of the lungs. Air-filled bronchi also are seen in contrast to the poorly aerated lungs. (Courtesy of the American College of Radiology, Reston, Virginia.)

are particularly in need of a low surface tension in the alveoli, and surfactant (an agent that lowers surface tension) provides this. Its deficiency results in alveolar collapse with widespread atelectasis. Chest radiographs demonstrate the *air-bronchogram sign*, characterized by bronchi surrounded by non-aerated alveoli (Fig. 3-24). Treatment consists of maintenance of a proper thermal environment and satisfactory levels of tissue oxygenation, which is monitored frequently via arterial blood gas measurements.

INFLAMMATORY DISEASES
Pneumonias

Pneumonia is the most frequent type of lung infection, resulting in an inflammation of the lung and compromising pulmonary function. The main causes of pneumonia are bacteria, viruses, and mycoplasms. Radiographically, pneumonias appear as soft, patchy, ill defined alveolar infiltrates or pulmonary densities. Alveolar infiltration results when the alveolar air spaces are filled with fluid or cells.

Pneumococcal lobar pneumonia is the most common bacterial pneumonia. This type of infection can affect anyone at any age and is generally preceded by an upper respiratory infection. Pneumococcal bacteria is present in healthy throats. When the body defenses

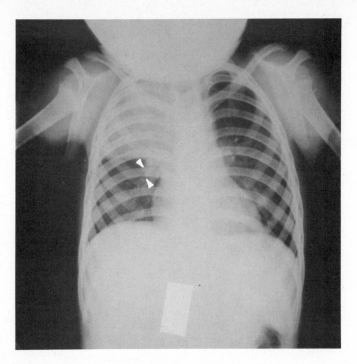

Fig. 3-25. Pneumococcal pneumonia with ''air-bronchogram sign'' in right lung created by consolidation within the lung that serves to outline the air-filled bronchi. The air-filled esophagus lies to the left of the spine. (Courtesy of the American College of Radiology, Reston, Virginia.)

are weakened, the bacteria multiply and work their way into the lungs, inflaming the alveoli. This disease is usually accompanied by chills, a cough, and a fever. Pneumococcal pneumonia generally affects the alveoli of an entire lobe of a lung, without affecting the bronchi themselves (Figs. 3-25 and 3-26). Chest radiographs demonstrate a collection of fluid in one or more lobes, with a lateral view serving to identify the degree of segmental involvement. Pleural fluid can often be seen in lateral decubitus views. Antibiotics (typically penicillin) and bed rest are the methods of treatment for pneumococcal pneumonia.

Far less frequent types of bacterial pneumonia are *staphylococcal* and *streptococcal* pneumonia. Staphylococcal pneumonia occurs sporadically except during epidemics of influenza when secondary infection with staphylococci is common. It is severe and may be fatal, especially in infants. A *pneumatocele,* a thin-walled, air-containing cyst, is the characteristic radiographic lesion and is more typically seen in children. These may enlarge and form abscesses in the later stages of the disease. Another characteristic sign is patchy, spreading areas localized in and around the bronchi (Fig. 3-27, p. 116). Drug therapy with particular chemotherapeutic agents is the treatment of choice.

Streptococcal pneumonias are even more rare, accounting for less than 1% of all hospital admissions for acute bacterial pneumonia. The radiographic appearance is local-

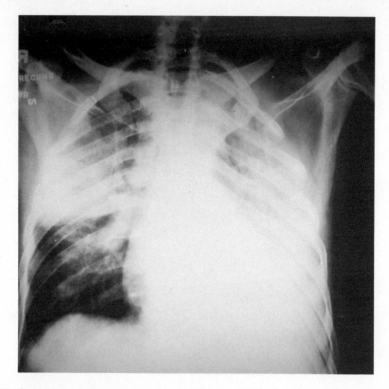

Fig. 3-26. Pneumococcal pneumonia in a 35-year-old male with severe head injuries. Relatively severe case demonstrates replacement of air by exudate and pus. (Courtesy of the American College of Radiology, Reston, Virginia.)

ized around the bronchi, usually of the lower lobes. Appropriate antibiotic therapy is the treatment of choice for this condition.

Legionnaires' disease is the name given to a severe, bacterial pneumonia that became known after causing the death of four persons attending an American Legion convention in Philadelphia, Pennsylvania in 1976. The causative bacteria (*legionella pneumophila*) was unknown at the time, and its explosive effects attracted significant attention. Now, it is thought to be responsible for less than 10% of all pneumonia cases occurring in the United States. Its radiographic appearance is similar to bacterial pneumonia, displaying patchy infiltrates throughout the lungs (Fig. 3-28, p. 116). Treatment consists primarily of antibiotic administration and oxygen therapy.

Mycoplasma pneumonia is caused by mycoplasmas, the smallest group of living organisms. They have characteristics of both bacteria and viruses. This disease is most common in older children and young adults. Radiographically, this disease demonstrates as a fine reticular pattern in a segmental distribution, followed by patchy areas of air space consolidation. In severe cases, the radiographic appearance may mimic tuberculosis. The morbidity rate associated with mycoplasma pneumonia is very low, even when the disease is not treated.

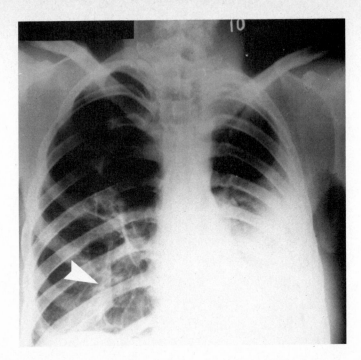

Fig. 3-27. Staphylococcal pneumonia in a 20-year-old male indicated by multiple large pneumatoceles in right lung and consolidation of the left lower lobe of the lung. An empyema in the lower left lung was later drained surgically. (Courtesy of the American College of Radiology, Reston, Virginia.)

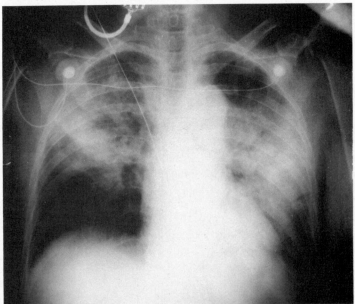

Fig. 3-28. Legionnaires' disease in a 55-year-old female showing rounded opacities in the upper half of the right lung and lower two thirds of the left lung. (Courtesy of the American College of Radiology, Reston, Virginia.)

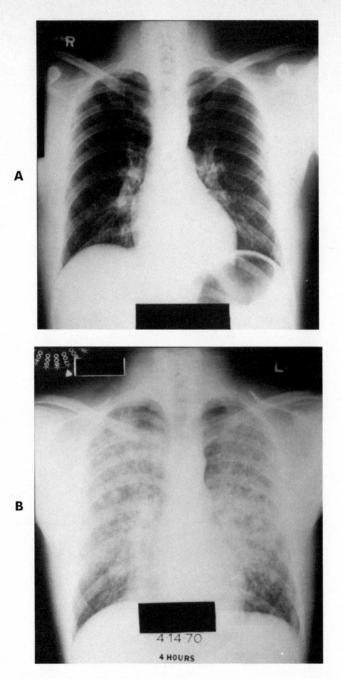

Fig. 3-29, *A.* ER admission film on a 34-year-old male working with paint remover in a closed environment. *B.* Chemical pneumonia, resulting from inhalation of paint remover, as displayed on film taken four hours later. Diffuse density with several areas of confluence are seen. (Courtesy of the American College of Radiology, Reston, Virginia.)

Aspiration (chemical) *pneumonia* is caused by acid vomitus aspirated into the lower respiratory tract, resulting in a chemical pneumonitis. This may follow anesthesia, alcoholic intoxication, or stroke caused by loss of the cough reflex. Chest radiographs reveal edema produced by the irritation of the air passages (Fig. 3-29), appearing as densities radiating from one or both hila into the dependent segments. The treatment of aspiration pneumonia is strictly supportive, including correction of hypoxia, control of secretions, and replacement of fluids. Further infection is treated by antimicrobial drugs based on laboratory results. *Viral* (interstitial) pneumonia can be caused by various viruses and is more common than bacterial pneumonia but less severe. This disease is spread by an infected person shedding the virus and a nonimmune individual receiving the infection. Most cases of viral pneumonia are mild, and the radiographic findings are often minimal. The diagnosis of this disease is based on clinical findings and serologic tests. Treatment usually focuses on relief of symptoms.

Bronchiectasis

Bronchiectasis is a permanent, abnormal dilatation of one or more large bronchi occurring as a result of destruction of the elastic and muscular components of the bronchial wall (Fig. 3-30). The basic pathogenesis is either congenital or an acquired weakness, typically from bacterial infection. Bronchography demonstrates this dilatation and can usually confirm the diagnosis. However, bronchography is not usually performed on patients with impaired pulmonary function.

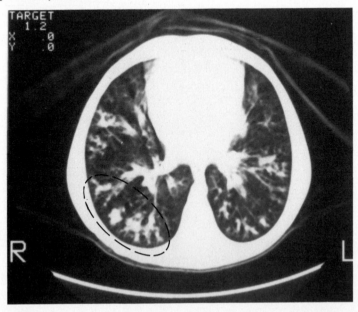

Fig. 3-30. Bronchiectatic changes are seen peripherally on this CT of the lungs from the 9-year-old patient with cystic fibrosis seen in Fig. 3-23. Compare the size of these bronchi with those seen in the normal chest CT (Fig. 3-5). (Courtesy of the American College of Radiology, Reston, Virginia.)

Since bacterial infection causes most forms of bronchiectasis, the treatment of choice is antimicrobial drugs.

Tuberculosis

Tuberculosis is an infection caused by inhalation of mycobacterium tuberculosis. Although it generally affects the lungs, it may also affect other areas of the body. Of great concern worldwide is the alarming increase in tuberculosis, and its rise in the United States where it was once considered nearly eradicated. An estimated 1.7 billion people worldwide (including 10 million Americans) carry the tuberculosis bacteria. Eight million develop active disease annually, and 3 million of these die.

Early pulmonary tuberculosis is asymptomatic, with signs appearing when the lesion is large enough to be seen on a chest radiograph. Lesions are most commonly seen in the apical region of the chest (Fig. 3-31); therefore, the apical lordotic projection of the chest is useful in the evaluation of tuberculosis.

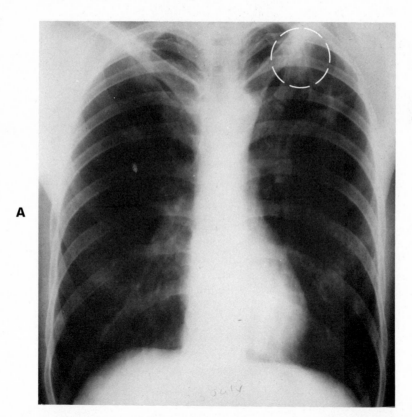

Fig. 3-31, *A.* Tuberculosis of left upper lobe in a 49-year-old male admitted with esophagitis and dull pain in the left subclavicular region. Subsequent tomography demonstrated a tuberculous, cavitary lesion. (Courtesy of the American College of Radiology, Reston, Virginia.)

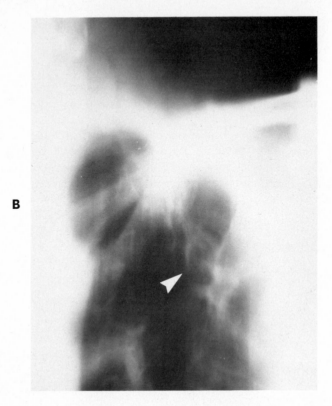

Fig. 3-31, *B.* Routine linear tomography of the left upper lobe reveals the tuberculous cavitary lesion. (Courtesy of the American College of Radiology, Reston, Virginia.)

Necrosis is a prominent feature of the disease because its infiltration affects lung parenchyma. This infiltration may expand and produce the formation of a cavity *(cavitation)* (Fig. 3-32). Chest tomograms are of great value in demonstrating the extent of these cavities. If these cavities spread to communicate with the bronchus, the bacteria is spread throughout the lung, producing bronchogenic spread of tuberculosis. If the blood stream picks up the tuberculosis, large numbers of bacteria are carried throughout the body, resulting in *miliary tuberculosis. Miliary* is a term derived from its characteristic appearance that is similar to millet seeds, which are small, white grains (Fig. 3-33, p. 122).

A positive response to intradermal injection of purified protein derivative (PPD), i.e., the *Mantoux test,* is the primary means of diagnosing tuberculosis. Because reading the results of this test is more an art than science, further testing may be necessary to confirm the diagnosis. Modern treatment of tuberculosis consists primarily of various chemotherapeutic agents. Historical treatments of bed rest, collapse therapy (i.e. artificial reduction in lung volume by one of several methods, including an artificial pneumothorax), and placement in a sanitarium are no longer practiced.

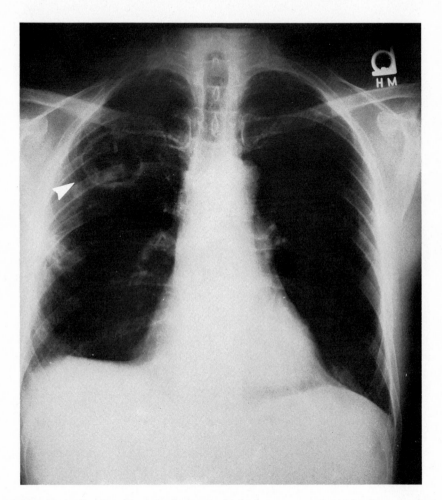

Fig. 3-32. Cavitation in the right lung resulting from expansion of tubercular lesion. (Courtesy of Riverside Methodist Hospitals, Columbus, Ohio)

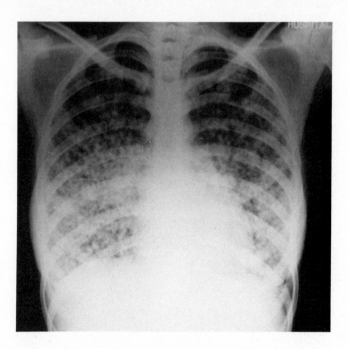

Fig. 3-33. Miliary tuberculosis resulting from hematogenous spread of tuberculosis, demonstrating small, distinct nodules throughout the lung fields. (Courtesy of the American College of Radiology, Reston, Virginia.)

Chronic Obstructive Pulmonary Disease

Chronic obstructive pulmonary disease (COPD) refers to a group of disorders that cause chronic airway obstruction. The most common forms of it are chronic bronchitis and emphysema, which frequently coexist and may be associated with varying degrees of asthma and bronchiectasis—two other causes of airway obstruction.

Since it may be difficult to determine whether the pulmonary obstruction is due to bronchitis, emphysema, or a combination of the two diseases, the designation of chronic obstructive pulmonary disease is commonly used. This disease is irreversible and results in limited airflow and decreased elastic recoil in the case of emphysema. Statistics show the mortality rate of COPD doubling approximately every 5 years.

Chronic bronchitis most often arises from long-term, heavy cigarette smoking, which irritates the mucous lining of the bronchial tree, increasing susceptibility to both bacterial and viral infections.

Persistent cough and *expectoration* (expulsion of mucus or phlegm from the throat) are the primary symptoms of chronic bronchitis. The effects of the disease develop slowly and progressively over months and years, gradually resulting in bronchial obstruction. Eventually the lungs remain in a chronically inflated state because more air is inhaled than is exhaled. No dependable radiographic criteria exist for a definitive diagnosis of chronic bronchitis.

Chest radiographs may demonstrate hyperinflation of the lungs. Bronchography may demonstrate an irregular, serrated appearance of the major bronchi. Elimination of the causative agent (e.g., cigarettes) is an important first step in treatment. Antibiotics can reduce the presence of infection; bronchodilators are used to reduce bronchospasm.

Emphysema is a condition in which the lung's alveoli become distended, usually from loss of elasticity or interference with expiration. It is characterized by an increase in the air spaces distal to the terminal bronchioles, with destruction of the alveolar walls.

The primary symptom of emphysema is dyspnea, which at first demonstrates only during exertion but eventually even at rest. In the early stages of emphysema, the patient may present with a normal chest radiograph. However, as the disease progresses, hyperinflation results (Fig. 3-34). This hyperinflation appears radiographically as a depressed or flattened diaphragm, abnormally radiolucent lungs, and an increased retrosternal air space (barrel-shaped chest). Large *bullae,* or blisters filled with air, may be visible on conventional chest radiographs (Fig. 3-35, p. 124), but smaller lesions are best demonstrated with lung tomograms.

Treatment of emphysema is much like that for chronic bronchitis. Goals are to improve symptoms, treat any reversible elements (e.g., infection), and prevent further progression of the disease as possible.

Because these two forms of COPD represent chronic deterioration of the pulmonary system, the continued problems eventually lead to heart failure. The heart begins to wear out over time in its effort to overcompensate blood flow for the decreased airflow caused by COPD. Eventually, *pulmonary edema* results and, if the patient lives long enough, *cor pulmonale* occurs. These conditions are both discussed in Chapter 8.

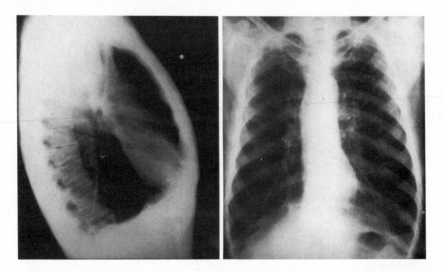

Fig. 3-34. PA and lateral views of the chest demonstrate pulmonary emphysema, a form of COPD, with its characteristic hyperinflation of the lungs, increased radiolucence, and the "barrel-shaped" appearance of the chest. (Courtesy of Riverside Methodist Hospitals, Columbus, Ohio.)

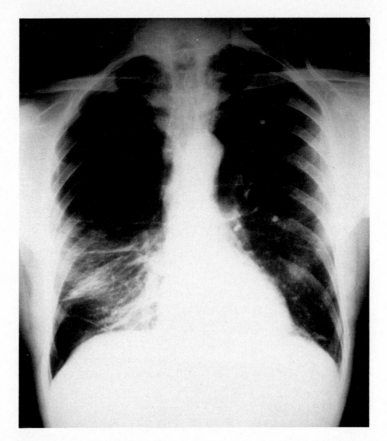

Fig. 3-35. Pulmonary emphysema with a giant emphysematous bleb occupying the upper half of the right lung. (Courtesy of the American College of Radiology, Reston, Virginia.)

Pneumoconioses

Pneumoconioses consist of a group of occupational diseases in which inhalation of foreign inorganic dust materials results in pulmonary fibrosis. The size of the dust particle inhaled is of particular importance in pneumoconioses. Most occupationally generated dusts and those occurring naturally are too large to cause pneumoconioses. Dusts greater than 10 microns are filtered out in the nasal passages or the mucous lining of the tracheo-bronchial tree. Those less than 1 micron generally remain suspended in air and are exhaled. Those most likely to be trapped are of the 1 to 5 micron size. In addition to the size criteria, exposure to a substance capable of causing disease and for a sufficient duration are factors required to cause a pneumoconiosis.

Radiography assists in the detection and follow-up of this disease group. Lesions produced by the different pneumoconioses vary, but they may include nodules, cavitation, and pleural thickening. The three primary types of pneumoconioses are silicosis, anthra-

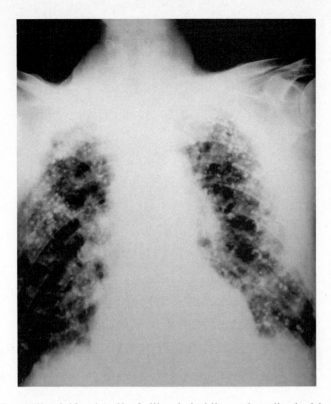

Fig. 3-36. "Eggshell calcifications" of silicosis in hilar and mediastinal lymph nodes of 70-year-old male stone cutter. Multiple small calcifications are also distributed throughout the lungs. (Courtesy of the American College of Radiology, Reston, Virginia.)

cosis, and asbestosis. Treatment of these disorders centers on preventing infection, relieving any respiratory symptoms, and maintaining adequate oxygenation.

Silicosis results from inhaling silica (quartz) dust and is common among miners, grinders, and sandblasters. This disease is characterized radiographically by multiple small, rounded opaque nodules throughout the lungs, visible on a chest radiograph. Sometimes these are peripheral calcifications that are referred to as "eggshell calcifications" (Fig. 3-36).

Anthracosis (more commonly referred to as "Black Lung Disease") results from inhalation of coal dust and is associated with coal workers (Fig. 3-37, pp. 126 and 127). As the coal dust is deposited in the lungs, "coal macules" develop around the bronchioles, later resulting in dilation of these bronchioles. This dilation does not affect the alveoli or the airflow.

Asbestosis results from the inhalation of asbestos dust. Radiographically, diaphragmatic pleural calcifications are very suggestive of asbestosis. Pleural changes in asbestosis are considered far more striking than parenchymal changes. Pleural thickening may also be present.

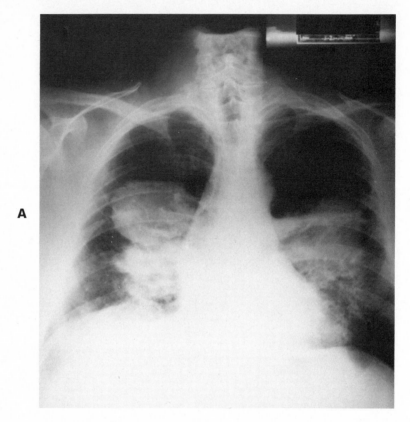

A

Fig. 3-37, *A.* Large, perihilar nodules without eggshell calcifications. Thoracotomy revealed heavy anthracotic pigmentation, with two largest nodules containing black fluid, consistent with anthracosis. (Courtesy of the American College of Radiology, Reston, Virginia.)

Fungal Diseases

Histoplasmosis is a systemic, fungal infection caused by a fungus that thrives in soil, especially that fueled by bird or bat excreta. Fungi are plants without chlorophyll and are widely found in nature. Histoplasmosis is particularly endemic to the Ohio and Mississippi River valleys. Most cases of histoplasmosis are sufficiently mild so that they go undiagnosed. Disseminated histoplasmosis that leads to cavitary formations is more serious. Dyspnea, cough, and fatigue may persist for months or even years, but recovery most often occurs. Chest radiographs eventually may reveal small calcifications as a late manifestation of the disease, although these do not usually appear for 4 or 5 years. Only a small portion (less than 1%) of those who acquire histoplasmosis require treatment because most forms of the disease are self-limiting and may evade diagnosis.

Coccidiomycosis is also a systemic, fungal infection caused by a fungus that thrives

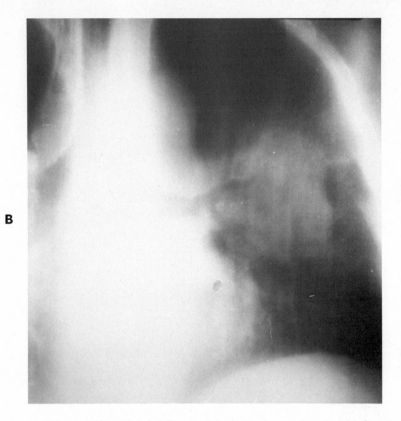

Fig. 3-37, *B.* Tomography of left hilar nodule in patient subsequently found to have anthracosis reveals air-bronchogram sign. (Courtesy of the American College of Radiology, Reston, Virginia.)

in semi-arid soil, particularly in the southwestern United States and northern Mexico. Infective spores in the soil become airborne from winds, digging, or other disruptions of the soil. For this reason, agriculture and construction workers are particularly at risk. Like histoplasmosis, most infections are mild, usually self-limited, and may go unrecognized. The most common radiographic finding, if present, is a small area of pulmonary consolidation (Fig. 3-38, p. 128). Lesions may form nodules of varying size that can simulate a malignant nodule, thus requiring biopsy or surgical excision. The typical treatment involves bedrest, since most occurrences are mild.

Lung Abscess

A *lung abscess* is a localized area of dead (necrotic) lung tissue surrounded by inflammatory debris. These abscesses may result from periodontal disease, pneumonias, neoplasms or other organisms that invade the lungs. Radiographically, an abscess generally

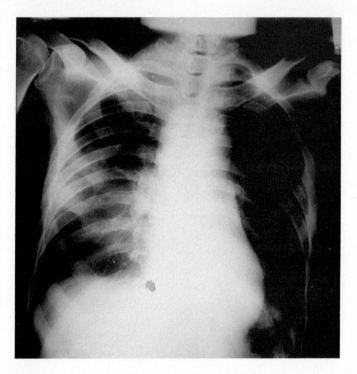

Fig. 3-38. Coccidiomycosis with diffuse fine military infiltration, especially in right lung. (Courtesy of the American College of Radiology, Reston, Virginia.)

appears as a consolidation that becomes globular in shape as pus accumulates (Fig. 3-39) or it may appear as a round, thick-walled capsule containing air and fluid. Tomography may be used to detect cavity formations. Bronchography should not be performed to demonstrate any bronchiectatic changes until the abscess has cleared or stabilized. *Empyemas* consist of an accumulation of pus in the pleural cavity, usually caused by some primary lung infection. They may be caused by the invasion of a lung abscess, resulting in a bronchopleural fistula.

Treatment of an abscess and empyema centers on treatment of the primary condition causing it, including antibiotic therapy and possible drainage of fluids.

Pleurisy

Inflammation of the pleura is loosely termed *pleurisy*, a word often used to indicate inconsequential thoracic pain. True pleurisy is often indicative of serious conditions such as pneumonia, pulmonary embolism, tuberculosis, or malignant disease. Pain, varying in intensity, is usually distributed to one side or the other and along the intercostal nerve roots. Since the parietal layer of the pleura contains sensory receptors (while the visceral layer does not), pain felt indicates that the parietal layer is involved in the inflammatory process.

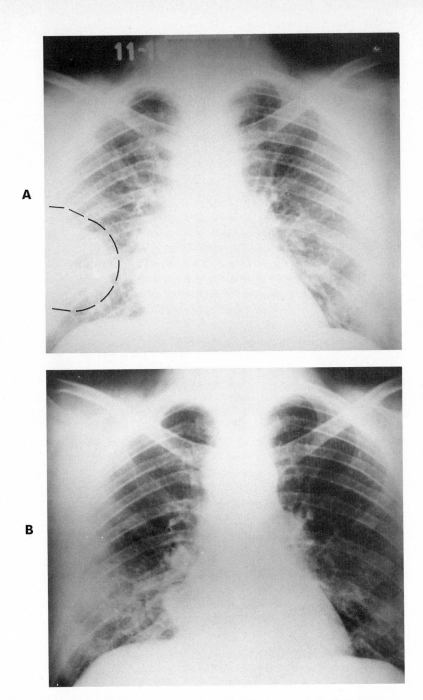

Fig. 3-39, *A*. Tuberculous abscess in a 33-year-old male seen in the lateral segment of the right middle lobe before treatment. *B.* Aggressive chemotherapeutic management reduces the tuberculous abscess significantly in size after 7 weeks of treatment. (Courtesy of the American College of Radiology, Reston, Virginia.)

Chest radiographs do not generally demonstrate pleurisy, but they are helpful in confirming the presence of pleural fluid associated with the disease. Diagnosis and treatment of any underlying condition is important in relieving the symptoms of pleurisy.

Pleural Effusion

Pleural effusion results when excess fluid collects in the pleural cavity and is a frequent manifestation of serious thoracic disease, usually pulmonary or cardiac in origin. It should be regarded not as a disease entity, but rather as a sign of an important underlying condition. Pleural effusion may be caused by inflammation, renal disease, surgery, or chest trauma. A pleural effusion containing blood is called a *hemothorax*. The radiographic signs of pleural effusion include a blunting of the costophrenic angles (Fig. 3-40), which is often best demonstrated on an erect lateral chest radiograph. Lateral decubitus chest radiographs are also of great value in the diagnosis of pleural effusions (Fig. 3-41). Thoracocentesis, sometimes with fluoroscopic or sonographic guidance, is used to remove excess fluids for symptom alleviation and laboratory analysis.

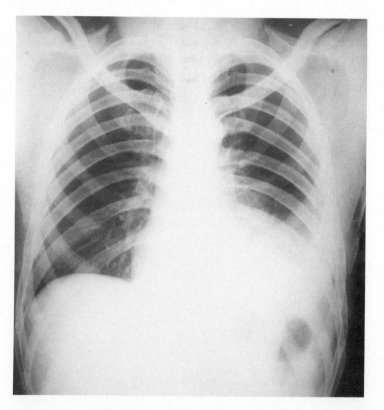

Fig. 3-40. Left pleural effusion on erect PA chest of 40-year-old male recovering from acute pancreatitis. (Courtesy of the American College of Radiology, Reston, Virginia.)

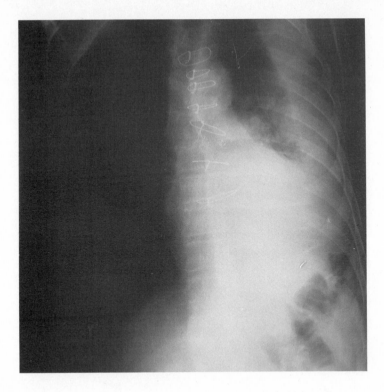

Fig. 3-41. Left lateral decubitus chest shows free pleural fluid layering out against the chest wall. Phototiming for correct density in area of interest has resulted in overexposure of the superior right lung. (Courtesy of Riverside Methodist Hospitals, Columbus, Ohio.)

Sinusitis

The communication with the nasal cavities subjects the paranasal sinuses to infection and inflammation called *sinusitis*. The ethmoid sinuses tend to be the most commonly affected because of their proximity to the nose. Common causes of sinusitis are exposure to extremes in humidity and temperature or a deviated septum. The symptoms of sinusitis include nasal discharge and a headache.

Radiography is important in the diagnosis of sinusitis. Upright sinus radiographs will demonstrate increased density and possible air-fluid levels in the affected sinuses (Fig. 3-42, p. 132). This increased density results from both mucosal swelling and fluid accumulation. CT is also useful in demonstrating sinusitis (Fig. 3-43, p. 133). Chronic sinusitis may result in the formation of nasal polyps.

Treatment of sinusitis typically involves antibiotic therapy and analgesics for pain relief. A deviated septum that contributes to sinusitis can be corrected surgically, if necessary.

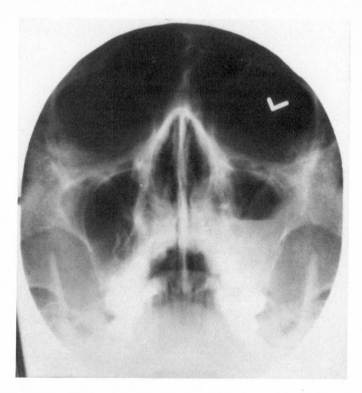

Fig. 3-42. Air-fluid level present in the left maxillary sinus reflects sinusitis in this 26-year-old female, secondary to an oral-antral fistula. (Courtesy of the American College of Radiology, Reston, Virginia.)

TRAUMATIC DISEASES
Atelectasis

Atelectasis means incomplete expansion of the lung as a result of partial or total collapse. *Compression atelectasis* occurs when pleural effusions, pneumothoraces, or other space-occupying lesions cause collapse (Fig. 3-44, p. 134). Air that is completely absorbed from alveoli beyond an obstructed bronchus results in *absorption atelectasis*.

Atelectasis itself is not a disease, but it is a sign of an abnormal process. The most common manifestation is bibasilar atelectasis, which is seen after thoracic or abdominal surgical procedures. A chest radiograph reveals the airless area of the lung, which may be segmental or lobar. If an entire lobe is affected, the mediastinum shifts to the affected side because of loss of volume of the affected lung. The chest radiograph can also demonstrate a decrease in the intercostal interspace, elevation of the hemidiaphragm of the affected side, and depression or elevation of the hilum, depending on which lobe is affected. If the atelectasis is segmental, the radiographic shadow appears triangular in shape, with the apex of the triangle pointing toward the hilum of the affected lung.

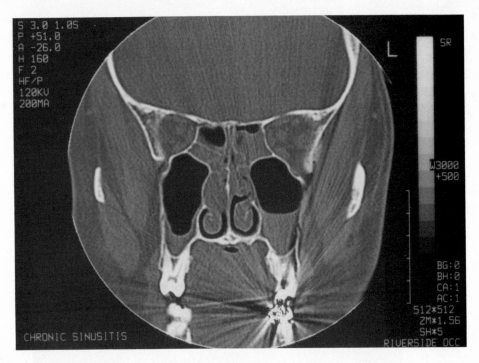

Fig. 3-43. Coronal CT view of the sinuses reveals sinusitis as shown by air-fluid levels in the maxillary sinuses and significant amounts of fluid in the maxillary sinuses. Obstruction seen in the nasal cavity is the cause of this sinusitis. (Courtesy of Riverside Methodist Hospitals, Columbus, Ohio.)

Plate-like atelectasis describes the radiographic appearance of one or more linear opacities, usually at the lung bases and parallel to the diaphragm (Fig. 3-45, page 135).

Treatment of acute atelectasis can be accomplished by appropriate respiratory therapy treatments such as coughing and deep breathing. Bronchoscopy can also be used to allow suctioning of secretions that are causing an obstruction. As mentioned with pleural effusions, thoracocentesis can be used to relieve the compression caused by an effusion.

Pneumothorax

A *pneumothorax* occurs when free air is trapped in the pleural space and compresses the lung tissue. This air may enter the pleural space from perforation of the visceral pleura, allowing gas to enter from the lung, penetration of the chest wall, or finally by generation of gas by gas-forming organs in an empyema.

Common causes of a pneumothorax include penetrating chest trauma (such as stab wounds (Fig. 3-46, p. 136), gunshot wounds, fractured ribs, or a thoracentesis needle) or

Text continued on page 136.

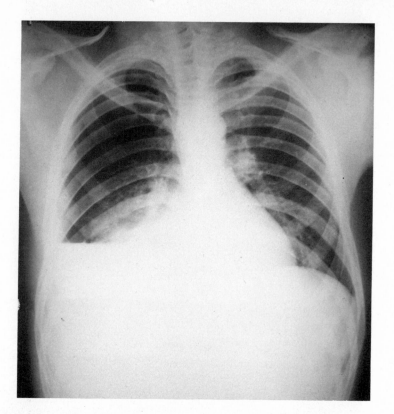

Fig. 3-46. Stab wound in the right chest of this 40-year-old male results in a pneumo-hemothorax. Fluid level in the right pleural space is blood, and the collapsed lung is outlined by its pleural margin in the upper chest. (Courtesy of the American College of Radiology, Reston, Virginia.)

a spontaneous blowout of a *bleb* (a flaccid vesicle, like a blister), resulting from some other pulmonary disease (Fig. 3-47). A pneumothorax may occur spontaneously as a result of trauma or as the result of some pathologic process. The typical manifestation of a spontaneous pneumothorax is sudden, one-sided chest pain followed by dyspnea.

Radiographically, a pneumothorax appears as a strip of radiolucency devoid of vascular lung markings, with separation of the visceral and parietal pleura (Fig. 3-48). It is best demonstrated on an erect expiration chest radiograph. Occasionally, wrinkles in the patient's skin produce artifacts that can mimic a pneumothorax. Such an artifact is called a *pseudopneumothorax*.

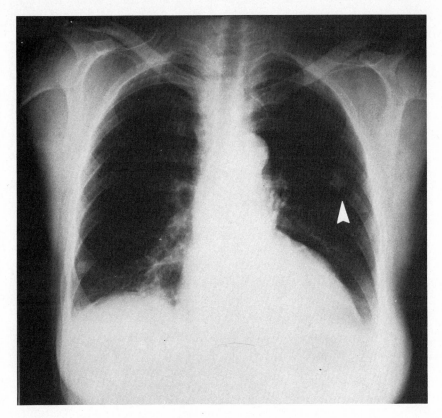

Fig. 3-52. Solitary lung nodule seen on PA projection represents a suspicious neoplasm, requiring further investigation. (Courtesy of Riverside Methodist Hospitals, Columbus, Ohio.)

The second most common radiographic presentation of a neoplasm consists of a solitary radiopaque lung nodule (Fig. 3-52), sometimes called a "coin" lesion. Tomography is used in the evaluation of calcium deposits within these lesions, although CT is increasingly the standard for nodule evaluation. Malignant lesions are rarely calcified, whereas benign lesions generally have a calcified center. Fluoroscopy also aids in the diagnosis of neoplasms of the lung. The patient may undergo percutaneous lung biopsy bronchoscopy, or brush biopsy. The latter is a procedure in which a device with tiny brushes is introduced through a bronchoscope or bronchial catheter to procure cells and tissues under fluoroscopic guidance. Although rarely used, pulmonary arteriography may assess obstruction of a pulmonary artery caused by an invasive tumor.

The prognosis is very poor for bronchogenic carcinoma, with only a 12% to 14% 5-year survival rate. Cigarette smoking is by far the most important etiologic factor. Exposure to potentially carcinogenic substances from air pollution and occupational exposure are also etiologic factors. This disease process may be treated with surgery, chemotherapy, radiation therapy, or any combination of the three modalities.

Metastases from Other Sites

Pulmonary metastases are much more common than primary lung neoplasms. Many malignancies develop pulmonary metastases, which are detectable on a chest radiograph (Fig. 3-53). The most common primary sites for these tumors are the breast, gastrointestinal tract, female reproductive system, and the kidneys.

Spreading of malignancy to the lungs from a primary site occurs via five different routes: 1. Through the bloodstream in *hematogenous metastases;* 2. Through the lymph system in *lymphogenous metastases;* 3. By direct extension in *local invasion;* 4. Through the tracheobronchial system in *bronchogenic metastases;* 5. Direct implantation from biopsies or other surgical procedures (although rarely). Radiographically, these metastatic lesions appear as single or multiple rounded opacities throughout the lungs (Fig. 3-54, *A* and *B*). CT is again more sensitive than conventional chest radiography in the detection of small metastatic lesions.

As in the case of bronchogenic carcinoma, treatment of pulmonary metastases is accomplished through surgery, chemotherapy, radiation therapy, or a combination of them, depending on the type of tumor and its likely primary site. For example, hormonal therapy of prostatic and breast carcinoma can cause pulmonary lesions to resolve. The field of oncology is growing, with new treatment options in research and ongoing development.

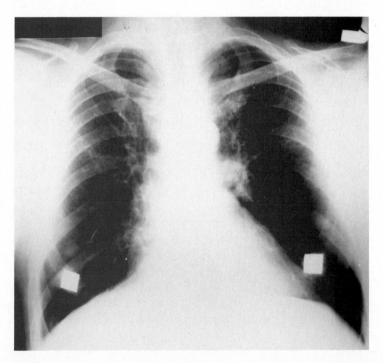

Fig. 3-53. Questionable densities seen on routine chest radiograph resulted in application of nipple markers. Film with markers demonstrated lesions above, which were found to be metastases secondary to colon carcinoma. (Courtesy of the American College of Radiology, Reston, Virginia.)

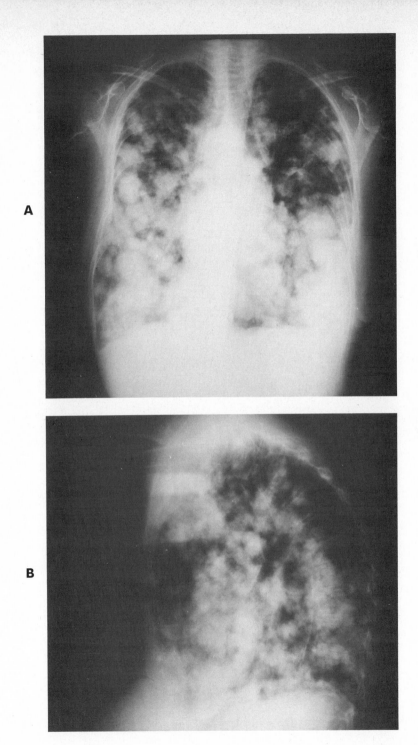

Fig. 3-54, *A.* Pulmonary metastases from uterine cancer demonstrates multiple lesions with characteristic ''cotton ball'' appearance. *B.* Lateral projection of pulmonary metastases resulting from uterine cancer. Courtesy of Riverside Methodist Hospitals, Columbus, Ohio.)

▼ QUESTIONS

1. Which of the following statements related to exposure conditions of chest radiography are true?
   1. Subtractive pathologies increase the difficulty of adequately penetrating the chest.
   2. Heart magnification is avoided in portable radiography by use of a 72-inch SID.
   3. An attractive feature of digital radiography is its wide exposure latitude.
      a. 1 and 2   **c.** 2 and 3
      b. 1 and 3   **d.** 1, 2, and 3

2. Because of its late development, which respiratory sinus would you *not* expect to see on radiographs of a 1-year-old child?
   a. ethmoid   **d.** sphenoid
   b. frontal   **e.** all of these are visible in a
   c. maxillary   1-year-old child

3. Bony structures such as the clavicles can be removed from the apices of the lung by use of which projection?
   a. AP   **c.** lordotic
   b. decubitus   **d.** oblique

4. Which of the following statements are true of a normal chest radiograph?
   1. Pectus excavatum, if severe enough, can cause displacement of the heart laterally.
   2. Visualization of 5 to 7 posterior ribs indicates achievement of adequate inspiration.
   3. Demonstration of the pectoral muscles on a chest film is expected and common.
      a. 1 and 2   **c.** 2 and 3
      b. 1 and 3   **d.** 1, 2, and 3

5. The "sail sign" in an infant is commonly associated with enlargement of the:
   a. heart   **c.** thymus
   b. pulmonary arteries **d.** thyroid

6. Which of the following types of tubes is readily visible on a chest radiograph and serves to maintain an adequate airway in a pulmonary-compromised patient?
   a. chest tube   **d.** Swan-Ganz catheter
   b. CVP line   **e.** none of the above
   c. endotracheal tube

7. A congenital condition that demonstrates gradually increasing bronchial secretions that lead to obstruction of the bronchial tree and infection is:
   a. cystic fibrosis   **c.** pectus excavatum
   b. hyaline membrane disease   **d.** pneumatocele

8. An infant born after only 6 months of gestation may likely suffer from:
   a. bronchogenic carcinoma   **c.** mediastinal emphysema
   b. cystic fibrosis   **d.** respiratory distress syndrome

9. Which of the following is the most common type of bacterial pneumonia?
   a. aspiration   **c.** pneumococcal
   b. Legionnaires'   **d.** streptococcal

10. A thin-walled, air-containing cyst is a(n):
    a. air-bronchogram   **c.** mycoplasma
    b. alveoli   **d.** pneumatocele

11. Loss of elasticity of the bronchial walls as a result of bacterial infection can result in:
    a. bronchiectasis   **c.** pneumococcal pneumonia
    b. bronchogenic carcinoma   **d.** tuberculosis

12. The presence of apical lesions and pulmonary cavitation are characteristics of which pulmonary inflammatory disease?
    a. atelectasis   **d.** tuberculosis
    b. bronchogenic carcinoma   **e.** none of the above
    c. pneumoconiosis

13. The most common forms of chronic obstructive pulmonary disease are chronic bronchitis and:
    a. asthma   **c.** emphysema
    b. atelectasis   **d.** tuberculosis

14. Which of the following would *not* be seen radiographically in the case of pulmonary emphysema?
    a. abnormally lucent lungs   **d.** high, rounded diaphragms
    b. abnormally large lungs   **e.** all are seen in emphysema
    c. barrel-chested appearance

15. Pulmonary fibrosis resulting from occupationally inhaled dusts is characteristic of a(n):
    a. atelectasis   **c.** pleural effusion
    b. chronic bronchitis   **d.** pneumoconiosis

16. Which of the following fungal diseases is more commonly found in semi-arid regions and places agriculture and construction workers particularly at risk?
    a. asbestosis   **c.** histoplasmosis
    b. coccidiomycosis   **d.** silicosis

17. An accumulation of pus in the pleural cavity is known as a(n):
    a. coin lesion   **c.** pleural effusion
    b. empyema   **d.** pleurisy

18. Incomplete expansion of a lung as a result of partial or total collapse defines:
    a. atelectasis   **c.** pleurisy
    b. empyema   **d.** pneumothorax

19. Acute atelectasis can often be relieved by:
    a. antibiotic administration   **c.** coughing and deep breathing
    b. chemotheraphy   **d.** endotracheal tube insertion

20. Spontaneous blowout of a bleb could lead to a(n):
    a. atelectasis   **c.** pleurisy
    b. emphysematous lesion   **d.** pneumothorax

21. Demonstration of a pneumothorax is best accomplished by making the exposure:
    - **a.** in an erect, lateral position
    - **b.** in a lateral decubitus position
    - **c.** on expiration
    - **d.** on inspiration

22. The most common radiographic presentation of bronchogenic carcinoma is a(n):
    - **a.** coin lesion
    - **b.** pleural effusion
    - **c.** pneumothorax
    - **d.** unilateral hilar mass

23. The most common etiologic factor in bronchogenic carcinoma is:
    - **a.** auto emission
    - **b.** cigarette smoking
    - **c.** dust
    - **d.** iatrogenic treatment

24. Which of the following statements are true about pulmonary neoplasms?
    1. Bronchial adenomas are usually considered benign, but can metastasize.
    2. Primary lung neoplasms are much more common than pulmonary metastases.
    3. CT is more sensitive than chest radiography in detection of small chest lesions.
    - **a.** 1 and 2
    - **b.** 1 and 3
    - **c.** 2 and 3
    - **d.** 1, 2, and 3

25. A stab wound to the chest could easily result in an acute:
    - **a.** empyema
    - **b.** emphysema
    - **c.** pneumothorax
    - **d.** viral pneumonia

4

The Abdomen and Gastrointestinal System

▼

Upon completion of Chapter 4, the reader should be able to:

- Describe the anatomical components of the abdomen and gastrointestinal system and how they are visualized radiographically.

- Compare and contrast the various imaging modalities used in evaluation of the abdomen and its contents.

- Identify the tubes and catheters related to the gastrointestinal system by type and briefly explain their use.

- Characterize a given condition as congenital, inflammatory, traumatic, neurogenic, or neoplastic.

- Identify the pathogenesis of the gastrointestinal pathologies cited and typical treatments for them.

- Describe, in general, the radiographic appearance of each of the given pathologies.

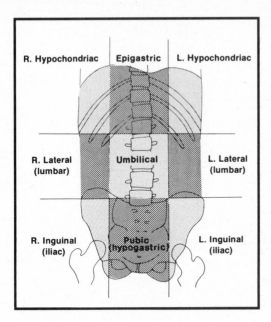

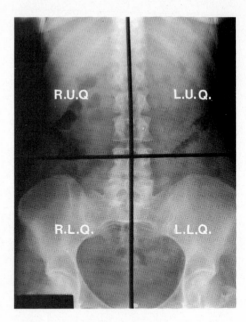

Fig. 4-1, left. The nine regions of the abdomen. (From Bontrager KL: *Textbook of Radiographic Positioning and Related Anatomy,* ed 3, St Louis, 1993, Mosby.)

Fig. 4-2, right. The four quadrants of the abdomen. (From Bontrager KL: *Textbook of Radiographic Positioning and Related Anatomy,* ed 3, St Louis, 1993, Mosby.)

ANATOMY AND PHYSIOLOGY REVIEW

• THE ABDOMEN

The abdomen comprises the abdominal and pelvic cavities and is often divided into nine anatomical regions: right hypochondriac, epigastric, left hypochondriac, right lumbar, umbilical, left lumbar, right iliac, hypogastric, left iliac (Fig. 4-1). It may also be described in terms of quadrants: right-upper (RUQ), right-lower (RLQ), left-upper (LUQ), and left-lower (LLQ) (Fig. 4-2). The abdominal cavity contains organs of the digestive system (stomach and intestines), the hepatobiliary system (liver, gallbladder, and pancreas), the urinary system (kidneys and ureters), and the circulatory system (spleen). The pelvic cavity contains the bladder, portions of the intestines, and the reproductive organs.

The abdominal cavity is lined by the peritoneum, a serous membrane. (Fig. 4-3, *A*). The serous lining attached to the abdominal organs is the visceral peritoneum. The peritoneum attached directly to the abdominal wall is the parietal peritoneum. The mesentery is a double fold of parietal peritoneum projecting from the posterior abdominal wall in the lumbar region (Fig. 4-3, *B*). Most of the small bowel is attached to the outer edge of the mesentery.

The greater omentum is a double fold of peritoneum that attaches to the duodenum, stomach, and transverse colon. It hangs loosely over the intestines. The lesser omentum is a fold of peritoneum that attaches the liver to the lesser curvature of the stomach and the duodenum (Fig. 4-4, p. 150).

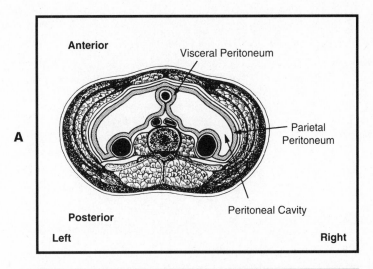

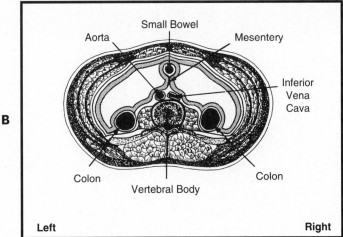

Fig. 4-3, *A.* A cross-sectional drawing of the abdomen demonstrates the peritoneum. *B.* A cross-sectional drawing of the lower abdomen demonstrates the mesentery. (From Bontrager KL: *Textbook of Radiographic Positioning and Related Anatomy,* ed 3, St Louis 1993, Mosby.)

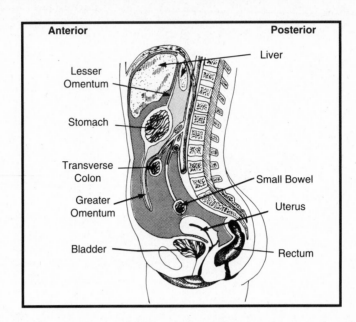

Fig. 4-4. A cross-sectional drawing of the abdominal cavity demonstrates the omentum. (From Bontrager KL: *Textbook of Radiographic Positioning and Related Anatomy,* ed 3, St Louis, 1993, Mosby.)

• THE GASTROINTESTINAL SYSTEM

A major portion of the gastrointestinal (GI) system is the *alimentary tract,* which serves to digest and absorb food. Extending from the mouth to the anus, the alimentary tract comprises the mouth, pharynx, esophagus, stomach, small and large bowel, and the rectum.

The esophagus is the first part of the GI system. It is approximately 10 to 12 inches in length and extends from the posterior pharynx to the stomach (Fig. 4-5). While the upper esophagus is midline, it courses to the left to pass behind the aortic arch, which indents the esophagus. Other indentations occur at the level of the left mainstem bronchus and at the gastroesophageal junction. As it passes downward, the esophagus follows the curvature of the thoracic spine and thoracic descending aorta.

The stomach occupies the body's left-upper quadrant, with the cardiac orifice at the level of the tenth or eleventh thoracic vertebra, and the pyloric canal just to the right of the first or second lumbar vertebra (Fig. 4-6). Peristalsis churns the gastric content and propels it toward the pylorus. Gastric emptying of liquids is accounted for by the peristalsis initiated in the fundus of the stomach; gastric emptying of solids requires a to-and-fro action of the antrum and pylorus. In the presence of masses, inflammation, or diabetes, the peristaltic activity may be diminished. When filled with barium, the curvatures of the stomach visualize as generally smooth contours. The mucosae appear as longitudinal ridges within the stomach.

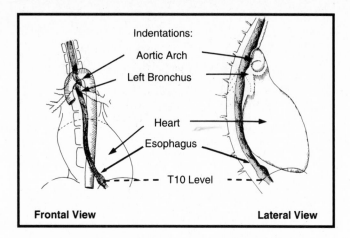

Fig. 4-5. The esophagus in the mediastinum. (From Bontrager KL: *Textbook of Radiographic Positioning and Related Anatomy,* ed 3, St Louis, 1993, Mosby Year Book)

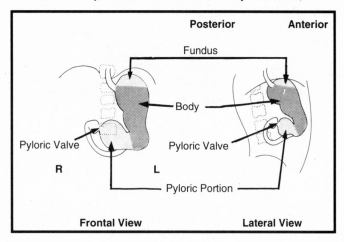

Fig. 4-6. The stomach depicted in its average orientation when empty. (From Bontrager KL: *Textbook of Radiographic Positioning and Related Anatomy,* St Louis 1993, Mosby.)

The small bowel includes the duodenum, jejunum, and the ileum. It arises from the stomach at the duodenal bulb and courses to the ileocecal valve (Fig. 4-7, p. 152), over a length of nearly 21 feet. The duodenal C-loop moves posteriorly from the gastric antrum to its ending at the ligament of Treitz. The jejunum begins here and coils in the left-upper quadrant before terminating into the ileum in the right-upper quadrant. The ileum then courses through the right- and left-lower quadrants to terminate at the ileocecal junction. When filled with barium, the segments of the small bowel are distinguishable by their appearance. Duodenal mucosa is indicated by its transverse rigid appearance. Jejunal mucosa appears delicate and feathery. Ileal folds appear similar to those of the duodenum, though not as large.

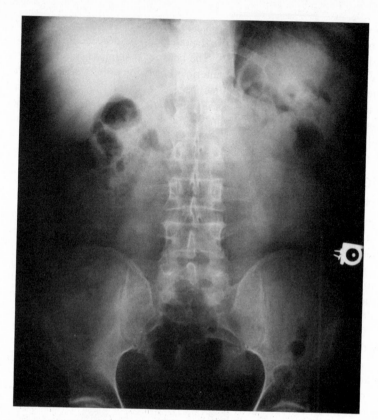

Fig. 4-9. Radiographic appearance of a normal abdomen, demonstrating kidney shadows, liver shadow, psoas muscles, and transverse processes of the lumbar spine. (Courtesy of Riverside Methodist Hospitals, Columbus, Ohio.)

• THE GASTROINTESTINAL SYSTEM

Some contents of the abdomen can be seen without contrast media, as explained. However, most of the GI tract cannot be examined directly. The internal surfaces of both ends can be visualized through *endoscopy,* the use of lighted instruments with optics to visualize disease of the esophagus, stomach and duodenum, or rectum and distal colon, and occasionally the terminal ileum. Endoscopy is seeing significant growth in health care as the instrument technology continues to improve, allowing more detailed studies and improved patient comfort. Abnormal areas can be visualized, biopsied, and examined histologically. Those areas unable to be directly examined are studied radiographically.

Radiographic investigation of the GI system commonly consists of a combination of fluoroscopy and radiography. Fluoroscopy provides dynamic information, whereas radiographs provide a permanent static record of the examination. Radiographic examination of the gastrointestinal system requires the use of positive and negative contrast agents for visualization of the body parts. Barium sulfate is generally used as the positive contrast agent but is contraindicated in cases of GI tract perforation. If a perforated bowel is suspected, a water-soluble contrast agent should be used. Although infrequently used, a negative contrast agent (e.g., air or carbon dioxide) may be used to distend the stomach and bowel for better visualization of the mucosal lining.

The Esophagus

Most upper GI studies begin with the patient in an erect position to evaluate air-fluid levels present in the alimentary tract. An esophageal study may be performed to demonstrate anomalies and abnormalities of the esophagus. Transport of the food or liquid bolus through swallowing is the sole function of the esophagus. If studied as part of a GI tract examination, thin barium may be used. Thick barium is used if the esophagus is the single object of study. Most patients presenting for a traditional esophagram have a chief complaint of *dysphagia,* or difficult swallowing. The causes for dysphagia are numerous and are discussed in this chapter.

Radiographs are typically taken of a barium-filled esophagus in an erect or prone position. They include a PA, right lateral, and an right anterior oblique (RAO) (Fig. 4-10) to visualize the esophagus between the spine and the heart.

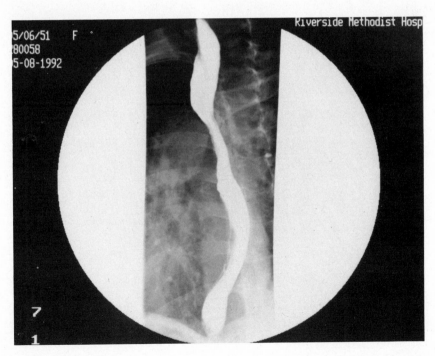

Fig. 4-10. Normal esophagus as seen on this RAO digital spot film on a 21-year-old female. (Courtesy of Riverside Methodist Hospitals, Columbus, Ohio.)

During fluoroscopy, the radiologist can visualize mechanical problems presented while the patient is swallowing the barium sulfate mixture. Esophageal studies are also used to study the contour of the heart, as described in Chapter 9 of this text.

The Stomach

One of radiology's most common procedures is an "upper GI," in which barium flows from the esophagus and into the stomach and small bowel. Once the barium reaches the stomach, the radiologist evaluates the stomach contour, position, rugae, and the peristaltic changes occurring as the stomach fills and empties.

In the event the radiologist wishes to diminish peristalsis, glucagon is given to relax the stomach musculature. Occasionally, a gas-producing substance is used along with the barium to produce a double-contrast examination. The purpose of this is to expand the stomach and promote coating of the stomach mucosa. The duodenal bulb is studied as it fills with barium and empties into the small bowel. Compression may be used for better visualization of specific anatomic areas of the upper GI tract.

A series of radiographs is taken following fluoroscopy, with the projections differing from one institution to another. Typical patient positions include a recumbent PA projection to demonstrate the entire stomach and duodenal bulb, RAO to highlight the pyloric canal and duodenal bulb (Fig. 4-11), right lateral to show the duodenal bulb and loop, and the LPO to demonstrate the gastric fundus. Proper positioning relates significantly to the

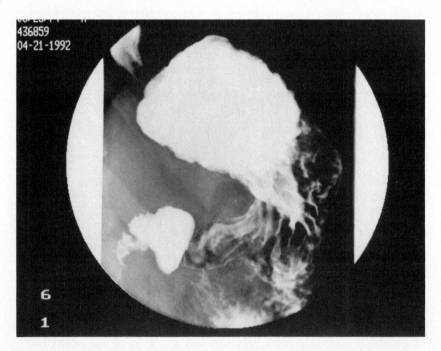

Fig. 4-11. Normal stomach as seen on this digital spot film on an 18-year-old male. (Courtesy of Riverside Methodist Hospitals, Columbus, Ohio.)

patient's body habitus. Generally, the more hypersthenic a patient is, the more his or her stomach tends to lie transversely and higher. The stomach is more J-shaped for other body habiti (i.e., sthenic, hyposthenic, and asthenic), lying lower and closer to the spine.

The Small Bowel

In some instances, the barium may be followed as it progresses through the small intestines. Radiographs are exposed at set intervals to determine GI motility and to demonstrate abnormalities within the small bowel. Once the contrast agent reaches the ileocecal valve, the small bowel study is complete, typically within 2 to 3 hours (Fig. 4-12).

The small intestines may also be studied radiographically by means of enteroclysis, a small bowel enema. This is accomplished by advancing an intestinal tube through the patient's mouth to the end of the duodenum at the ligament of Treitz. Contrast agents, both positive and negative (barium and methylcellulose, respectively), are directly injected into the small bowel.

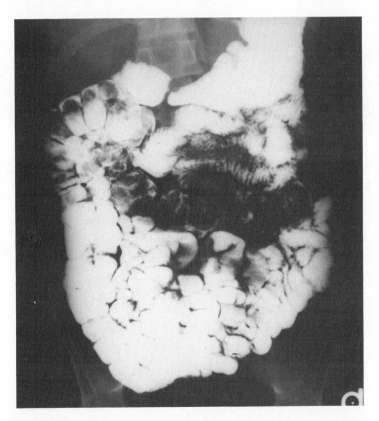

Fig. 4-12. Small bowel film taken 75 minutes after the examination began on this 18-year-old male, demonstrating passage through the ileocecal valve into the colon, with no mucosal abnormalities or dilated loops of small bowel. (Courtesy of Riverside Methodist Hospitals, Columbus, Ohio.)

The Large Bowel

The lower GI tract is examined by administering a barium enema through the rectum. This examination demonstrates abnormalities of the large bowel and intraluminal neoplasms. The barium enema can be performed in a single contrast fashion using only barium or as a double-contrast study mixing barium with a negative contrast agent (e.g., air). The negative contrast agent distends the lumen, allowing improved visualization of the mucosal lining (Fig. 4-13), especially small polyps and intraluminal tumors. In either case, the radiologist typically exposes a series of spot films with the patient in various positions to highlight certain areas of the colon (e.g., flexures). The technologist may also expose a series of radiographs per the radiologist's instructions (Fig. 4-14). Following evacuation of the barium, the technologist takes a "post-evacuation" film to visualize colon contraction and demonstrate mucosa.

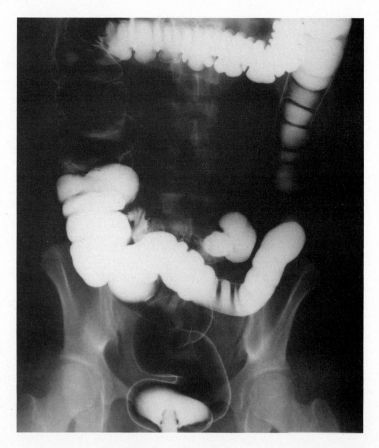

Fig. 4-13. Normal air-contrast enema on this 19-year-old female with a history of low hemoglobin, as demonstrated on this PA projection. (Courtesy of Riverside Methodist Hospitals, Columbus, Ohio.)

If a patient has had a surgical enterostomy procedure, the contrast media may be administered through the opening in the abdominal wall to the specific area of the GI system. A *colostomy* is a procedure in which a stoma is surgically created to the abdominal wall to allow drainage of bowel contents into a closed pouch hung outside the body. Those found in the sigmoid and descending colon are most frequently placed because of rectal or sigmoid cancer. Those placed in the transverse or ascending colon are often for indications that allow for the colostomy to be placed for temporary purposes for diversion of flow of colonic contents (e.g., sigmoid diverticulitis, rectovaginal fistula, colon obstruction).

Ileostomies are similar openings but placed from the ileum, with the most common indication being ulcerative colitis. As with colostomies, patient problems with ileostomies include proper skin protection and odor control. Proper fit of the appliance for drainage is essential to prevent problems caused by excoriating digestive enzymes. Other enterostomies (i.e., jejunostomies and duodenostomies) are more rarely used and only under very specific circumstances because of the loss of electrolytes that occurs before their absorption through the small bowel. These patients often require total parenteral nutrition (TPN) to maintain life.

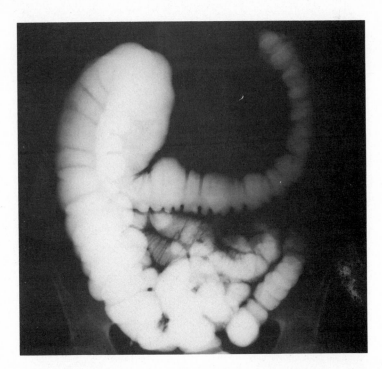

Fig. 4-14. Normal barium enema on a 23-year-old female with a history of irritable bowel and severe constipation as demonstrated on this PA projection. (Courtesy of Riverside Methodist Hospitals, Columbus, Ohio.)

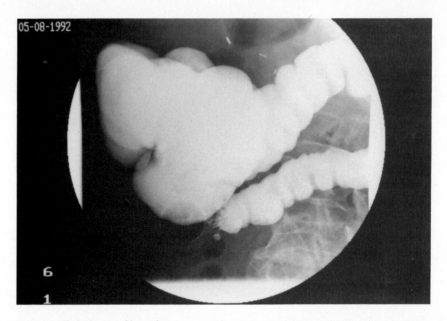

Fig. 4-15. A digital spot film of an enema through a colostomy in the descending colon on this 72-year-old male. The ostomy is clearly indicated by its circular opening into the bowel. Also seen is a small diverticulum just adjacent to the colostomy site and an inverted cecum. (Courtesy of Riverside Methodist Hospitals, Columbus, Ohio.)

If a patient has had a surgical enterostomy procedure, the contrast agent may be administered through the opening in the abdominal wall to the specific area of the GI system (Fig. 4-15).

Other Studies

Computer tomography (CT) is an important modality used for abdominal survey examination, as well as playing a significant role in the examination of the GI system. Because CT can visualize small differences in tissue density, it clearly demonstrates abdominal organs that are normally not apparent on conventional abdominal radiographs without the use of contrast agents. Upon CT examination, the liver, spleen, pancreas and kidneys appear as homogeneous soft tissue densities, making any alteration in the density from pathologic conditions readily visible, even without the use of contrast media. Abscesses and solid and cystic masses all have a respective range of densities between water and normal soft tissue densities. CT is also quite useful in the evaluation of retroperitoneal pathologies such as lymph node enlargement resulting from neoplastic disease or infection. Finally, it has become the accepted modality for following the progress of GI malignancies and also plays a role in the diagnosis of inflammatory conditions (e.g., abscess).

The role of MRI in the abdomen and GI tract is still evolving as current scan times and bowel motion are still limiting factors, although emerging developments may allow it to play a larger role. Along with ultrasound, CT and MRI are useful in demonstrating the presence of any retroperitoneal masses that may impinge on the GI tract. In nuclear medicine, GI bleed scans are useful in demonstrating GI bleeding and help direct angiographers to the site of bleeding if therapeutic intervention is to be performed.

Digital fluoroscopy has emerged as a substantive improvement over traditional fluoroscopy for a number of reasons. Sophisticated on-line image processing allows enhancement of selective image quality parameters relevant to diagnosis not possible with conventional spot-film devices. Radiologists can view the images throughout the procedure rather than waiting for film processing at the end of the study. This immediate availability has altered the practice of fluoroscopy in terms of its speed and efficiency. Hard copy film production is available at the touch of a button with no interruptions for changing of cassettes. Anatomical motion can be captured as it occurs, instead of the radiologist trying to synchronize the timing of their filming with, for example, esophageal swallowing. Serial filming capability further enhances this and allows several images per second to be exposed. Diagnosis is often made in midprocedure, allowing hard copies to be produced later for historical purposes. Many sites are reporting that fewer hard copies are necessary and film costs are consequently reduced. Radiation dose is therefore also reduced.

As earlier noted, endoscopy is the use of tubular fiber optic devices to look inside the GI tract and other hollow organs or cavities of the body. As its sophistication and specificity have increased, it is assuming a greater role in diagnosis and therapy of the GI tract. Upper endoscopy is capable of seeing down into the esophagus, stomach, duodenum (including the Ampulla of Vater), and even into the proximal jejunum. Colonoscopy can allow visualization retrograde through the rectum as far as the terminal ileum. The small bowel is still largely out of reach through endoscopy. Photographic views of the interior of the body provide readily diagnosable information (Figs. 4-16 and 4-17). Therapeutic

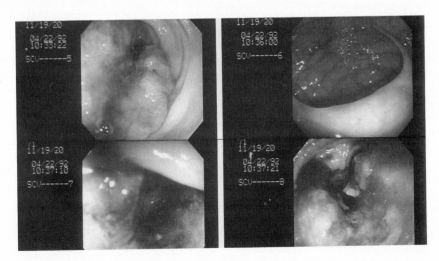

Fig. 4-16. Endoscopic image of a sigmoid colon mass in a 72-year-old female seen as a mass bulging into the lumen of the colon. (Courtesy of Riverside Methodist Hospitals, Columbus, Ohio.)

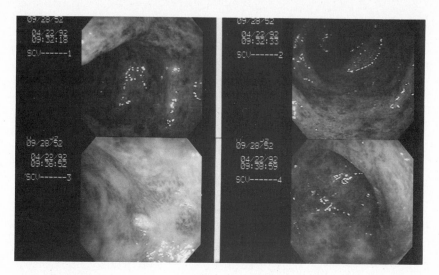

Fig. 4-17. Endoscopic image of diffuse colitis with a bacterioetiology in this 40-year-old male indicated by the splotchiness of the bowel mucosa. (Courtesy of Riverside Methodist Hospitals, Columbus, Ohio.)

applications of endoscopy are numerous. They include polyp removal, electrocautery to stop hemorrhaging, sclerosing of esophageal varices, lesion biopsy, sealing of tracheoe-sophageal fistulas, stone removal, esophageal prosthesis insertion, and laser tumor re-moval (both generally for palliative purposes).

• ABDOMINAL TUBES AND CATHETERS

As with the chest, a variety of tubes and catheters can be placed within particular portions of the abdomen. It is important for the technologist to be familiar with each type of tube and exercise great caution in attempting to move patients with abdominal tubes in place. The technologist should also ask the patient's nurse or consult the chart before altering the patient's position. In addition, some abdominal tubes/catheters allow entry into body systems that are normally sterile and require special care to avoid infection.

Gastric tubes may be placed (generally through the nose) for a variety of diagnostic and therapeutic purposes. They may be indicated for aspiration of gastric contents, to help control nausea and vomiting, for decompression and removal of gastric contents because of bowel dysfunction or surgery, and for nutritional support tube feedings (gastric gavage) or medication administration. A *Levin tube* is the most common nasogastric tube. It is a fairly small, single-lumen tube with a plain tip and it may be visualized radiographically. Proper placement is commonly assessed through aspiration of gastric juices and listening for proper placement within the stomach via a stethoscope. If a nasogastric tube is placed for feeding, the patient's head must remain elevated to prevent the tube from becoming displaced, leading to aspiration of the gastric contents. If an emergent condition exists that requires large amounts of gastric contents to be aspirated quickly (gastric lavage), an

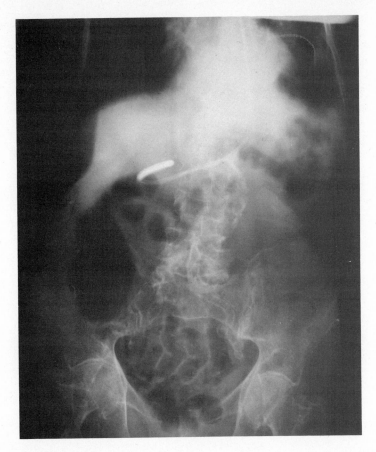

Fig. 4-18. Radiographic appearance of a Dobhoff tube being checked for placement in this 93-year-old female. It is placed in the antrum of the stomach. Also seen are extensive vascular calcifications. (Courtesy of Riverside Methodist Hospitals, Columbus, Ohio.)

Ewald or *Edlich tube* may be used. These tubes are placed through the mouth, are wider than a Levin tube, and contain several openings that allow quicker aspiration. A *Levacuator tube* may also be used for evacuation of gastric contents. This is a wide, double-lumen tube placed through the patient's mouth with the larger lumen used for gastric lavage, while the smaller lumen allows instillation of an irrigant.

An *enteral tube* is a small caliber tube used to deliver a liquid diet directly to the duodenum or jejunum. It most commonly has a weighted end to hold the tube in the proper placement. The *Dobhoff tube* is a common radiopaque enteral tube (Fig. 4-18).

Nasoenteric decompression tubes are used to remove gas and fluids in the prevention and treatment of abdominal distention. These tubes have a balloon or rubber bag at one end filled with air, mercury, or water to stimulate peristalsis and facilitate passage through the pylorus into the intestinal tract. The *Miller-Abbott tube* is a common type of double-

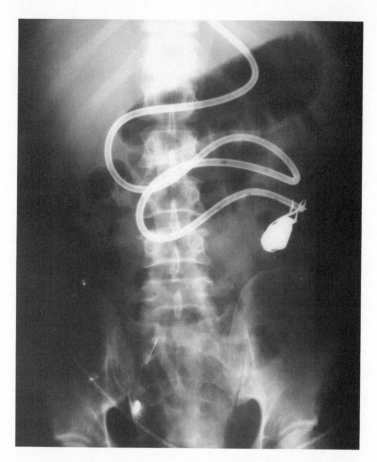

Fig. 4-19. Radiographic appearance of a Cantor tube. Placed 4 hours earlier in this 50-year-old male with a mechanical bowel obstruction, it is now advanced into the second portion of the duodenum. (Courtesy of Riverside Methodist Hospitals, Columbus, Ohio.)

lumen decompression tube. It is passed through the nose, pharynx, and esophagus with the balloon uninflated. Once the end of the tube reaches the stomach, the balloon is inflated and the tube is pulled back until it stops at the cardiac sphincter. The patient is then placed on his or her right side in a semi-erect position, the air is withdrawn from the balloon and replaced with mercury. Progress of the tube is assessed by taking abdominal radiographs at regular intervals. *Harris and Cantor tubes* are other types of decompression tubes. Unlike the Miller-Abbott tube, however, the Cantor (Fig. 4-19) and Harris tubes contain a single lumen.

Levin tubes or *Foley catheters* may also be surgically placed in any portion of the GI system. A gastrostomy tube indicates the tube is placed in the stomach, whereas a duodenostomy tube or jejunostomy tube is specific to that portion of the intestines. These tubes provide a direct route for administering liquid feedings.

CONGENITAL/HEREDITARY ANOMALIES
Atresia

Esophageal atresia is a congenital anomaly in which the esophagus fails to develop past some point (Fig. 4-20). The symptoms of this are visible soon after birth and include excessive salivation, choking, gagging, dyspnea, and cyanosis. Immediate surgery is required to alleviate the problem. Usually coincident with atresia is a tracheoesophageal fistula. This consists of an atresia at the level of the fourth thoracic vertebra with a fistula, an abnormal tubelike passage from one structure to another, to the trachea (Fig. 4-21, p. 166). Such a condition is incompatible with life for more than 2 to 3 days.

Duodenal atresia is a congenital anomaly in which the lumen of the duodenum does not exist, resulting in complete obstruction of the GI tract at the duodenum. While a rare occurrence (1 in approximately 20,000 births), it is evident soon after birth when vom-

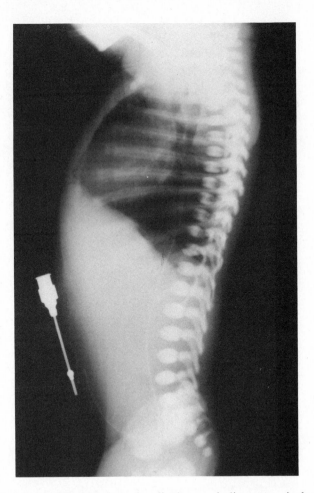

Fig. 4-20. Lack of any GI air below the diaphragm indicates an isolated esophageal atresia. (Courtesy of the American College of Radiology, Reston, Virginia.)

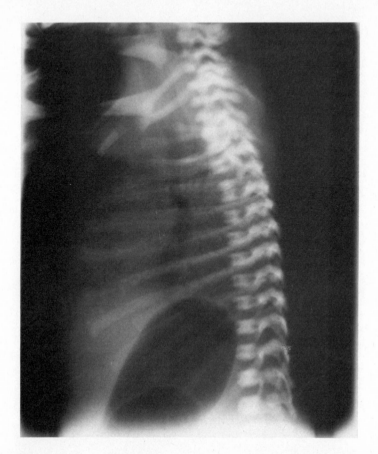

Fig. 4-21. Lateral view of the chest on a 1-day-old premature infant demonstrates distention of the distal esophagus with air and in continuity with the trachea. Marked gastric distention is also present. Appearance is consistent with esophageal atresia and a tracheosophageal fistula. (Courtesy of the American College of Radiology, Reston, Virginia.)

iting begins and the epigastrium becomes distended. The ''double bubble sign'' is a radiographic indication of duodenal atresia, and consists of gaseous distention of the stomach and proximal duodenum (Fig. 4-22). Treatment consists of surgery to open the duodenum for connection to the pylorus. During surgery, it is common to examine the other areas of the small and large bowel for other sites of atresia and malrotation, which often accompany duodenal atresia.

Colonic atresia is a congenital failure of development of the distal rectum and anus, which can occur to a variable extent (Fig. 4-23, pp. 169–170). A frequent complication of this is fistula formation to the genitourinary system, which often can be repaired surgically.

Text continued on p. 171.

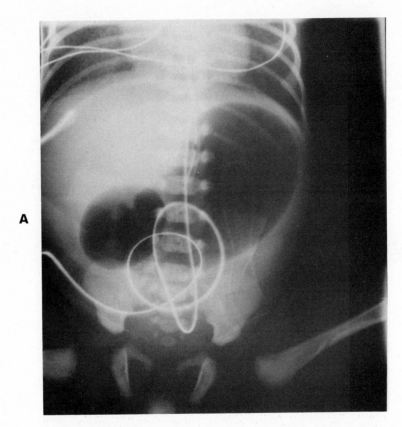

Fig. 4-22, *A.* Marked distention of the stomach and duodenal bulb with bowel gas distal to the duodenum. Visualization of the classic ''double-bubble sign'' indicates duodenal atresia. (Courtesy of Riverside Methodist Hospitals, Columbus, Ohio.)

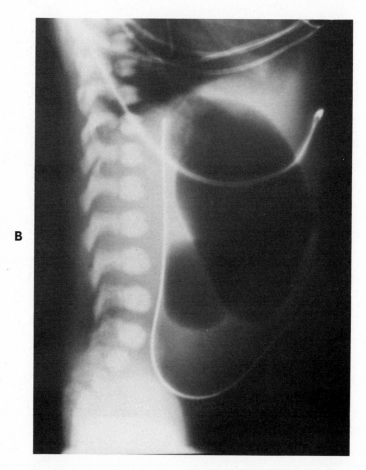

Fig. 4-22, *B.* The "double-bubble sign" seen in a lateral projection of the same 1 day-old infant. (Courtesy of the American College of Radiology, Reston, Virginia.)

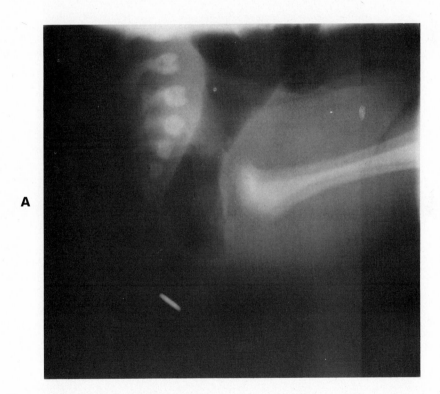

Fig. 4-23, *A.* Visualization of the rectal air column extending to within centimeters of the perineum (indicated by lead marker) in a 15-hour-old newborn with abdominal distention. (Courtesy of the American College of Radiology, Reston, Virginia.)

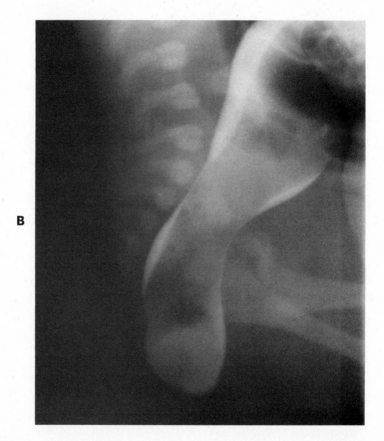

Fig. 4-23, *B.* A transperineal percutaneous water-soluble contrast study of the rectum reveals a blind distal colon pouch, evidence of colonic atresia. No genitourinary fistulas were noted as is common with this condition. (Courtesy of the American College of Radiology, Reston, Virginia.)

Hypertrophic Pyloric Stenosis

Hypertrophic pyloric stenosis is a congenital anomaly of the stomach where the pyloric canal leading out of the stomach is greatly narrowed because of hypertrophy of the pyloric sphincter (Fig. 4-24). The exact etiology of this is unknown, but it seems genetically related. It occurs 3 to 4 times more often in male children and most often in the first-born male. Typically, the first sign of the condition is projectile vomiting at 3 to 5 weeks of age. A surgical procedure is used to incise the hypertrophied muscle fibers, increasing the opening of the pyloric channel.

Malrotation

Aberrations of the normal process of intestinal rotation in utero can result in anomalous position of the small and large bowel, with abnormal fixations predisposing the patient to internal herniation and volvulus.

Malrotation exists when the intestines are not in their normal position (Fig. 4-25, p. 172), occurring in an equal male-to-female ratio. There are varying degrees of mal-

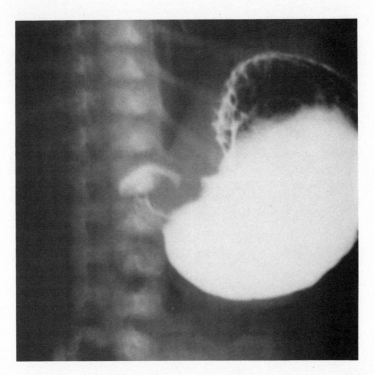

Fig. 4-24. A thin column of barium flowing from the stomach into the pylorus in this 1-month-old male with projectile vomiting indicates hypertrophic pyloric stenosis. (Courtesy of the American College of Radiology, Reston, Virginia.)

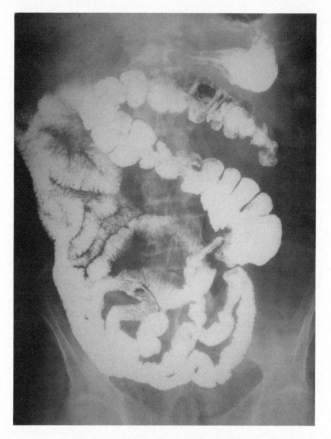

Fig. 4-25. Malrotation of the bowel indicated by the position of the small bowel in the right abdomen and the colon in the left. Note how the terminal ileum enters the cecum from the right. (Courtesy of the American College of Radiology, Reston, Virginia.)

rotation of the intestinal tract, ranging from failure of fixation of the cecum in the right-lower quadrant, to complete *transposition* of the bowel, a condition where the small bowel is on the right and the colon is on the left. While such errors of fixation are often symptomless, they may lead to bowel volvulus, or incarceration of bowel in an internal hernia. Surgery is the choice for correction of a volvulus or bowel incarceration, with resection of the involved bowel required to relieve infarction of the intestine.

Complete reversal of all abdominal organs, although rare, is known as *situs inversus*.

Imperforate Anus

Imperforate anus is a congenital disorder in which there is no anal opening to the exterior. This condition is corrected surgically shortly after birth.

INFLAMMATORY DISEASES
Esophageal Strictures

Esophageal strictures can occur in varying degrees, with the symptoms displayed differing according to the amount of obstruction produced. Strictures can be secondary to the ingestion of caustic materials (Fig. 4-26) or from any factor that inflames the mucosa and creates scarring.

Strictures can be differentiated radiographically from normal peristalsis by their unchanging appearance; peristalsis is transitory. The mucosa of a benign stricture appears normal with a smooth contour, while the contour of a malignant stricture typically appears ragged.

Reflux esophagitis, the backward flow of gastric acids into the esophagus, is the primary cause of esophageal inflammation. Reflux is not necessarily abnormal, and *heartburn,* symptomatic reflux, has been experienced by most people. It is only when the

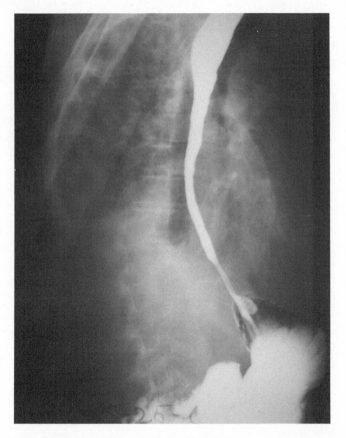

Fig. 4-26. Long-standing esophageal stricture in a 78-year-old male due to accidental ingestion of a caustic agent at age 3. (Courtesy of the American College of Radiology, Reston, Virginia.)

normal event leads to chronic symptoms and complications such as a stricture that it becomes of concern. Treatment includes use of antacids to wash gastric acids out of the esophagus for pain relief and medical therapy using a variety of medicines to inhibit their production or prokinetic agents to enhance motility.

Surgery as a treatment is the last option and is usually used for those whose symptoms have failed to respond to medical therapy.

Esophageal Varices

Varicose veins are abnormally lengthened, dilated, and superficial veins; those in the esophagus are referred to as *esophageal varices*. They occur in the esophagus because of portal hypertension. Conditions that cause a resistance to the normal blood flow through the liver (such as cirrhosis) cause a bypass of the normal venous drainage mechanism. Instead, the blood is directed through the esophageal and gastric collateral veins. The increase in blood flow through these channels results in venous dilatation.

Esophageal varices are best demonstrated in a recumbent position because gravity causes poor visualization in an erect position. A thin barium mixture will radiographically demonstrate the varices as wormlike defects within the column of barium (Fig. 4-27). Use of thick barium may be counterproductive because it may cover the varices. Patients with esophageal varices are subject to their rupture and hemorrhage, which may be massive and often is fatal. An erect film taken for this situation should be done with great caution as the patient's blood loss may be significant. The resultant reduced blood pressure along with the elevation may cause them to faint.

Treatment for esophageal varices may consist of infusion of vasopressin, a natural hormone useful in stopping hemorrhage. Compression of the varices through balloon tamponading may be occasionally used. Shunts applied in surgery may be used to help redirect liver blood flow, thus reducing portal hypertension and easing venous pressure in the esophageal and gastric collateral circulation.

Peptic Ulcer

A *peptic ulcer* is an erosion of the mucous membrane of the lower end of the esophagus, stomach, or duodenum. The most likely site of development is in the duodenal bulb and on the lesser curvature of the stomach. Males are more frequently affected than females by both duodenal and gastric ulceration; duodenal ulceration is up to 10 times more frequent while gastric ulceration is about 4 times more frequent in males.

The etiology of peptic ulcers generally relates to hypersecretion of acidic gastric juice (hydrochloric acid) and pepsin, a protein-digesting enzyme. The normal function of these agents is to digest meat and other proteins that reach the stomach. A small, superficial erosion of the mucosa, whose cause is not yet fully understood, becomes larger as the gastric acid and pepsin begin digesting deeper tissues. In addition to hypersecretion of gastric juice and pepsin, certain drugs (e.g., aspirin) have been shown to contribute to gastric and duodenal ulcers.

The main symptom of a peptic ulcer is pain, usually above the epigastrium and radiating to all parts of the abdomen. Food ingestion or antacids provide temporary relief, but the pain usually returns when the stomach is empty. In some patients, food may

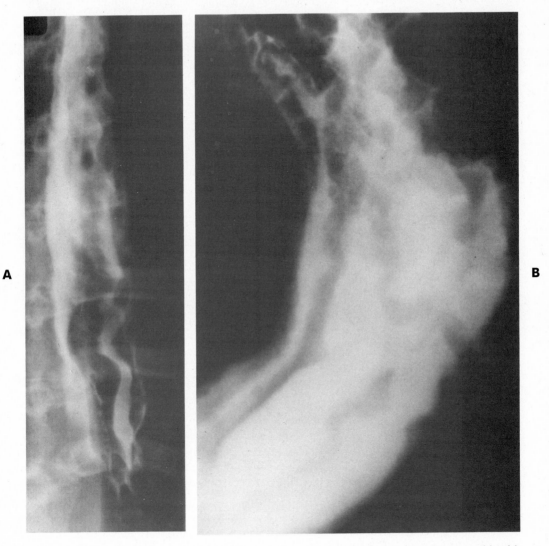

Fig. 4-27, *A.* Long, serpentine filling defects in the esophagus of a 41-year-old with chronic alcoholism, indicative of esophageal varices. (Courtesy of the American College of Radiology, Reston, Virginia.) *B,* Similar filling defects seen in the cardia of the stomach of the same patient, indicative of gastric varices. (Courtesy of the American College of Radiology, Reston, Virginia.)

actually increase pain as it stimulates peristalsis, which irritates the ulcer.

Intermittent healing in the midst of continuing digestion leads to considerable scarring at the base of the ulcer. Based on the pattern of scarring, certain radiographic features suggest the benign or malignant nature of an ulcer. Benign ulcers generally display as radiating spikelike wheels of mucosal folds that run to the edge of the crater (Fig. 4-28). Seen *en face,* the edge of this ulcer appears round and regular (Fig. 4-29, p. 178). Also, benign ulcers usually occur on the lesser curvature and rarely on the greater curvature of the stomach. Malignant ulcers, on the other hand, show mucosal folds that are obliterated at some distance from the edge of the ulcer crater edge. In profile, such an ulcer does not usually project beyond the original lumen as does a benign ulcer. Seen en face the edge of the malignant ulcer is irregular. Ulcers can occur anywhere, but those in the proximal stomach and on the greater curvature are particularly suspicious for malignancy.

Ulcers should respond to treatment within a few weeks if they are benign. Although controversial, some experts argue that the most important aspect of treatment is to provide mental, physical, and gastric rest. Medication may be given to minimize acid production and intestinal spasm. Dietary adjustments are made to minimize irritating food substances (e.g., coffee, alcohol, and aspirin), and avoidance of stress factors is also encouraged. Failure of such medical therapies may necessitate surgery. Surgical options include severing of the vagus nerve to eliminate stimulation of the gastric cells that produce the gastric acid. More involved procedures, including gastrectomy and variants of it, are used if additional complications arise from peptic ulceration.

Complications of an ulcer do occur and can include a pneumoperitoneum or peritonitis if the ulcer perforates into the abdomen. Ulceration into an artery can produce life-threatening hemorrhage. Finally, the edema, spasm, and scarring produced by ulceration can result in bowel obstruction.

Gastroenteritis

A number of inflammatory disorders of the stomach and intestine fall into a general grouping of *gastroenteritis:* inflammation of the mucosal lining of the stomach and small bowel (Fig. 4-30, pp. 179–180). Acute gastroenteritis may be caused by excessive alcohol intake, viral infection, food allergy, and specific infectious diseases. Ingestion of foods contaminated with salmonella or staphylococcal bacteria may also result in gastroenteritis. Diarrhea associated with it is a threat to the normal electrolytic balance of the body.

Changes resulting from gastroenteritis are not easily seen by gastroscopy and are poorly visualized radiographically. A good patient history can often point out the offending agent, and treatment consists of proper fluid management and relief of nausea and vomiting.

Malabsorption Syndrome

Malabsorption syndrome is a group of diseases of various causes in which there is interference with normal digestion and absorption of food through the small bowel. The best known small bowel malabsorption disorder is *celiac disease,* which occurs as a result of sensitivity to gluten, an agent found in wheat products such as bread. With such a

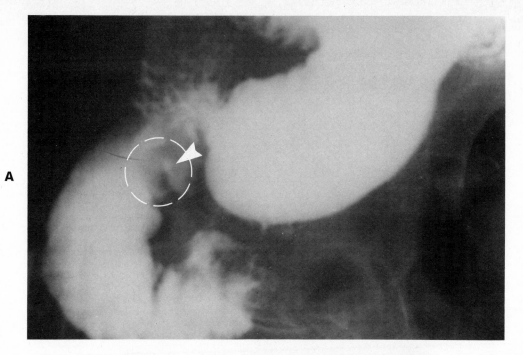

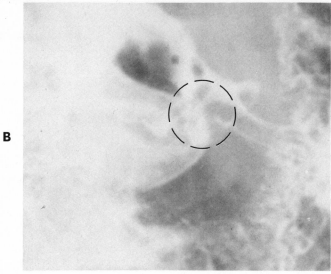

Fig. 4-28, *A.* Prone RAO projection of the duodenal bulb demonstrates a dense collection of barium in an ulcer crater, suggesting that it is on the anterior duodenal wall. *B.* Persistent collection of barium in the middle portion of the duodenal bulb indicating a superficial ulcer crater, with radiating folds extending from the ulceration. An *incisura* (fold) along the lower bulb margin points toward the ulcer. (Courtesy of the American College of Radiology, Reston, Virginia.)

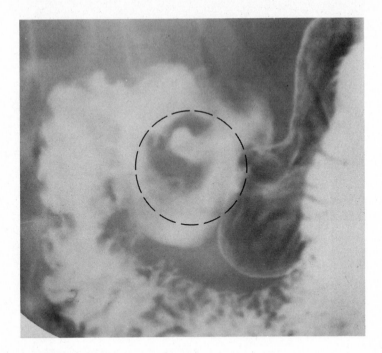

Fig. 4-29. A duodenal ulcer in a 25-year-old male, evidenced by an ulcer crater surrounded by edema represented by the radiolucent halo. (Courtesy of the American College of Radiology, Reston, Virginia.)

condition, the bowel dilates, mucosal folds atrophy, and peristalsis slows or stops. Radiographic changes generally seen with malabsorption syndrome are segmentation of the barium column, flocculation (resembling tufts of cotton), and edematous mucosal changes (Fig. 4-31, p.181). Treatment of celiac disease consists of avoidance of substances containing gluten and dietary substitution of other products. Vitamin therapy is also used to ensure adequate amounts of nutrients not available because of the malabsorption occurring in the small bowel.

Lactose insufficiency is another form of the malabsorption syndrome, affecting about 60% of the nonwhite population and 20% to 30% of the white population. With this condition, the small bowel lacks sufficient quantity of the enzyme lactase, which is used to digest lactose into simple sugars that can be absorbed. The result is that lactose stays in the bowel and acts as an osmotic agent, causing fluid to weep into the bowel lumen from the wall and creating cramping and diarrhea. Lactose mixed with barium shows the barium moving quickly through the bowel and becoming diluted in the distal ileum and colon (Fig. 4-32, p. 182). Patients affected by this condition avoid symptoms through avoidance of dairy products.

Text continued on p. 183.

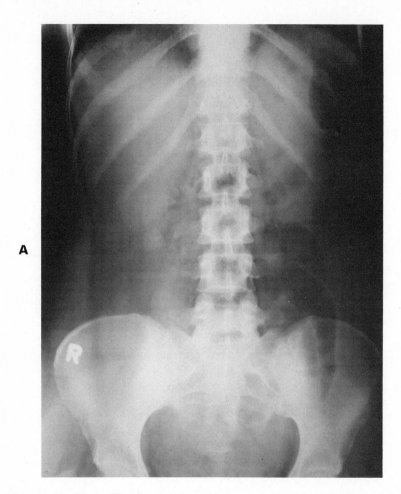

Fig. 4-30, *A.* Air-filled, dilated small bowel loops seen on this abdominal plain film are suggestive of an obstruction in this 30-year-old patient with abdominal pain, nausea, and vomiting. (Courtesy of the American College of Radiology, Reston, Virginia.)

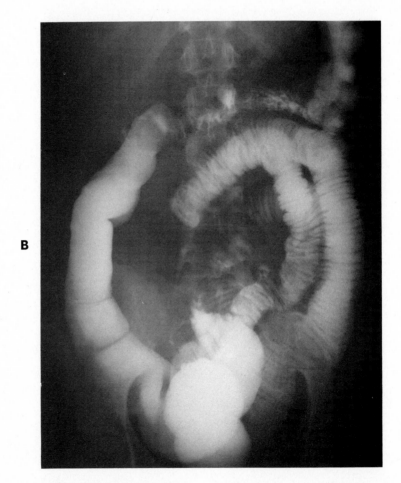

Fig. 4-30, *B.* Barium readily refluxes from a barium enema into the distal ileum, demonstrating dilatation without obstruction. The dilatation was due to inflammation caused by gastroenteritis. (Courtesy of the American College of Radiology, Reston, Virginia.)

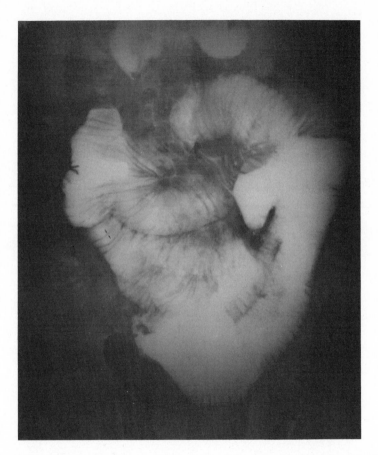

Fig. 4-31. Celiac disease in a 15-year-old patient with a history of diarrhea, indicated on this small bowel study by dilated bowel loops, thickened folds, a grayish appearance of the barium (due to excess fluid in the bowel), and a delayed transit time. (Courtesy of the American College of Radiology, Reston, Virginia.)

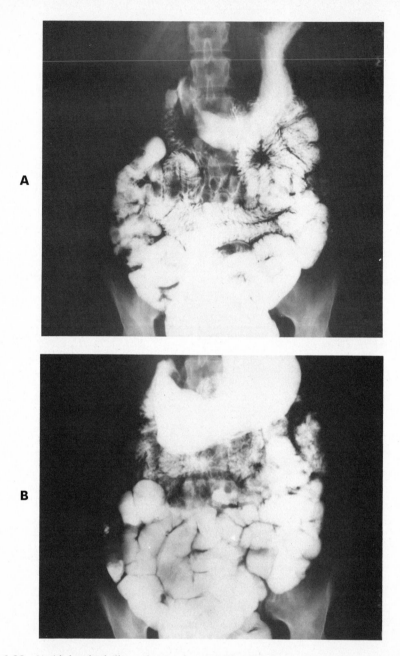

Fig. 4-32, *A.* Abdominal distension, pain, and diarrhea led to this small bowel examination, diagnosed as normal for this 35-year-old patient. *B.* Mixing of lactose with barium on a repeat study led to mild bowel dilatation, rapid transit time, and dilution of barium in the distal small bowel, indicative of lactase insufficiency. (Courtesy of the American College of Radiology, Reston, Virginia.)

Regional Enteritis

Regional enteritis, also known as Crohn's Disease or granulomatous colitis, is a chronic inflammatory disease of unknown etiology. It is typically located in the lower ileum but may be seen anywhere throughout the bowel. Over half of all cases involve the colon. This disease typically affects young adults in their twenties and thirties, with symptoms suggestive of appendicitis or acute bowel obstruction. Emotional stress is thought to be an important causative factor of bowel dysfunction, in general.

Regional enteritis starts as mucosal inflammation with ulceration of the bowel wall. It eventually affects all layers of the bowel wall. The bowel wall thickens in response to the inflammation and may form fistulas to adjacent loops of bowel, skin, or other abdominal viscera. Subsequent fibrotic scarring may give rise to mechanical obstruction of the bowel. The combination of mucosal edema and criss-crossing fine ulcerations gives the bowel a "cobblestone" radiographic appearance. The "string sign" (Fig. 4-33) is demonstrated where the terminal ileum is so diseased and stenotic that the barium mixture can only trickle through a small opening that looks like a string. Presentation of the disease in two or more areas with normal intervening bowel between is identified as "skip

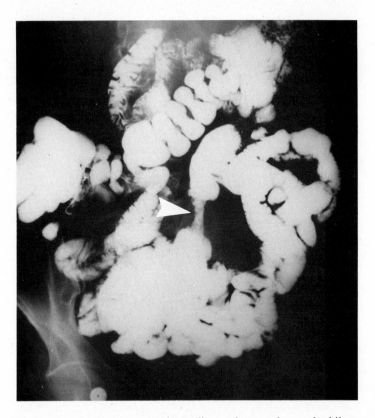

Fig. 4-33. The "string sign" demonstrating a diseased, stenotic terminal ileum. (Courtesy of Riverside Methodist Hospitals, Columbus, Ohio.)

areas'' (Fig. 4-34). Treatment of regional enteritis centers on management of pain, relief of diarrhea, and treatment of infection. Occasionally bowel resection is used to remove the involved section of the intestine, particularly if perforation or hemorrhage is present. Recurrence of the disease in other areas of the bowel, however, is common.

Appendicitis

Appendicitis is an inflammation of the vermiform appendix, generally resulting from an obstruction caused by a fecalith (Fig. 4-35) or neoplasm. The obstruction leads to inflammation and distention and affects the blood supply to this portion of the bowel. Venous blood return is decreased, which in turn results in deoxygenation of the tissue. All of these factors leave the appendix susceptible to infection from bacteria, such as *Escherichia coli* (*E.coli*), normally found within the intestinal tract. Poor blood supply can also lead to gangrene, perforation, and possible rupture. Once the vermiform appendix ruptures, the infection spreads to the peritoneum, leading to general peritonitis that could result in death.

Appendicitis is one of the most common GI diseases and may occur at any age, but it most frequently affects individuals between the ages of 15 to 24 years. Signs and symptoms include initial pain in the epigastrium that moves to the right lower quadrant and becomes persistent. Nausea and vomiting may occur as a reflex symptom because the vagus nerve supplies both the stomach and appendix. Individuals also carry a low-grade fever, have a sudden onset of constipation, and present with an elevated white blood cell count. The elevation of white blood cells helps to distinguish appendicitis from other colicky abdominal disorders.

Surgical removal of the appendix is the most common treatment and in cases of early surgical intervention, the mortality is low. However, complications such as abscess formation or perforation and peritonitis place the individual at a greater risk and greatly increase the recovery period.

Ulcerative Colitis

Ulcerative colitis is an inflammatory lesion of the colon mucosa. Its etiology is unknown but it is thought to be an autoimmune disease. Typically, it affects young individuals who present with symptoms of excessive diarrhea, blood, pus, and mucus in the stools. The disease generally starts in the rectum and spreads to the sigmoid, sometimes involving the entire colon.

Inflammation of the mucosa and submucosa cause abscesses to form, separating them from their blood supply and leading to ulceration. Gradually, the mucosa is replaced by fibrous tissue whose crevices give a rough, cobblestone appearance to the involved colon.

Colon strictures are a rare complication of ulcerative colitis. Another complication of ulcerative colitis is *toxic megacolon,* an acute dilatation of the colon from colonic paralytic ileus (Fig. 4-36, p. 186). The dilated bowel is particularly susceptible to rupture, causing a barium enema to be absolutely contraindicated. The incidence of carcinoma is greatly increased with ulcerative colitis in comparison with the general population.

Sigmoidoscopy and colonoscopy are the usual means of diagnosing ulcerative colitis. Barium enemas are used to assess the progression of the disease and its complications.

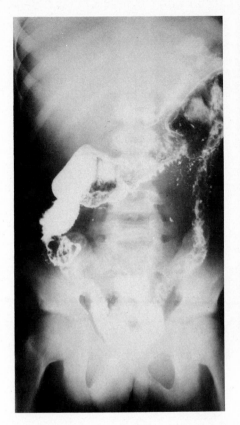 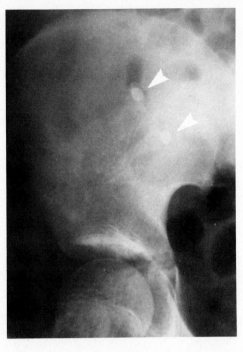

Fig. 4-34, left. Regional enteritis in an 11-year-old patient demonstrated by the "cobble-stone" appearance of the cecum and left colon, with "skip" areas of normal bowel between. (Courtesy of the American College of Radiology, Reston, Virginia.)

Fig. 4-35, right. Spot film of a fecalith within the appendix, a common cause of appendicitis. (Courtesy of the American College of Radiology, Reston, Virginia.)

When filled with barium, the normally smooth colon outline becomes irregular due to the ulceration present. *Pseudopolyps* are islands of unaffected mucosa that become visible when surrounded by affected mucosa. Another radiographic indication of ulcerative colitis is an easily recognized loss of colon haustration.

Certain characteristics of ulcerative colitis help distinguish it from regional enteritis (Crohn's Disease). Ulcerative colitis is a disease of the mucosa of the colon, while regional enteritis affects all layers of the bowel wall. Also, ulcerative colitis typically begins at the anus and ascends, often results in megacolons and bowel perforations, and frequently progresses to cancer. Regional enteritis usually begins in the terminal ileum and cecum and descends through the bowel, often with skip areas. It rarely produces megacolon or bowel perforations, and seldom progresses to cancer.

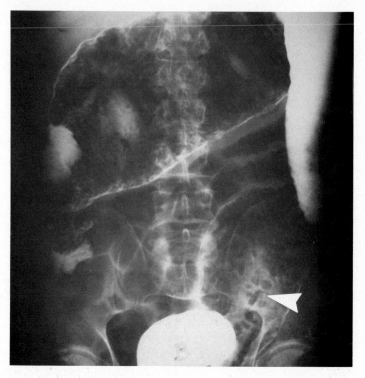

Fig. 4-36. Barium enema on a 61-year-old male demonstrates toxic megacolon secondary to ulcerative colitis. Pseudopolyps are seen in the descending colon. (Courtesy of the American College of Radiology, Reston, Virginia.)

Treatment of ulcerative colitis is initially medical in nature and usually involves steroid therapy. Development of an obstruction or neoplasm may require surgical intervention. Usually, this involves removal of the colon from cecum to sigmoid with establishment of an ileostomy or ileorectal or ileoanal anastomosis.

DEGENERATIVE DISEASES
Herniation

A *hernia* is a protrusion of a loop of bowel through a small opening, usually in the abdominal wall. It is also popularly referred to as a "rupture" and occurs because of an anatomic weakness. As the bowel loop herniates, it pushes the peritoneum ahead of it. An *inguinal hernia* is common in men and occurs when a bowel loop protrudes through a weakness in the inguinal ring (Fig. 4-37) and may descend downward into the scrotum. Femoral and umbilical herniation (Fig. 4-38) occur in both sexes.

If a herniated loop of bowel can be pushed back into the abdominal cavity, it is said

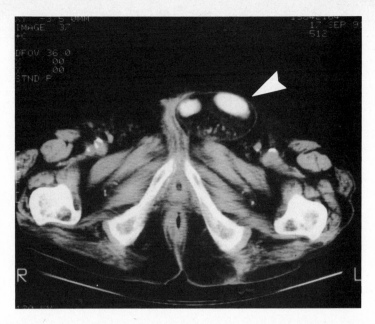

Fig. 4-37. Moderate left inguinal hernia (*arrow*) on this CT image of a 96-year-old male. Also well-defined are *1*, the femurs, showing the lesser trochanters projecting posteriorly, and *2*, the ischial tuberosities. (Courtesy of Riverside Methodist Hospitals, Columbus, Ohio.)

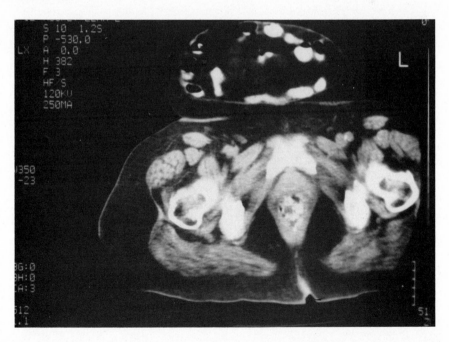

Fig. 4-38. CT demonstration of a large anterior abdominal hernia containing multiple loops of small bowel and possibly some large bowel, without evidence of obstruction in this 70-year-old male. (Courtesy of Riverside Methodist Hospitals, Columbus, Ohio.)

to be reducible. If it becomes stuck and cannot be reduced, it is an *incarcerated hernia*. As described previously, this can result in a bowel obstruction (Fig. 4-39). If the constriction through which the bowel loop has passed is tight enough to cut off blood supply to the bowel, it is called a *strangulated hernia*. Prompt surgical intervention is required in this case to avoid necrosis of that portion of the bowel. Bowel that has already necrosed can generally be surgically resected.

Hiatal Hernia

A *hiatal hernia* is a weakness of the esophageal hiatus, which permits some portions of the stomach to herniate into the thoracic cavity. Hiatal hernias are common to about half of the population over the age of 50 years. In its early stages, a hiatal hernia is reducible. Chronic herniation can lead to complications such as reflux esophagitis.

A direct, or sliding hiatal hernia occurs when a portion of the stomach and gastroesophageal junction are both situated above the diaphragm (Fig. 4-40, p. 190). This type of hernia comprises the outstanding majority of all hiatal hernias. A *Schatzki's ring* is often visible with this condition (Fig. 4-41, p. 191) and consists of a mucosal ring that protrudes into the lumen. Such a ring is thought to develop as a result of gastric reflux. It is, however, generally of no clinical significance unless it produces narrowing sufficient to cause dysphagia, usually less than 13 mm in diameter.

Although far less common, another type of hiatal hernia is a rolling, or paraesophageal hiatal hernia. This occurs when a portion of the stomach or adjacent viscera herniates above the diaphragm, while the gastroesophageal junction remains below the diaphragm (Fig. 4-42, pp. 191–192) if all of the stomach slides above the diaphragm, an *intrathoracic stomach* (Fig. 4-43, p. 193) results.

While most hiatal hernias are asymptomatic, some are accompanied by reflux. Most patients experiencing reflux complain of a full feeling in the chest, particularly after meals. Some reflux of gastric contents leads to complaints of heartburn. An upper GI examination is useful in pinpointing the herniation and distinguishing the cause of reflux esophagitis. Treatment of hiatal herniation is generally conservative, and is centered on efforts to reduce reflux esophagitis and minimize discomfort. This includes modification of eating habits, weight loss, avoidance of smoking, medication to decrease acid, and elevation of the head of the bed.

BOWEL OBSTRUCTIONS

Both the small and large bowels of the normal patient are nearly always active in peristalsis. Many lesions of various types (e.g., inflammatory, degenerative) can interfere with this action and cause an obstruction of either small or large bowels. The resultant obstruction can be either *mechanical,* as occurs from a blockage of the bowel lumen, or a *paralytic ileus,* as results from a failure of peristalsis. There are gradations of each, and both may be present at the same time.

General signs and symptoms of a bowel obstruction include vomiting, abdominal distention, and abdominal pain. Radiography helps to determine the diagnosis and to locate the level of the obstruction in individuals with mechanical obstructions. Most commonly, gas confined to the small bowel with multiple air-fluid levels visible on an

Text continued on p. 192.

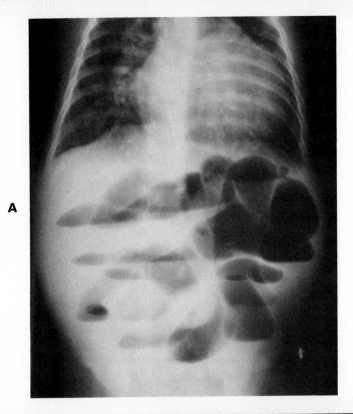

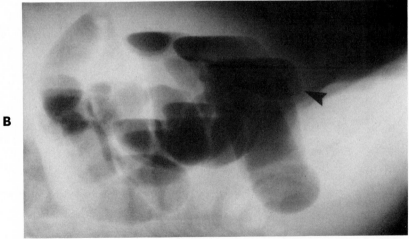

Fig. 4-39, *A.* Upright abdomen on a 3-month-old indicates multiple dilated loops of bowel with air-fluid levels present, suggesting a mechanical bowel obstruction. *B.* A prone cross-table lateral view shows the small bowel forming a beaklike projection at the point of obstruction at the internal inguinal ring in this incarcerated hernia. (Courtesy of the American College of Radiology, Reston, Virginia.)

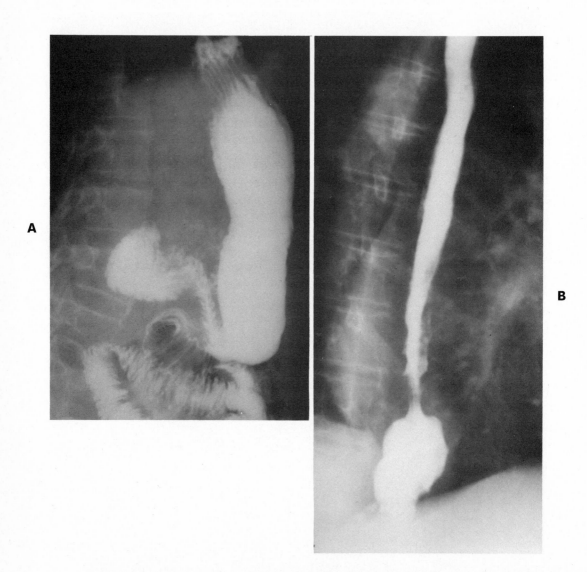

Fig. 4-40, *A.* Demonstration of contrast material above the hemidiaphragm on an upper GI series of this 51-year-old female. *B.* The esophagus narrows to the stomach, which is seen to empty passively, above the hemidiaphragm in this sliding hiatal hernia. (Courtesy of the American College of Radiology, Reston, Virginia.)

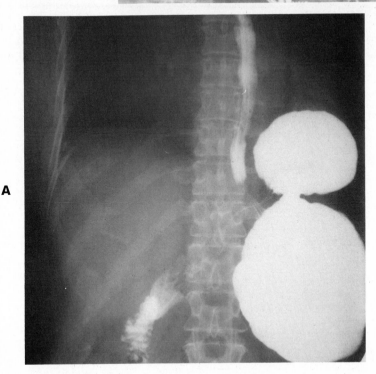

Fig. 4-41. Schatzki's ring as demon as demon as demonstrated in the case of a sliding hiatal hernia. (Courtesy of Riverside Methodist Hospitals, Columbus, Ohio.)

A

Fig. 4-42, *A.* Paraesophageal hiatal hernia, demonstrating narrowing in the fundus. (Courtesy of the American College of Radiology, Reston, Virginia.)

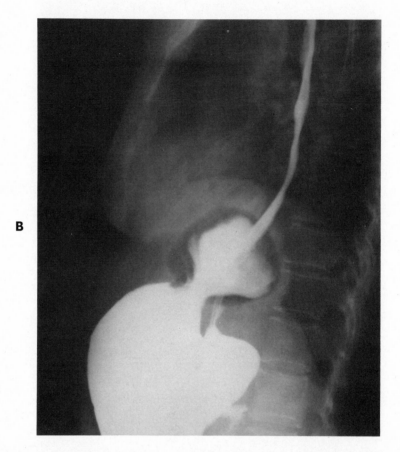

B

Fig. 4-42, *B.* A lateral view of the same patient demonstrates the cardioesophageal junc-tion in its normal place below the hemidiaphragm. The fundus is highlighted by the radiolucency of the lung. (Courtesy of the American College of Radiology, Reston, Virginia.)

erect abdominal radiograph indicates a mechanical obstruction, whereas gas distributed throughout both the large and small bowel is indicative of paralytic ileus. Physical signs are also helpful in distinguishing the type of obstruction present. *Bowel sounds,* the normal sounds of a bowel in motion as heard on auscultation, are absent with an ileus; they are present with a mechanical obstruction, and are often hyperactive and high pitched. Emesis containing bile is also indicative of a mechanical obstruction.

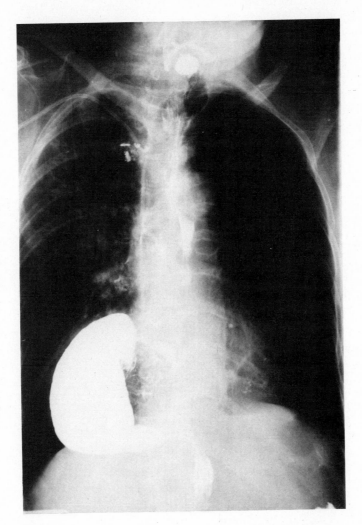

Fig. 4-43. Intrathoracic stomach indicated by the presence of the entire stomach above the diaphragm, also with malrotation of the stomach. (Courtesy of Riverside Methodist Hospitals, Columbus, Ohio.)

Mechanical Bowel Obstruction

A *mechanical bowel obstruction* (Fig. 4-44) is one in which the lumen of the bowel becomes occluded, as might occur for a variety of reasons, most often postoperatively from adhesions. Generally these require surgical intervention to correct. Nearly half of all mechanical bowel obstructions are caused by an incarcerated (i.e., trapped) hernia, a condition discussed earlier in this chapter as a degenerative disease. Entrapment of a hernia, usually involving the small bowel, causes impairment of blood flow and swelling of the affected tissues. The resultant edema affects the arterial blood flow to the bowel and may lead to ischemic necrosis, perforation, and peritonitis. Prompt surgical intervention and reduction is required to relieve an incarcerated hernia.

Gallstone ileus is another cause for a mechanical bowel obstruction and is a condition in which a gallstone can erode from the gallbladder and create a fistula to the small bowel. This leads to an obstruction, usually when the gallstone reaches the ileocecal valve.

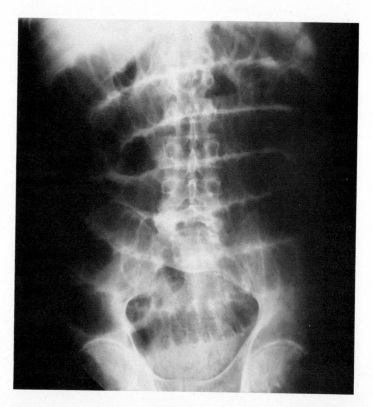

Fig. 4-44. Abdominal radiograph demonstrating a mechanical bowel obstruction, with numerous loops of dilated bowel seen within the midabdomen. The patient had an acute onset of abdominal pain, nausea, and vomiting. (Courtesy of the American College of Radiology, Reston, Virginia.)

Radiographic signs of this include air-fluid levels or air in the biliary tree (Fig. 4-45). The gallstone itself may also be visible, often in the terminal ileum where it causes the obstruction.

A *volvulus* is a twisting of a bowel loop about its mesenteric base, usually at either the sigmoid or ileocecal junction (Fig. 4-46, p. 196). This most commonly occurs in the elderly and is identifiable on a plain abdomen radiograph as a collection of air conforming to the shape of the affected, dilated bowel. Surgical untwisting and resection, if needed, is the method of treatment for a volvulus.

An *intussusception* occurs when a segment of bowel, constricted by peristalsis, telescopes into a distal segment and is driven further into the distal bowel by peristalsis. Recall that the bowel is connected to the mesentery, so as the bowel telescopes into itself, the mesentery (with its rich blood supply) is also involved. Intussusception is responsible for approximately 5% of all mechanical obstructions and most frequently affects the ileocecal valve (Fig. 4-47, p. 197). It is more common in children and infants than in

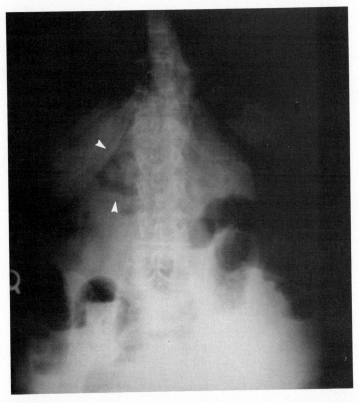

Fig. 4-45. Abdominal radiograph of a 43-year-old female demonstrating air within the biliary ductal system and an overall density (gallstone) in the right lower abdomen. (Courtesy of the American College of Radiology, Reston, Virginia.)

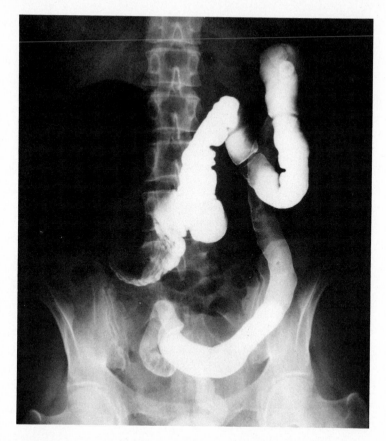

Fig. 4-46. A barium enema radiograph depicting a cecal volvulus. Note how the column of barium stops at the level of the volvulus. (Courtesy of the American College of Radiology, Reston, Virginia.)

adults. Its presence in an adult generally signifies an accompanying intraluminal mass and is generally reduced surgically so that the physician can search for the cause of the intussusception and correct the condition. In children and infants, an intussusception can often be reduced by an enema, sparing a surgical intervention.

Other causes of small bowel obstruction beside these include adhesions, tumors, Crohn's disease, and appendicitis.

Paralytic Ileus

Paralytic ileus is a failure of normal peristalsis and may result from a variety of factors. The most common causes are following surgery, especially that requiring manipulation of the bowel, and intraperitoneal or retroperitoneal infection. It may also be associated with bowel ischemia, certain drugs, electrolyte imbalance, pancreatitis, or simply as a reaction

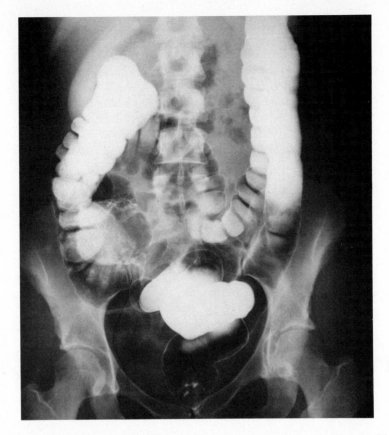

Fig. 4-47. Pediatric barium enema demonstrating intussusception at the ileocecal junction. (Courtesy of the American College of Radiology, Reston, Virginia.)

to any stressful medical illness. Paralytic ileus generally lasts no longer than 3 days with proper medical treatment. The absence of peristalsis causes the lumen of both the small and large intestines to fill with gas and fluid with the resultant dilatation extending to the rectum (Fig. 4-48, p. 198). Treatment for paralytic ileus generally consists of medical stimulation of the bowel to restore peristalsis.

NEUROGENIC DISEASES
Achalasia

Achalasia is a neuromuscular abnormality of the esophagus that results in failure of the lower esophageal sphincter of the distal esophagus to relax, leading to dysphagia. Radiographically, the condition demonstrates as a dilated esophagus with little or no peristalsis. The distal esophagus itself is often described as having a "beaked" appearance (Fig. 4-49, p. 198). Because the distal esophagus only opens intermittently when the pressure is high enough, food residue may be seen in the distal esophagus or even on a

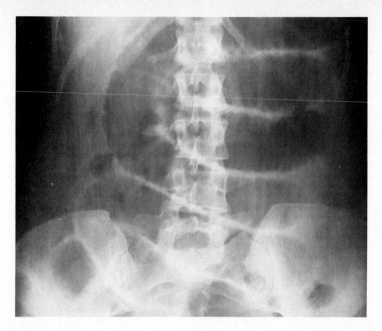

Fig. 4-48. Abdominal radiograph on a postoperative patient demonstrating paralytic ileus. Note the dilated bowel loops extending through the large intestine. (Courtesy of Riverside Methodist Hospitals, Columbus, Ohio.)

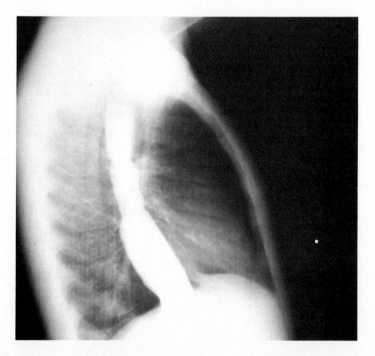

Fig. 4-49. Dilated esophagus in a 10-year-old patient that demonstrated no normal peristalsis on filling, indicating achalasia. The distal esophagus terminates into a "beaked" appearance. (Courtesy of the American College of Radiology, Reston, Virginia.)

chest radiograph. Since the esophageal contents act as a water seal, the normal gastric gas bubble may be absent.

Initial treatment of achalasia is conservative. Affected patients have sometimes learned on their own what induces pain and prevents it, and they have modified their eating habits accordingly. Most patients, however, require other interventions for treatment, including medication, a pneumatic dilation done endoscopically, and surgical myotomy.

Hirschsprung's Disease

Hirschsprung's Disease is an absence of neurons in the bowel wall, typically in the sigmoid colon, and is also known as *congenital megacolon*. Occurring in approximately 1 in 5000 births, this defect is a familial disease, primarily affecting males. The absence of neurons in the bowel wall prevents the normal relaxation of the colon and subsequent peristalsis, resulting in gross dilatation to the point of narrowing and constriction.

This generally becomes apparent shortly after birth when the affected infant passes little meconium, and the abdomen becomes distended. As the patient ages, the continued effects are severe constipation and recurrent fecal impactions. Barium enemas demonstrate a transition from the narrow, distal rectum to a dilated proximal colon (Fig. 4-50, p. 200). Initial treatment in an infant may consist of a temporary colostomy until surgical resection is possible later.

DIVERTICULAR DISEASE
Esophageal Diverticuli

A *diverticulum* is a pouch or sac of variable size that occurs normally or is created by herniation of a mucous membrane through a defect in its muscular coat. Esophageal diverticula occur when mucosal outpouchings penetrate through the muscular layer of the esophagus. The two primary types of esophageal diverticula are pulsion and traction.

A *pulsion diverticulum* involves the mucosa only and results from a motility disorder of the esophagus, which allows the mucosa to herniate outward. This type of diverticulum appears radiographically as a rounded projection with a narrow neck and occurs more frequently in the upper and lower thirds of the esophagus. A *Zencker's diverticulum* is a pulsion-type found at the pharyngoesophageal junction at the upper end of the esophagus (Fig. 4-51, pp. 201–202). An *epiphrenic diverticulum* is another pulsion-type but is found in the distal esophagus just above the hemidiaphragm (Fig. 4-52, p. 203).

A *traction diverticulum* involves all layers of the esophagus and results from adjacent scar tissue that pulls the esophagus toward the area of involvement (Fig. 4-53, p. 203). Such a diverticulum occurs more frequently in the middle third of the esophagus at the carina and appears radiographically as a triangle whose apex points toward the disease.

Usually, diverticula are asymptomatic until they reach a relatively large size at which time complications may occur. For example, food and secretions can collect in the diverticulum and cause a mechanical obstruction of the esophagus. Such contents can also be aspirated by a recumbent patient, resulting in a chemical pneumonia. Failure to control the effects of diverticula through diet modifications may result in the need for surgical removal, dependent on the amount of food retention in the diverticulum.

Text continued on p. 204.

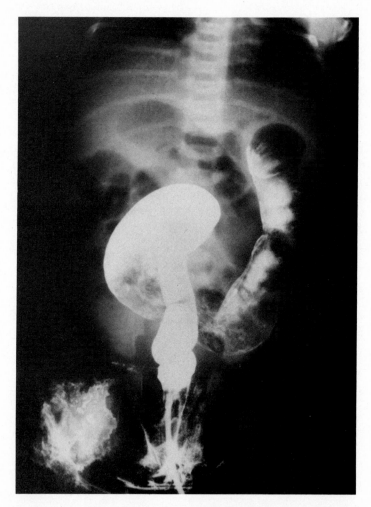

Fig. 4-50. Barium enema on a 6-day-old infant demonstrates a normal rectosigmoid leading to a distended large bowel consistent with Hirschsprung's disease. (Courtesy of the American College of Radiology, Reston, Virginia.)

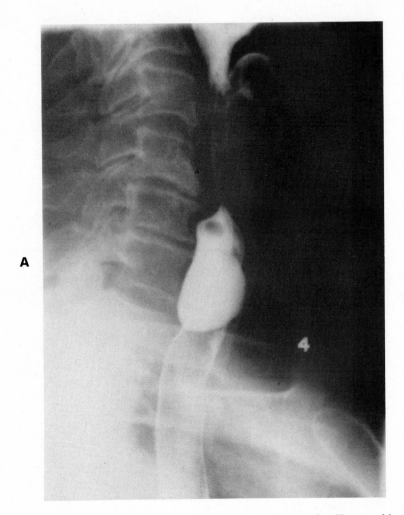

Fig. 4-51, *A.* Large Zencker's diverticulum in the esophagus of a 67-year-old male with complaints of swallowing over the past 6 months. (Courtesy of the American College of Radiology, Reston, Virginia.)

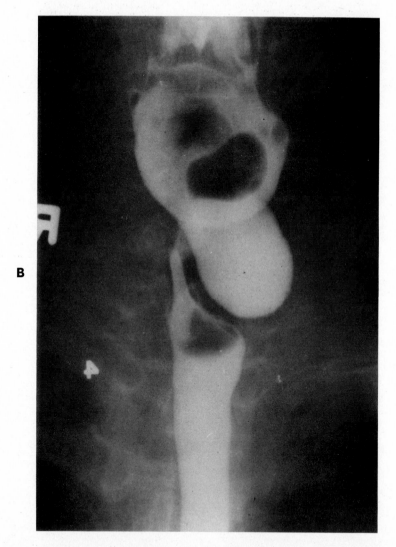

Fig. 4-51, *B.* Zencker's diverticulum in the same patient as seen on a magnified view. (Courtesy of the American College of Radiology, Reston, Virginia.)

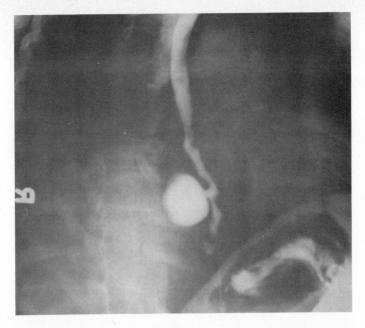

Fig. 4-52. An epiphrenic diverticulum shown as a large collection of barium connected and adjacent to the lower esophagus. (Courtesy of the American College of Radiology, Reston, Virginia.)

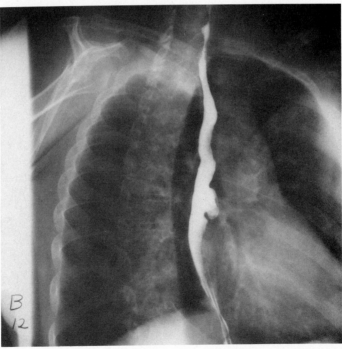

Fig. 4-53. Traction diverticulum indicated by the outpouching of the esophagus at the level of the carina seen in an esophagram of a 47-year-old female with a history of ulcer disease. (Courtesy of the American College of Radiology, Reston, Virginia.)

Colonic Diverticula

Diverticulosis, the presence of diverticula without inflammation, is seen in all parts of the colon, most frequently in the sigmoid colon, and particularly among the elderly (Figs. 4-54 and 4-55). Diverticula are associated with hypertrophy of the muscular layer of the bowel and are thought to be caused by a refined diet with little dietary bulk. They generally occur where the terminal branches of the mesenteric vessels pierce the bowel wall.

Inflammation of a diverticulum is termed *diverticulitis*. The inflammation is exacerbated by feces lodging in the diverticulum. This condition can lead to bowel obstruction, perforation, and fistula formation. A barium enema examination may be indicated to demonstrate the affected diverticulum, most commonly in the distal colon. Radiographic signs of diverticulitis on barium enema include extraluminal and/or intraluminal contrast. Spasm may be seen as well, and the underlying colonic mucosa appears intact.

Treatment of diverticulitis centers on reduction of inflammation and infection. Complications such as peritonitis can result if perforation of a diverticulum occurs, and these, of course, must be treated. Surgical resection of the bowel may be used to remove the diseased portion.

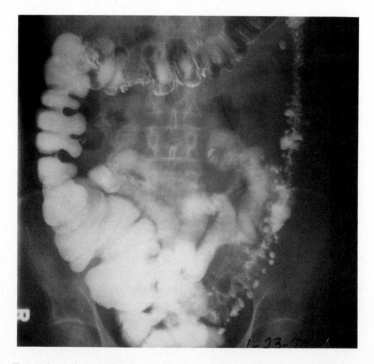

Fig. 4-54. Extensive diverticulosis of the descending and sigmoid colon in the barium enema of a 69-year-old female. (Courtesy of the American College of Radiology, Reston, Virginia.)

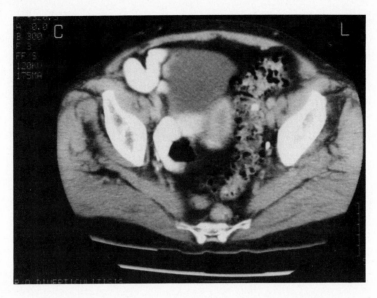

Fig. 4-55. Extensive diverticular disease seen as air-filled translucencies in the sigmoid colon on this CT film of an 87-year-old female. Also well-defined are the *1*, bladder, and *2*, sacrum. (Courtesy of Riverside Methodist Hospitals, Columbus, Ohio)

TRAUMATIC DISEASE
Foreign Bodies in the Esophagus

Unintentional swallowing or poor mastication may cause foreign bodies to become lodged in the esophagus. The affected patient may be asymptomatic or may complain of pain on swallowing. Radiopaque foreign bodies are easily demonstrated (Fig. 4-56, p. 206), but nonopaque foreign bodies may be much more difficult to detect. A swallowed foreign body can become imbedded in the esophageal mucosa, producing pain on swallowing. This action may eventually tear the esophagus. A barium swallow is commonly used in the case of acute esophageal obstruction to locate the site of the obstruction. Soft tissue neck radiographs may also be indicated in cases of radiopaque foreign bodies. Surgical excision or endoscopic removal may be necessary to remove the cause of obstruction.

Abdominal Trauma

Abdominal trauma can cause serious injury not only to the GI tract, but also to abdominal organs (e.g., liver, spleen, kidneys, and pancreas), the spine, retroperitoneum, and pelvic organs. CT has proven to be the best means of diagnosing GI trauma and is capable of visualizing lacerations, hematomas, and ruptures. Even small amounts of intraabdominal hemorrhage can be readily detected.

The duodenum is the portion of the GI tract most often damaged by blunt trauma. Because of its relationship to the spine, the duodenum can be compressed between the abdominal wall and the spine, resulting in a duodenal hematoma. Penetrating abdominal wounds, as would occur with a gunshot, may produce free air if the bowel has been injured. The initial inspection of the abdominal trauma may be followed by specific studies involving the urinary tract (Fig. 4-57) or by angiography. Some of the common conditions seen radiographically posttrauma are fractures of the spine, pelvis, or ribs; obliteration of normal fat planes and visceral margins; accumulation of peritoneal fluid such as blood; and the presence of free peritoneal air (Fig. 4-58).

Intraperitoneal Air

In the normal patient, the peritoneum is a closed cavity (except for the female reproductive system), containing only small amounts of serous fluid. The presence of free air in this cavity, a *pneumoperitoneum*, is usually abnormal and can indicate perforation of the GI tract. Large amounts of air are likely due to colon perforation, whereas small amounts of air are more indicative of duodenal perforation.

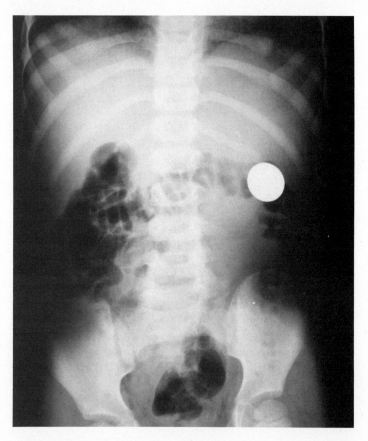

Fig. 4-56. Ready demonstration of a quarter that has been swallowed into the stomach of this child. (Courtesy of Riverside Methodist Hospitals, Columbus, Ohio.)

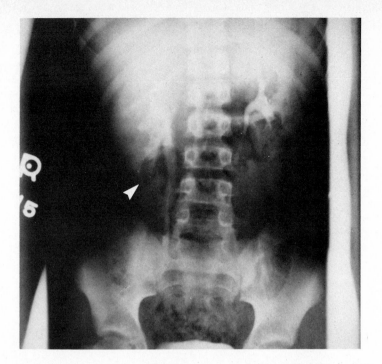

Fig. 4-57. An intravenous urogram demonstrating a fractured right kidney after a football injury. (Courtesy of Riverside Methodist Hospitals, Columbus, Ohio.)

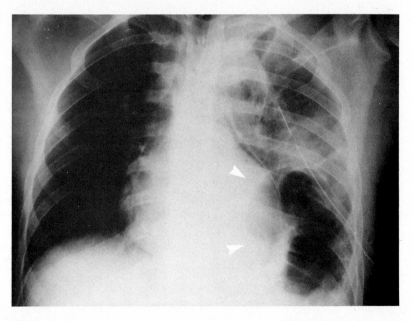

Fig. 4-58. A chest radiograph demonstrating a traumatic diaphragmatic hernia resulting from a motor vehicle accident. (Courtesy of The Ohio State University Hospitals, Columbus, Ohio.)

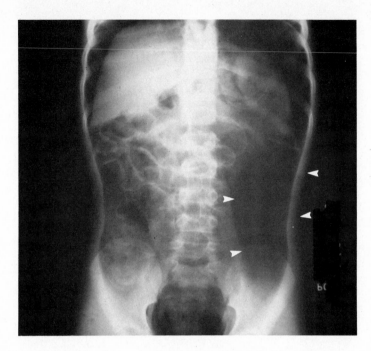

Fig. 4-59. An abdominal radiograph of a 5-year-old child with a passive pneumoperito-neum resulting from perforation of the stomach during anesthesia. Note how the free air outlines the outer border of the bowel, liver, and spleen. (Courtesy of the American College of Radiology, Reston, Virginia.)

The common causes of a *pneumoperitoneum* (Fig. 4-59) include the perforation of a peptic ulcer (either gastric or duodenal), carcinoma of the stomach or colon, cecum perforation from distal colon obstruction, colonic diverticula perforation, or traumatic rupturing of the stomach or intestines. In response to perforation, an intense inflammatory response develops and may eventually wall off the perforation into an abscess.

Free air is best demonstrated radiographically with the patient in an erect position. Often, it is well seen on a chest radiograph because of the proximity of the central ray to the diaphragms. Free air will ascend and accumulate under the diaphragm on one or both sides. Amounts as small as 1 cc of air can be demonstrated on an erect projection. Much larger amounts of air must be present to be visualized on a supine radiograph. Left lateral decubitus radiographs can be substituted for the erect projection, with any free air present accumulating over the lateral aspect of the liver and the lateral aspect of the pelvis. The patient should remain on the left side for approximately 10 minutes before the exposure to allow sufficient time for the air to ascend.

In the supine position, the ''football sign'' may be demonstrated as an indicator of a pneumoperitoneum. This is a lucent, oval-shaped gas collection that corresponds to the anterior peritoneal cavity. The pattern of gas resembles the shape of a football with the ''seam'' of the football being the falciform ligament outlined by free air. Visualization of this sign requires a relatively large amount of free air to demonstrate such a pattern.

NEOPLASTIC DISEASES
Tumors of the Esophagus

While benign and malignant tumors can occur anywhere in the esophagus, tumors of the lower third are the most common. Benign tumors are almost always a *leiomyoma,* which is a smooth muscle tumor, although these have an incidence of less than 10% that of malignant tumors of the esophagus. Many are discovered on x-ray examination for complaints not related to esophageal problems. These benign lesions demonstrate as an intramural defect in the barium-outlined esophageal wall (Fig. 4-60). Treatment of a leiomyoma consists of surgical removal through a thoracic or abdominal incision, sparing esophageal resection.

Most cancers arising in the body of the esophagus are squamous cell carcinomas; those at the esophogastric junction are typically adenocarcinomas. Chronic irritation of

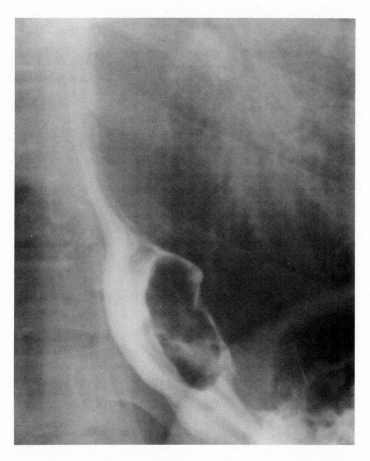

Fig. 4-60. Sharply defined filling defect in the distal esophagus indicative of a benign, esophageal leiomyoma. (Courtesy of the American College of Radiology, Reston, Virginia.)

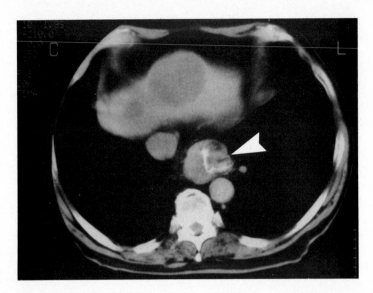

Fig. 4-61. A CT scan with contrast demonstrates an increased thickening of the esophageal wall and distortion of the lumen (*arrow*), compatible with a gastroesophageal junction malignancy. Also seen are *1*, a large metastatic lesion in the superior portion of the liver, and *2*, the aorta. (Courtesy of Riverside Methodist Hospitals, Columbus, Ohio.)

the esophagus is thought to be a predisposing factor, with particular agents causing irritation, including reflux, alcohol and smoking, and disorders such as achalasia and esophageal diverticula. The primary symptom of esophageal cancer is dysphagia.

Malignant tumors of the esophagus occur more often in males, usually after the age of 40 years. The radiographic appearance of a malignant tumor may include mucosal destruction, ulceration, narrowing, and a sharp demarcation between normal tissue and the malignant tumor.

Metastasis to mediastinal structures and hematogenous spread to the liver, lung, and bone occur readily (Fig. 4-61). Surgery is used as a treatment, with the goal to excise the tumor and regional metastasis. The rapid spread of esophageal cancer, however, requires the goal to be palliation in many cases.

Tumors of the Stomach

Benign tumors account for less than 10% of all stomach tumors. Those that are clinically significant are quite rare. Most stomach tumors are malignant, and the outstanding preponderance of these are *adenocarcinomas*. The incidence of gastric cancer varies strikingly by geographic area, race, diet, heredity, and sex. For example, the rate is nearly five times greater in Japan than in the United States. Factors that predispose an individual to gastric carcinoma include being male; being part of a fish-eating population; a salty, spicy, or high cabbage diet; being black; and having type A blood.

Most gastric carcinomas develop in the pyloric and antrum regions, particularly along the lesser curvature, although they can be present anywhere (Fig. 4-62). Gastric ulcers are

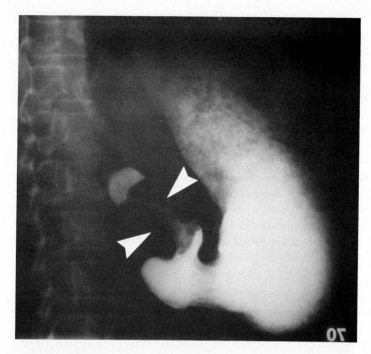

Fig. 4-62. Adenocarcinoma of the stomach in a 66-year-old female, resulting in gastric outlet obstruction. Note the area of narrowing and the abrupt transition between normal stomach and the acutely narrowed area. (Courtesy of the American College of Radiology, Reston, Virginia.)

particularly suspicious, as they may represent a carcinoma. Stomach carcinoma metastasizes fairly readily outside the stomach to involve the omentum, liver, pancreas, and colon. Liver involvement creates the possibility of discharge into the bloodstream and dispersal throughout the body.

Patients who complain of persistent GI pain should have a thorough workup, with the primary diagnostic study being the GI series. Symptoms of gastric tumors are often vague, but include bleeding, vomiting, loss of appetite, weight loss, and early satiety. Tumors are radiographically indicated by a relative rigidity of peristalsis and *filling defects* on compression. Filling defects demonstrate as areas of total or relative radiolucency within the barium column.

Surgical removal of gastric cancer has been the only successful treatment; a subtotal gastrectomy is the usual procedure. Resection of the stomach to attach to the jejunum via a gastrojejunostomy usually accompanies this procedure. Results of radiation therapy and chemotherapy treatments for stomach carcinoma have been less effective.

Small Bowel Neoplasms

Small bowel tumors represent less than 2% of all benign and malignant GI neoplasms. The incidence of malignancy for this small amount is about 50%. The low overall incidence is surprising, considering that the small bowel composes 75% of the entire GI

Colon Cancer

Carcinoma of the colon is one of the most common malignancies in males and is generally *adenocarcinoma*. The incidence of colon cancer rises significantly after age 40 and doubles with each decade, reaching a peak at about age 75. Predisposing factors include a family history of juvenile polyps and ulcerative colitis. Environmental factors also seem to correlate with colorectal cancer as countries with higher intakes of sugar and animal fats (e.g., the United States) have a higher incidence than countries with a higher fiber intake.

Adenocarcinoma is a cancer derived from the glandular epithelium of the colon. It is characterized by infiltration of the colon wall, as opposed to being a bulky, intraluminal mass. Although the incidence of proximal colon cancers is increasing, nearly 50% still occur below the mid-descending colon. Most of these occur in the rectosigmoid area and are readily detectable by flexible sigmoidoscopy.

Right colon lesions differ considerably from left colon lesions in terms of symptoms produced. Lesions in the right colon may produce no early symptoms, often becoming quite large, ulcerating, and even bleeding without significant symptoms. They also tend to penetrate and extend into surrounding tissues without causing obstruction. Such patients often present initially with anemia and blood in their stools. Left colon lesions, on the other hand, present more often with obstruction and bleeding, largely because of a smaller lumen and an annular (ring-like) growth pattern.

Diagnostic means of evaluating colon cancer include screening tests for fecal blood, proctosigmoidoscopy, colonoscopy, and the barium enema. An air-contrast enema has been noted to produce more accurate diagnoses than the traditional single-contrast study. The radiographic appearance of adenocarcinoma has led to its designation as the ''napkin-ring'' carcinoma or the ''apple-core'' lesion, as the edges of the lesion tend to overhang and form acute angles with the bowel wall (Fig. 4-65). While it may be difficult to distinguish between carcinoma and an inflammatory lesion (e.g., regional enteritis or ulcerative colitis), a carcinoma generally has a more clearcut transition between malignant and normal mucosa. In addition, the length of involved bowel is usually shorter with carcinoma as compared with an inflammatory lesion.

Without treatment, invasion of local tissue spreads the cancer via the lymphatics to the mesenteric nodes and on to the liver (Fig. 4-66) and lungs. Fortunately, the lesion does not metastasize early, leading to a good prognosis. The primary means of treatment are surgical excision of the primary tumor and its margins, and resection of the bowel as possible. A colostomy may be required, depending on the site of the tumor. Radiation therapy is generally given before and after surgery. For inoperable tumors, the radiation therapy is given to reduce the tumor size and its resultant complications (e.g., obstruction) and also to provide pain relief. Chemotherapy is given when the cancer has metastasized.

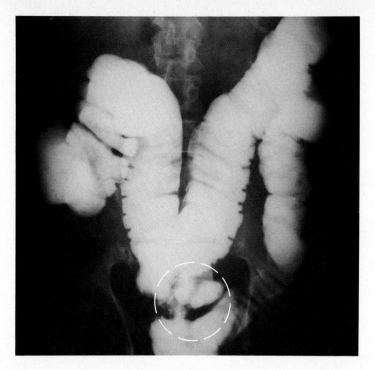

Fig. 4-65. The ''apple core lesion'' of the rectosigmoid colon consistent with adenocarcinoma, with characteristic appearance of abrupt change from normal to abnormal colon, and shelflike appearance of overhanging edges caused by the mass. (Courtesy of the American College of Radiology, Reston, Virginia.)

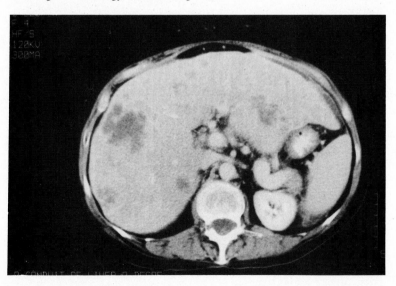

Fig. 4-66. CT demonstration of extensive metastatic disease from the colon to both lobes of the liver, ranging from punctate to up to 5 cm in this 50-year-old female. (Courtesy of Riverside Methodist Hospitals, Columbus, Ohio.)

▼ QUESTIONS

1. Dysphagia is the chief complaint of patients scheduled for a(n):
   a. barium enema   c. esophogram
   b. enteroclysis   d. small bowel study

2. Esophageal atresia is classified as a(n) _____ condition of the GI system.
   a. congenital   c. inflammatory
   b. degenerative   d. neurologic

3. The use of glucagon during an upper GI procedure serves to:
   a. create a double-contrast study   c. expand the stomach confines
   b. enhance stomach coating   d. slow peristalsis

4. Radiographically, the esophagus appears grossly dilated in cases of:
   a. achalasia   c. leiomyoma
   b. esophageal atresia   d. reflux esophagitis

5. An outpouching of the bowel wall caused by a weakening in its muscular layer is a(n):
   a. atresia   c. diverticulum
   b. carcinoma   d. polyp

6. Which term best applies to the condition in which the entire stomach slides into the thorax?
   a. diaphragmatic   c. intrathoracic
      stomach   stomach
   b. hiatal hernia   d. sliding hernia

7. Esophageal varices are likely to occur because of obstructive disease of the:
   a. bowel, large or small   d. stomach
   b. liver   e. all of the above
   c. spleen

8. Which of the following statements are true of peptic ulcers:
   1. Its etiology relates to hyposecretion of acidic gastric juice and pepsin.
   2. Likely sites for development are duodenal bulb and lesser curvature.
   3. The pattern of scarring gives indications to benignancy vs. malignancy.
   a. 1 and 2   c. 2 and 3
   b. 1 and 3   d. 1, 2, and 3

9. Ulcers found on which of the following are particularly suspicious for malignancy?
   a. antrum   c. greater curvature
   b. duodenum   d. lesser curvature

10. Ingestion of food contaminated with salmonella or excessive intake of alcohol can result in:
    a. gastroenteritis   c. peptic ulceration
    b. malabsorption syndrome   d. ulcerative colitis

11. Which of the following are typically associated with Crohn's disease?
   a. begins at anus and ascends   **d.** produces toxic megacolon
   b. disease of the colon mucosa   **e.** none of the above
   c. frequently progresses to cancer

12. The radiographic ''string sign'' is associated with which disease?
   a. achalasia   **c.** regional enteritis
   b. adenocarcinoma   **d.** ulcerative colitis

13. Celiac disease is a type of:
   a. atresia   **c.** malabsorption syndrome
   b. herniation   **d.** ulcerative colitis

14. Which of the following statements are true of GI herniation?
   1. Hernias generally result from some anatomic weakness in tissues.
   2. A hernia that cannot be reduced is said to be ''incarcerated.''
   3. Inguinal herniation may result in bowel descent into the scrotum.
   a. 1 and 2   **c.** 2 and 3
   b. 1 and 3   **d.** 1, 2, and 3

15. The appearance of a Schatzki's ring is associated with a(n) _____ hernia.
   a. inguinal   **c.** sliding
   b. rolling   **d.** umbilical

16. Which type of esophageal diverticulum results from scar tissue pulling the esophagus toward the area of involvement?
   a. epiphrenic   **c.** traction
   b. pulsion   **d.** Zencker's

17. A neurogenic disease of the GI system characterized by an absence of neurons in the bowel wall is:
   a. achalasia   **c.** Hirschprung's disease
   b. diverticulosis   **d.** toxic megacolon

18. Smooth muscle tumors of the esophagus that are almost always benign are:
   a. adenocarcinoma   **c.** polyposis
   b. leiomyoma   **d.** regional enteritis

19. The least amount of all GI tumors, both benign and malignant, occur in the:
   a. colon   **c.** large bowel
   b. esophagus   **d.** small bowel

20. Which of the following statements are true of colon cancer?
   1. The majority of adenocarcinoma of the colon occurs in the rectosigmoid area.
   2. The appearance of the ''apple core'' lesion is indicative of colon cancer.
   3. The prognosis with colon cancer is generally poor because of its early metastasis.
   a. 1 and 2   **c.** 2 and 3
   b. 1 and 3   **d.** 1, 2, and 3

21. Mechanical bowel obstructions are generally treated by:
    a. antibiotic therapy   c. radiation therapy
    b. chemotherapy   d. surgery

22. A twisting of bowel about its mesenteric base best refers to a(n):
    a. ascites   c. intussusception
    b. incarcerated hernia   d. volvulus

23. What clinical sign helps to distinguish appendicitis from other colicky abdominal disorders?
    a. chronic constipation   c. high white blood cell count
    b. high fever   d. nausea and vomiting

24. Which portion of the GI system is most frequently damaged by blunt trauma of the abdomen?
    a. cecum   c. ileum
    b. duodenum   d. jejunum

25. The condition in which a gallstone erodes from the gallbladder and creates a fistula to the small bowel is:
    a. gallstone ileus   c. intussusception
    b. incarcerated hernia   d. volvulus

5

The Hepatobiliary System

▼

Upon completion of Chapter 5, the reader should be able to:

- Describe the anatomical components of the hepatobiliary system and how they are visualized radiographically.
- Discuss the role of other imaging modalities in imaging of the hepatobiliary system, particularly ultrasound and CT.
- Characterize a given condition as inflammatory, metabolic, or neoplastic.
- Identify the pathogenesis of the pathologies cited and the typical treatments for them.
- Describe, in general, the radiographic appearance of each of the given pathologies.

ANATOMY AND PHYSIOLOGY REVIEW

The hepatobiliary system is composed of the liver, gallbladder, and biliary tree (Fig. 5-1, p. 220). The pancreas is closely related and shares a portion of the biliary ductal system, hence its inclusion here. These organs are considered as "accessory" organs of digestion, although this implies that an individual can live without them. Clearly this is not the case with the liver or pancreas.

The Liver

The liver is the largest organ in the body and is sheltered by the ribs in the right upper quadrant of the abdomen. It is kept in position by peritoneal ligaments and intraabdominal

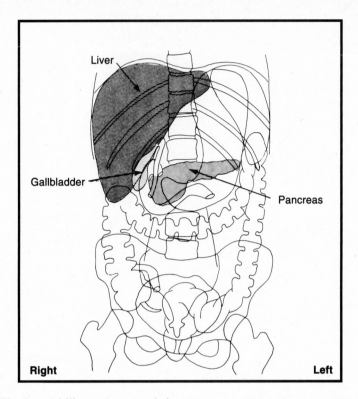

Fig. 5-1. The hepatobiliary system and the pancreas.   (From Bontrager KL: *Textbook of Radiographic Anatomy and Related Positioning,* ed 3, St Louis, 1993, Mosby.)

pressure from muscles of the abdominal wall. The functions of the liver are multiple, including metabolism of substances delivered via its portal circulation, synthesis of substances including those concerned with blood clotting, storage of vitamin B_{12} and other materials, and detoxification and excretion of various substances.

The liver has a double supply of blood, coming from both the hepatic artery and the portal vein. The hepatic artery usually originates from the celiac axis and takes oxygenated blood to the liver. The portal vein is also of significance. It is located within the liver and serves to filter venous blood from the abdominal viscera to remove impurities. Any interference with blood flow, such as might occur with liver disease, results in consequences elsewhere in the abdominal viscera.

The Biliary Tree

A system of ducts act to drain bile produced in the liver into the duodenum (Fig. 5-2). Bile from the liver's two main lobes is drained by the right and left hepatic ducts. These unite to form the common hepatic duct, which is joined in its midportion by the cystic duct from the gallbladder. Together, the cystic duct and the common hepatic duct form the common bile duct.

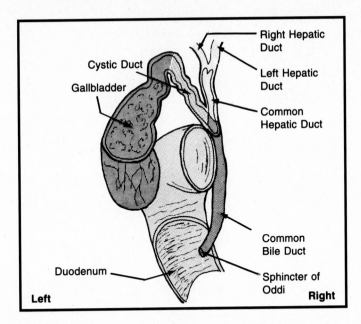

Fig. 5-2. The biliary system. (From Bontrager KL: *Textbook of Radiographic Anatomy and Related Positioning,* ed 3, St Louis, 1993, Mosby.)

The common bile duct descends posterior to the descending duodenum to enter at its posteromedial aspect. Before its entrance into the duodenum, the common bile duct may be joined by the pancreatic duct from the head of the pancreas. The short part of the common bile duct, after joining the pancreatic duct, is known as the hepatopancreatic ampulla, or more commonly as the Ampulla of Vater.

The flow of both bile and pancreatic juice into the duodenum is regulated by the hepatopancreatic sphincter, more commonly known as the sphincter of Oddi. The release of bile into the duodenum is triggered by cholecystokinin, a hormone released by the presence of fatty foods in the stomach. The purpose of bile is to emulsify fats so that they may be absorbed.

The Gallbladder

The gallbladder is a pear-shaped sac located on the undersurface on the right lobe of the liver. Normally the walls are quite thin, but they often thicken in the presence of inflammation. The sole function of the gallbladder is to store and concentrate bile that has been produced in the liver.

The Pancreas

The pancreas is an elongated, flat organ that crosses the left side of the abdomen behind the stomach; it is a powerful digestive organ. Its functions are both exocrine and endocrine. Composed of two parts, the first is concerned with production of digestive enzymes. These are discharged through the pancreatic duct into the duodenum. The other part of the pancreas consists of multiple clusters of specialized cells known as the islets of Langerhans. Their function is to produce insulin, which is discharged directly into the blood from the pancreas. Insulin serves to regulate carbohydrate metabolism.

IMAGING CONSIDERATIONS
Plain Films

A conventional abdominal radiograph may contain information about the hepatobiliary system through the demonstration of faint calcifications that might otherwise be obscured by contrast media. A plain radiograph of the gallbladder may demonstrate *"milk of calcium"* as a semiliquid sludge (Fig. 5-3) composed of calcium carbonate mixed with bile in the gallbladder. The hazy radiopacity is due to a settling of bile as a result of an obstruction at the neck of the gallbladder.

Gas may occasionally be seen in the wall or lumen of the gallbladder because of the presence of gas-forming organisms in the gallbladder walls. This is most generally seen in patients with poorly controlled diabetes. Gas visualized in the biliary tree may also be seen as a result of a spontaneous fistula, as might be seen in gallstone ileus, or postoperative biliary anastomosis (Fig. 5-4).

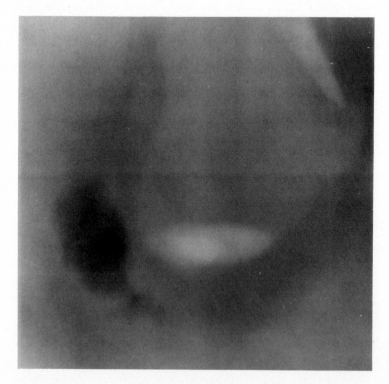

Fig. 5-3. "Milk of calcium" bile as seen in the bottom of this gallbladder in an erect spot film. (Courtesy of Riverside Methodist Hospitals, Columbus, Ohio.)

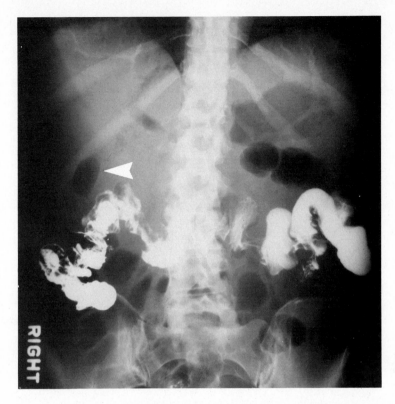

Fig. 5-4. Gas in the lumen of the gallbladder as a result of postsurgical fistula development to the bowel as seen on plain film. (Courtesy of the American College of Radiology, Reston, Virginia.)

Contrast Studies

An examination formerly widely used to study the biliary system is an oral cholecystogram, although it has been largely replaced by ultrasound. It still has use, however, in certain clinical situations. In this examination, the contrast media is absorbed in the small bowel and passes through the portal vein to the liver. The contrast agent is then excreted from the liver with bile and is stored in the gallbladder (Fig. 5-5, p. 224). Unfortunately, about 25% of all patients gallbladders fail to visualize on the first attempt at oral cholecystography. The reasons for this are diverse, but pathologically, the most common causes of nonvisualization are an obstruction of the cystic duct secondary to a stone, or chronic cholecystitis, with poor concentration of the contrast agent.

A percutaneous transhepatic cholangiogram is used sparingly as a means of visualizing the biliary tree and involves insertion of a needle into the biliary tree by puncture

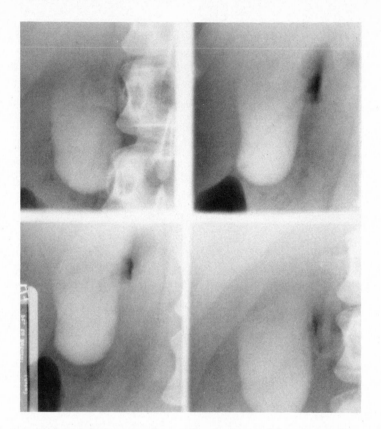

Fig. 5-5. A normal oral cholecystogram, with no evidence of stones as demonstrated on this standard 4-on-1 spot film in various projections. (Courtesy of Riverside Methodist Hospitals, Columbus, Ohio.)

directly through the wall of the abdomen. The subsequent injection of contrast media is useful in distinguishing medical jaundice, caused by hepatocellular dysfunction, from surgical jaundice, which results from biliary obstruction. Also, the examination is useful for detecting the presence of calculi or a tumor in the distal common bile duct.

An endoscopic retrograde cholangiopancreatogram (ERCP) is a means of visualizing the biliary system and main pancreatic duct, which provides drainage for the pancreatic enzymes into both the digestive tract and the common bile duct. A fiberoptic endoscope is passed through the duodenal C-loop to visualize the Ampulla of Vater. A thin catheter is then directed into the orifice of the common bile duct or pancreatic duct, followed by an injection of contrast media (Fig. 5-6). In many cases, the ERCP has replaced the transhepatic cholangiogram and is often supplemented with an ultrasonic examination or CT investigation of the pancreas.

T-tube cholangiography is used after a cholecystectomy to demonstrate patency of the

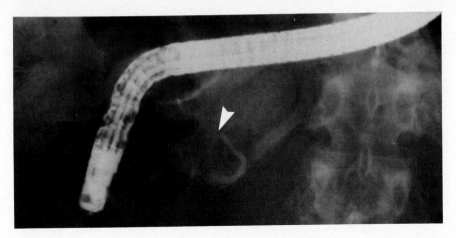

Fig. 5-6. An ERCP showing abrupt termination of the pancreatic duct about 4 cm from its opening. Compare with Fig. 5-21. (Courtesy of Riverside Methodist Hospitals, Columbus, Ohio.)

common bile duct and to check for calculi. With a T-shaped tube already inserted into the common bile duct, contrast media is injected to verify removal of all calculi. Care must be taken by the radiologist not to inject air bubbles because they may give the radiographic appearance of radiolucent calculi.

Other Studies

Diagnostic medical sonography is now the modality of choice for visualization of gallbladder disease (Fig. 5-7, p. 226). It is also an excellent tool for determining the presence of common bile duct obstruction, evaluation of the intrahepatic biliary ductal system, and abscesses. Advances in Doppler flow technology allow for clear analysis of portal blood flow. Ultrasound is also increasingly used for needle-directed biopsies of the hepatobiliary systems, and in cases where respiratory motion is a problem, it is preferred to CT-directed biopsy.

The role of CT in the hepatobiliary system is similar to that in the GI tract. It is the accepted modality for following malignancies and assessing masses, particularly of the liver and pancreas. Lacerations and resultant abdominal bleeding are readily detected (Fig. 5-8, p. 226). CT-guided biopsy procedures for the liver (Fig. 5-9, p. 227), pancreas, and kidney allow for analysis and drainage and offer significant advantages vs. conventional surgical biopsy and drainage. MRI is not used as often as CT currently, although its role will likely expand in the future.

Hepatobiliary scans performed in nuclear medicine are very useful to confirm cholecystitis, and they may be useful for distinguishing acute from chronic cholecystitis (Fig. 5-10, pp. 227–228). White cells labeled with radioactive indium are useful in locating sites of infection to allow for treatment.

Text continued on p. 228.

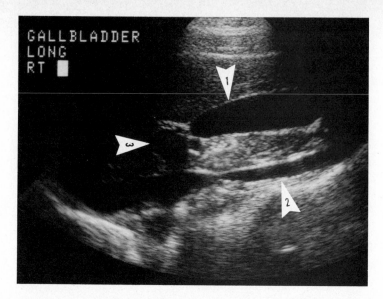

Fig. 5-7. Sonography of a normal gallbladder readily demonstrates *1*, the gallbladder, *2*, inferior vena cava, and *3*, the portal vein. (Courtesy of Riverside Methodist Hospitals, Columbus, Ohio.)

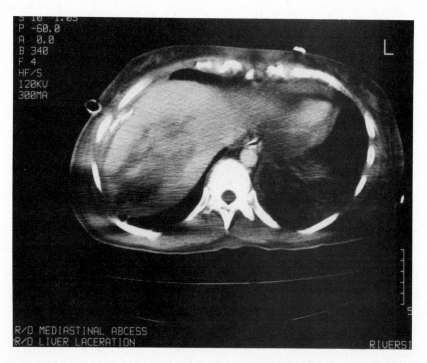

Fig. 5-8. CT of this 39-year-old female after a car accident reveals large lacerations to the liver. (Courtesy of Riverside Methodist Hospitals, Columbus, Ohio.)

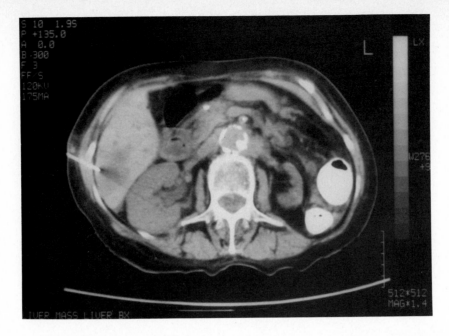

Fig. 5-9. CT of needle biopsy in this 87-year-old female clearly demonstrates the needle in the liver. (Courtesy of Riverside Methodist Hospitals, Columbus, Ohio.)

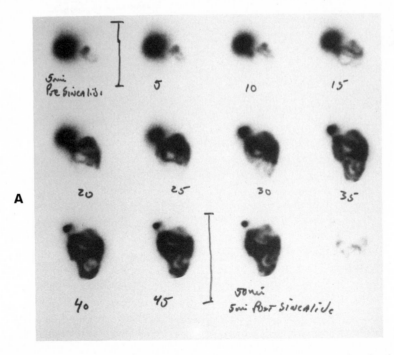

Fig. 5-10, *A.* Nuclear medicine hepatobiliary scan demonstrates ready ejection of the radionuclide from the gallbladder (large in upper left image) through sequential images into the duodenum (large in lower right image) in this 44-year-old female. (Courtesy of Riverside Methodist Hospitals, Columbus, Ohio.)

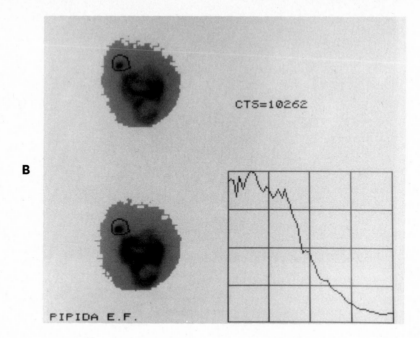

Fig. 5-10, *B.* Computer analysis of the accompanying data generates a graph showing 95% ejection of the agent. Above 50% is considered acceptable. (Courtesy of Riverside Methodist Hospitals, Columbus, Ohio.)

INFLAMMATORY DISEASES
Cirrhosis

Cirrhosis is a chronic liver condition in which the liver parenchyma and architecture is destroyed, fibrous tissue is laid down, and regenerative nodules are formed. In its early stages, it is usually asymptomatic, as it can take months or even years before damage becomes apparent. Thus, cirrhosis is considered an ''end-stage'' condition resulting from liver damage by chronic alcohol abuse, drugs, autoimmune disorders, metabolic and genetic disease, chronic viral infections, cardiac problems, and chronic biliary tract obstruction.

The scarring and formation of regenerative nodules associated with cirrhosis can have serious complications for the afflicted individual. The two functional impairments caused by cirrhosis are impaired liver function, generally resulting in jaundice, and portal hypertension. Because of interference of portal blood flow through the liver, portal hypertension may lead to development of collateral venous connections to the vena cavae. Most commonly, such connections involve the esophageal veins, which dilate to become esophageal varices, as described in the preceding chapter. These are best evaluated with endoscopy but may be seen on an esophagram. Also, the patient with cirrhosis has a tendency to bleed because the liver is unable to make the necessary clotting factors found

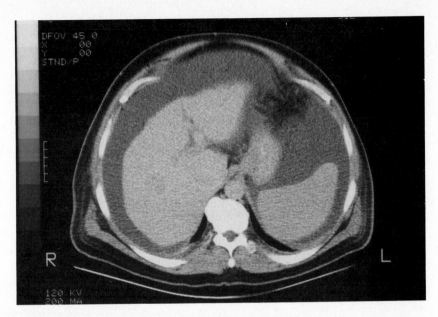

Fig. 5-11. Cirrhosis of the liver as indicated on this CT scan showing a shrunken liver with significant ascites around it within the abdomen. (Courtesy of Riverside Methodist Hospitals, Columbus, Ohio.)

in plasma or as a result of an esophageal variceal rupture. Such hemorrhaging may be, in fact, the first indication of portal hypertension.

Ascites, the accumulation of fluid within the peritoneal cavity (Fig. 5-11), is also seen as a result of portal hypertension and the leakage of excessive fluids from the portal capillaries. Much of this excess fluid is composed of hepatic lymph "weeped" from the liver surface. Ascites may also result from chronic hepatitis, congestive heart failure, renal failure, and certain cancers. When the cause of ascites is uncertain, diagnostic paracentesis may be conducted with sonographic guidance. This involves removal of 50 to 100 ml of peritoneal fluid for analysis. Patients with ascites generally complain of nonspecific abdominal pain and dyspnea. Medical treatment of ascites includes bedrest, dietary restrictions of sodium, use of diuretics to avoid excess fluid accumulation, and treatment of the underlying cause.

It is important for the technologist to be aware of the clinical diagnosis of ascites because the fluid accumulation can make it difficult to adequately penetrate the abdomen. An increase in exposure factors is necessary to obtain a diagnostic quality radiograph. Radiographically, large amounts of ascitic fluid give the abdomen a dense, gray, "ground glass" appearance. In a supine position, the fluid accumulates in the pelvis and ascends to either side of the bladder to give it a "dog-eared" appearance. Gradually the margins of the liver, spleen, kidneys, and psoas muscles become indistinct as the volume of fluid increases. Loops of bowel filled with gas float centrally, and a lateral decubitus radiograph will demonstrate the fluid descending with the gas-filled loops of bowel floating on top.

Although sonography is helpful in determining the presence of liver cirrhosis, the diagnosis is generally accomplished through a biopsy of liver tissue. Radiographic signs of cirrhosis are few and not specific. However, radiography is useful in diagnosis of the complications arising from cirrhosis, most notably ascites as noted previously and hepatocellular carcinoma. Treatment of cirrhosis depends on the extent of liver damage and the involvement of other organs (e.g., the esophagus and stomach). The primary goal of treatment is to eliminate the underlying causes of the disease and to treat its complications.

Viral Hepatitis

Hepatitis is a relatively common liver condition, with an estimated 70,000 cases reported annually. A virus causes acute inflammation of the liver and interferes with the liver's impaired ability to excrete bilirubin, the orange or yellowish pigment in bile. Evidence of the disease is seen clinically by nausea, vomiting, discomfort, and tenderness over the liver area, and laboratory results indicating a disturbance in liver function. Jaundice may also be present because of the disturbance of bilirubin excretion.

Two different viruses give rise to the two primary types of viral hepatitis, with their names describing the usual methods of transmission. Hepatitis A, infectious hepatitis, is excreted in the GI tract in fecal material and is spread by contact with an infected individual, normally through ingestion of contaminated food or water. It is the more common form of the two and is highly contagious. The incubation period of the disease is relatively short, and its course is usually mild. Hepatitis B, serum hepatitis, is transmitted parenterally in infected serum or blood products. Its incubation period is much longer, with the effects more severe than those seen in Hepatitis A. Toxic chemicals, alcohol, or allergic reactions are also known to produce hepatitis. A third type of viral hepatitis, Hepatitis C, is non-A, non-B, and is caused by a yet unidentified virus.

The diagnosis of viral hepatitis is usually made through laboratory testing because the disease is carried in the bloodstream during the acute phase. Evidence of hepatitis may be seen radiographically on a plain film of the abdomen that demonstrates *hepatomegaly,* enlargement of the liver, although this is a nonspecific finding. Cellular necrosis can be confirmed through nuclear medicine scanning of the liver, CT, or a liver biopsy under fluoroscopic guidance. Ultrasound is also useful in distinguishing characteristics of the liver.

Viral hepatitis is usually mild; the majority of patients recover without complications. Treatment generally consists of bed rest and medication to fight nausea and vomiting. In a healthy individual, the liver regenerates after hepatitis damage and complete recovery is gained. A few patients do, however, progress into a chronic state, harboring the virus in their blood and becoming chronic carriers. In some, the disease may become progressive and lead to liver failure.

Cholelithiasis

The incidence of *cholelithiasis* (gallstones) is fairly common, with at least 10% of all persons developing them in their lifetime. Females are more likely than males to have them. Their occurrence is also greater in diabetics, the obese, and in parous women. Heredity, also, seems to play a role in their development. Although most commonly found

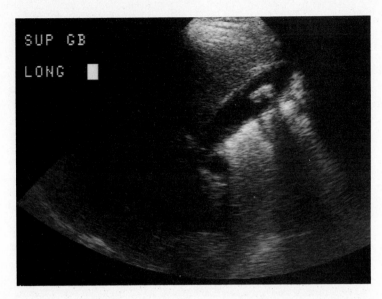

Fig. 5-12. Cholelithiasis as seen in this sonogram of the gallbladder in this young female with ready visibility of a single stone. (Courtesy of Riverside Methodist Hospitals, Columbus, Ohio.)

in the gallbladder, they can be located anywhere in the biliary tree.

The characteristics of gallstones are quite varied. They may occur as a single stone or as multiple stones. About 80% of all stones comprise a mixture of cholesterol, bile pigment (bilirubin), and calcium salts. The remaining 20% are composed of pure cholesterol and calcium-bilirubin mixture. Most stones are radiolucent since only about 10% of all stones contain enough calcium to be radiopaque. Those that are radiopaque may be difficult to distinguish from renal stones, but oblique radiographs help separate the two structures (kidney and gallbladder) from each other, demonstrating the gallbladder anterior to the kidney. As noted before, sonography readily demonstrates the presence of cholelithiasis (Fig. 5-12).

Size of gallstones varies from the size of a pinhead to the size of a large marble. The small stones, commonly referred to as gravel, tend to travel into the biliary tree and may result in obstruction. This obstruction results in edematous accumulation in the walls of the gallbladder and causes its inflammation.

Cholecystitis is an acute inflammation of the gallbladder. It is characterized clinically by a sudden onset of pain, fever, nausea, and vomiting. Its diagnosis is clinically suspected and supported through an ultrasound examination or radionuclide hepatobiliary scan. Repeated attacks of acute cholecystitis cause damage to the gallbladder, resulting in thickening of the walls (Fig. 5-13, p. 232) and decreased function. Complications of untreated gallbladder disease include infarction and possible gangrenous state, prompting a rupture of the walls. If a rupture does occur, bile peritonitis may result and require immediate treatment. Occasionally a stone can erode through the wall of the gallbladder

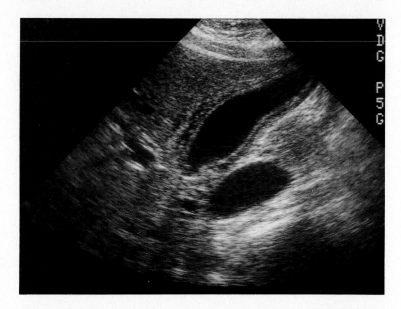

Fig. 5-13. Cholecystitis as indicated by the inflamed, thickened gallbladder walls in this 23-year-old female. (Courtesy of Riverside Methodist Hospitals, Columbus, Ohio.)

and create a fistula to the bowel. If it becomes impacted in the small bowel, the condition is referred to as *gallstone ileus* (Fig. 5-14).

Surgical removal of the gallbladder (cholecystectomy) is usually the treatment of choice, although laparoscopic diolecystectomy has replaced much of traditional cut-down cholecystectomies. The newer technique allows a less traumatic entry and laser excision and removal of the gallbladder, with a considerably shortened hospitalization and dramatically reduced costs. Radiographers are commonly called to the operating environment to film injections of contrast media into the exposed biliary duct to determine if all stones have been removed. If additional stones are suspected but not visualized, a T-tube may be inserted to allow for later study as noted earlier. An alternative treatment method, shock wave lithotripsy of gallstones, has not proven as successful in the gallbladder as it has in the kidneys for kidney stones. Investigation of it as an alternative in the United States continues, although it is used to some extent elsewhere in the world.

Pancreatitis

An acute or chronic inflammation of the pancreatic tissue is known as *pancreatitis*. Its causes include an excessive and chronic alcohol consumption, an obstruction of the Ampulla of Vater by a gallstone or tumor, and even the injection of contrast media during an ERCP has been known to cause pancreatitis. Once activated by any of these causes, trypsin, the pancreatic enzyme that is normally excreted through the ducts into the duodenum begins to autodigest the organ itself. This can be quite serious and carries a high mortality rate. Hemorrhagic pancreatitis is a complication of pancreatitis and consists of

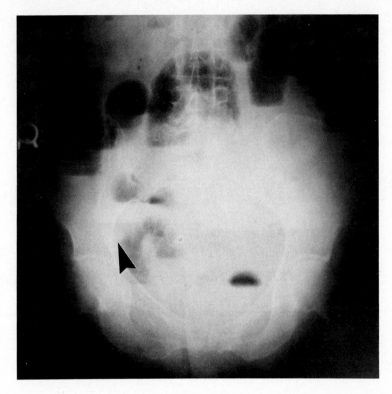

Fig. 5-14. Gallstone ileus in a 43-year-old female as a result of cholecystitis. The gallstone is in the lower right abdomen *(arrow)* with the small bowel air pattern as a result of the resultant bowel obstruction. (Courtesy of the American College of Radiology, Reston, Virginia.)

erosion into local tissues and blood vessels, with subsequent hemorrhaging into the retroperitoneal space. A *pseudocyst* is a fluid collection caused by pancreatitis and is readily visualized by sonographic or CT examination (Fig. 5-15, p. 234).

Radiographic indications of pancreatitis are subtle and previously centered on displacement of the duodenal C-loop or the stomach by the diseased pancreas. An ERCP is of value in determining the reasons for acute recurrent pancreatitis, chronic pancreatitis, or the complications associated with pancreatitis. CT and ultrasound examination are also of significant value in assessing pancreatic disease. Laboratory testing is the most common way to diagnose pancreatitis, through evaluation of serum, and occasionally the urine amylase level.

Management of patients with pancreatitis consists of a pain-relieving drug in mild cases and maintaining proper fluid levels to prevent shock, a frequent occurrence in acute pancreatitis. Proper dietary restrictions (e.g., abstinence from alcohol) are also important. The role of surgery in chronic pancreatitis remains controversial in regard to the effectiveness of results.

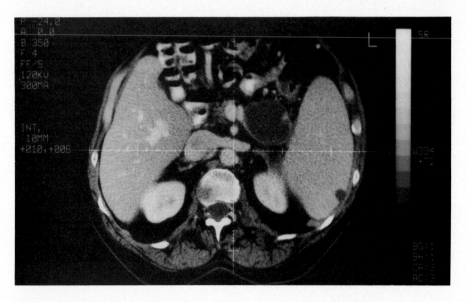

Fig. 5-15. Pancreatitis with demonstration of a 5 cm pseudocyst in the tail as seen on CT. (Courtesy of Riverside Methodist Hospitals, Columbus, Ohio.)

METABOLIC DISEASES
Jaundice

Jaundice, the yellowish discoloration of the skin and whites of the eyes, is not a disease itself but rather a sign of disease. The accumulation of excess bile pigments (i.e., bilirubin) in the body tissues "stains" the skin and eyes this yellowish color. Normally bile and its pigments are secreted into the bowel and eliminated. Bilirubin is a type of bile pigment that is produced when hemoglobin breaks down. Normal serum bilirubin levels are equal to or less than 1 mg/100 ml, but must exceed 3 mg/100 ml to be visible to the observer.

Medical (nonobstructive) *jaundice* occurs because of hemolytic disease in which too many red blood cells are destroyed or when the liver is damaged by cirrhosis or hepatitis. Its most common appearance is transient in the first few days after birth when more bile pigments are released than can be handled. If the liver is damaged from disease, it is simply unable to excrete the bilirubin in a normal fashion and it enters the bloodstream. *Surgical* (obstructive) *jaundice* occurs when the biliary system is obstructed, preventing bile from entering the duodenum. A common cause of this obstruction is blockage of the common bile duct caused by stones or masses. The longer the obstruction persists, the more likely it is that complications (e.g., liver injury, infection, or bleeding) will arise.

The jaundiced patient often undergoes an ultrasound examination of the liver, biliary tree, and pancreas to determine if the jaundice is obstructive or nonobstructive. The common bile duct is readily identified, and although simplified, a normal size implies nonobstructive jaundice and a dilated common bile duct suggests an obstruction. A variety of other methods may be used to diagnose the cause of jaundice, including plain abdominal radiographs, ERCP, and CT. An ultrasound or CT-directed needle biopsy may be used if an intrahepatic cause of the hepatitis is suspected. Treatment of jaundice centers on diagnosis and treatment of its underlying cause. In the case of obstructive jaundice, surgical excision of the obstructing body may be necessary. Endoscopic removal of common duct stones can be frequently used, and endoscopy also offers the opportunity to stent or bypass a tumor.

NEOPLASTIC DISEASES
Hemangioma

A *hemangioma* is the most common tumor of the liver. It is benign and composed of newly formed blood vessels. A port-wine stain on the face, a superficial purplish-red birthmark, is an example of a hemangioma elsewhere in the body. Hemangiomas can range in size from microscopic up to 10 to 15 cm in size. A hemangioma does not become malignant and is generally insignificant. It can, however, present symptoms as a result of tissue displacement or bleeding. Diagnosis can be complicated when it occurs with a known malignancy because its characteristics may be difficult to distinguish from metastasis. Nuclear medicine scans using labeled red blood cells that are attracted to the highly vascular tumor and MRI are useful in the diagnosis of hemangiomas (Fig. 5-16, p. 236).

Hepatoma

Hepatoma (hepatocarcinoma), a primary carcinoma of the liver, is uncommon in the United States, accounting for less than 2% of all cancers. An association between cirrhosis and hepatoma exists, with alcoholism and poor nutrition associated with each. Most primary hepatomas originate in liver parenchyma, creating a large central mass with smaller satellite nodules. Although vascular invasion is common, death occurs from liver failure, often without extension of the cancer outside the liver.

The liver is also a common site for metastasis from other primary sites, which makes sense, given its role in filtering blood that has traveled from these sites. Primary cancers located in the abdomen, especially those drained by the portal venous system, often metastasize to the liver (Fig. 5-17, p. 237).

Patients with cirrhosis and unexpected deterioration are suspect for hepatoma. Other symptoms include increased jaundice, abdominal pain, weight loss, ascites, and a rapid increase in liver size. Plain abdominal radiographs of patients with hepatoma may demonstrate hepatomegaly. Nuclear medicine liver scans are useful in distinguishing between primary and metastatic disease. CT and ultrasound are often used to reveal the extent of the tumor (Fig. 5-18, p. 237). Arteriography can readily demonstrate the increased vascularity associated with a carcinoma.

Surgical resection of the hepatoma represents the only possibility for cure. Those hepatomas that are diffuse or have multiple nodules generally preclude surgery. The general lack of radiosensitivity of these tumors makes radiotherapy ineffective. Patients treated with chemotherapy demonstrate tumor shrinkage and an addition of a few months to their lives. The disease, however, is generally fatal except for those who have had successful resection of a single liver mass.

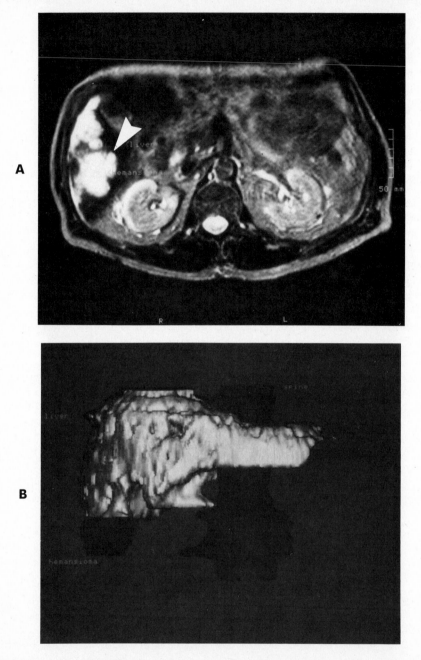

Fig. 5-16, *A*. An axial MRI slice through the liver reveals a hemangioma. *B*. Reconstruction isolates the liver and the hemangioma in this lateral view of the liver. (Courtesy of Riverside Methodist Hospitals, Columbus, Ohio.)

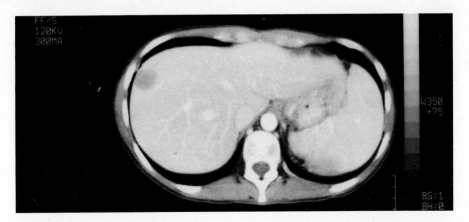

Fig. 5-17. CT scan after duodenal cancer resection in a 21-year-old female demonstrates local recurrence and metastases to the liver on its lateral border in this slice. (Courtesy of Riverside Methodist Hospitals, Columbus, Ohio.)

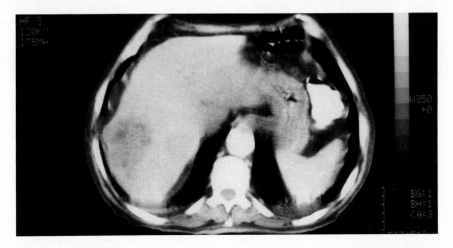

Fig. 5-18. Large, inhomogeneous lesion in the liver as consistent with hepatoma. (Courtesy of Riverside Methodist Hospitals, Columbus, Ohio.)

Carcinoma of the Gallbladder

Carcinoma of the gallbladder is very rare and is more common in women and the elderly. As a result of chronic cholecystitis, the gallbladder walls may assume a ''porcelain'' appearance (Fig. 5-19, p. 238), indicating a tendency to develop into gallbladder carcinoma. Gallstones exist in about 75% of all cases. Unfortunately, the prognosis with gallbladder carcinoma is often poor, since metastases to the liver usually occur before the primary disease is diagnosed (Fig. 5-20, p. 239).

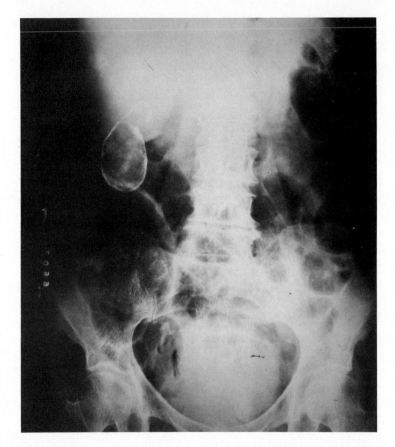

Fig. 5-19. A "porcelain" gallbladder in a 70-year-old male with a history of recurrent indigestion. (Courtesy of the American College of Radiology, Reston, Virginia.)

Carcinoma of the Pancreas

Pancreatic cancer is usually rapidly fatal. Its diagnosis is difficult because of the location of the pancreas and lack of symptoms before extensive local spread. In most cases, the tumor is well advanced before the diagnosis is made. Its incidence is greater in men than in women and in blacks than in whites; a clearcut association with cigarette smoking has been demonstrated. Most tumors arise as epithelial tumors of the duct (adenocarcinoma) and cause pancreatic obstruction (Fig. 5-21). The rich supply of nerves to the pancreas results in pain being a prominent feature of this carcinoma. Radical surgery as a treatment mode carries a high mortality rate, and chemotherapy also produces poor results. Radiation therapy is difficult because of the proximity to very radiosensitive structures such as the spinal cord. The prognosis with pancreatic carcinoma is very poor, demonstrating only a 2% survival rate for 5 years.

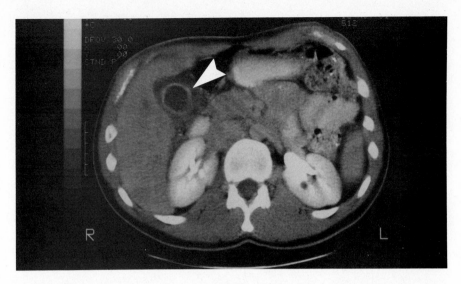

Fig. 5-20. Gallbladder carcinoma, resulting in metastasis to surrounding structures, as seen on this CT of a 23-year-old male. The gallbladder *(arrow)* is surrounded by metastasis, with significant metastasis into the pancreas area and right kidney. (Courtesy of Riverside Methodist Hospitals, Columbus, Ohio.)

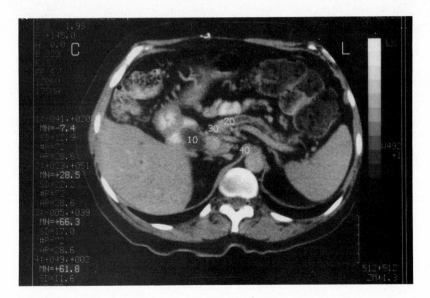

Fig. 5-21. Pancreatic carcinoma in the head of the pancreas, as indicated by atrophy of the pancreatic body and tail on this CT scan of the same patient shown in Fig. 6-6. Numbers shown are for density sampling, with *1, 2,* and *3* in the pancreas. (Courtesy of Riverside Methodist Hospitals, Columbus, Ohio.)

▼ QUESTIONS

1. Bile drains from the liver's right and left hepatic ducts directly into the:
   a. common bile duct
   b. common hepatic duct
   c. cystic duct
   d. duodenum

2. The modality of choice for visualization of gallbladder disease is:
   a. CT
   b. nuclear medicine
   c. radiography
   d. ultrasound

3. Which of the following statements are true about imaging of hepatobiliary disease?
   1. ''Milk of calcium'' demonstrated on a plain film suggests an obstruction.
   2. An ERCP allows for contrast injection into the neck of the gallbladder.
   3. CT is particularly useful for following the course of malignancies and masses.
   a. 1 and 2
   b. 1 and 3
   c. 2 and 3
   d. 1, 2, and 3

4. Impairment of normal liver function might result in:
   a. cirrhosis
   b. jaundice
   c. milk of calcium
   d. viral hepatitis

5. Which of the following statements are true of liver cirrhosis?
   1. As an ''end stage'' condition, damage may not be apparent for months or years.
   2. Portal hypertension can result from cirrhosis and cause esophageal varices.
   3. Ultrasound or CT needle-directed biopsy is useful in diagnosing cirrhosis.
   a. 1 and 2
   b. 1 and 3
   c. 2 and 3
   d. 1, 2, and 3

6. Patients with liver cirrhosis have a tendency to develop:
   a. ascites
   b. esophageal varices
   c. jaundice
   d. two of the above
   e. all of the above

7. Which of the following is more characteristic of Hepatitis A than Hepatitis B?
   a. effects are generally more severe
   b. excreted through blood products
   c. has a longer incubation period
   d. more common form of the two

8. The radiographic appearance of a porcelain gallbladder may be an indication of:
   a. biliary obstruction
   b. cholecystitis
   c. cirrhosis
   d. gallbladder carcinoma

9. The yellowish discoloration of the skin associated with jaundice is due to:
   a. an accumulation of milk of calcium
   b. infected fecal material transmission
   c. paralysis of the small bowel wall
   d. presence of bilirubin in the blood
   e. none of the above

10. Which of the following statements are true concerning cholelithiasis?
    1. Males are more likely to be afflicted with gallstones than are females.
    2. Most stones are radiolucent; only about 10% are radiopaque.

3. Cholecystitis refers to an acute inflammation of the gallbladder.

    a. 1 and 2   **c.** 2 and 3

    b. 1 and 3   **d.** 1, 2, and 3

11. A patient diagnosed with Hepatitis B is suffering from a(n) _____ condition.

    a. allergic   **c.** metabolic

    b. bacterial   **d.** viral

12. Pseudocysts are generally associated with:

    a. cholecystitis   **c.** hepatitis

    b. gallstone ileus   **d.** pancreatitis

13. Gallstone ileus refers to impaction of a gallstone in the:

    a. biliary tree   **c.** liver

    b. gallbladder   **d.** small bowel

14. Which of the following statements are true of hepatoma?

    1. Most primary hepatomas present as diffuse spreading throughout the liver.

    2. Patients with cirrhosis who deteriorate unexpectedly are suspect for the disease.

    3. Surgical resection of the liver represents the only real chance for cure.

    a. 1 and 2   **c.** 2 and 3

    b. 1 and 3   **d.** 1, 2, and 3

15. Enzymatic digestion of surrounding tissues is characteristic of which disease?

    a. cholecystits   **d.** medical jaundice

    b. cholelithiasis   **e.** none of the above

    c. hepatoma

16. Which of the following functions is *not* associated with normal liver function?

    a. detoxification of substances   **c.** production of insulin

    b. production of blood clotting   **d.** storage of vitamin B_{12}

      agents

17. The diagnostic imaging modality of choice for following the progress of a liver malignancy is:

    a. CT   **c.** radiography

    b. MRI   **d.** ultrasonography

18. Portal hypertension and the resultant leak of excessive fluids from the capillaries result in:

    a. ascites   **c.** hepatoma

    b. cirrhosis   **d.** jaundice

19. The release of the enzyme *trypsin* into surrounding tissues results in an inflammatory reaction known as:

    a. cirrhosis   **c.** pancreatitis

    b. hepatoma   **d.** viral hepatitis

20. The most common liver tumor is a(n):

    a. hepatitis   **c.** hepatoma

    b. hemangioma   **d.** jaundice

6

The Urinary
System

Upon completion of Chapter 6, the reader should be able to:

- Describe the anatomical components of the urinary system and their functions.
- Discuss the role of other imaging modalities in imaging of the urinary system, particularly ultrasound and computed tomography (CT).
- Discuss common congenital anomalies of the urinary system.
- Characterize a given condition as inflammatory, metabolic, or neoplastic.
- Identify the pathogenesis of the pathologies cited and the typical treatments for them.
- Describe, in general, the radiographic appearance of each of the given pathologies.

ANATOMY AND PHYSIOLOGY REVIEW

The urinary system consists of two kidneys, two ureters, a urinary bladder, and a urethra (Fig. 6-1). The urinary system forms urine to remove waste from the bloodstream for excretion. The kidneys are the site where urine is formed and excreted through remarkable processes of filtration and reabsorption, involving up to 180 liters of blood per day. Urine formed in this process amounts to about 1 to 1.5 liters per day and passes from the kidneys to the bladder through the ureters. Stored in the bladder, it is eventually excreted through the urethra.

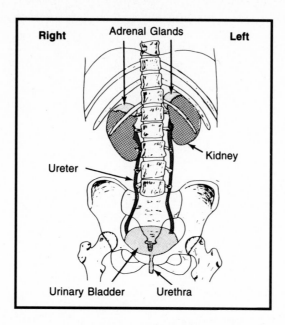

Fig. 6-1. The urinary system. (From Bontrager KL: *Textbook of radiographic positioning and related anatomy,* ed 3, St Louis 1993, Mosby.)

The kidneys are normally located between the twelfth thoracic vertebra and the third lumbar vertebra, with the right kidney lying slightly lower because of the presence of the liver superiorly. The notch located on the medial surface of each kidney is the hilus, the area where structures enter and leave the kidney. Microscopically, the nephron is the functional unit of the kidney responsible for forming and excreting urine (Fig. 6-2, p. 244). The nephron unit terminates into a collecting tubule, which helps to form a tube opening at the renal papilla into a minor calyx. Minor calyces terminate in the major calyces, which in turn terminate at the renal pelvis (Fig. 6-3, p. 244).

The ureters extend from the kidneys to the urinary bladder and are approximately 10 inches in length (Fig. 6-4, p. 245). They normally enter the bladder obliquely in the posterolateral portion of the bladder, equidistant from the urethral orifice in a triangular fashion. A number of variations of this can exist. The function of the ureters is to drain the urine from the kidneys to the bladder.

The bladder is located posterior to the symphysis pubis. It serves as a reservoir for urine before it is expelled from the body. The bladder is very muscular and capable of distention. Valves located at the junction of the ureters and bladder prevent the backflow of urine.

The urethra is a tube leading from the urinary bladder to the exterior of the body. In the male it also serves as a part of the reproductive system by receiving watery fluid via prostatic ducts that open into the urethra from the prostate.

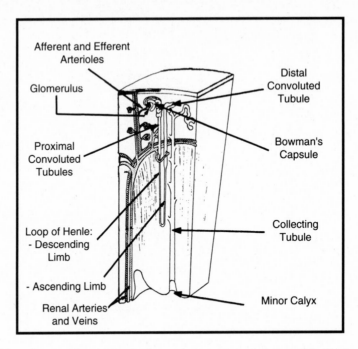

Fig. 6-2. The microscopic structure of a nephron. (From Bontrager KL: *Textbook of radiographic positioning and related anatomy,* ed 3, St Louis 1993, Mosby.)

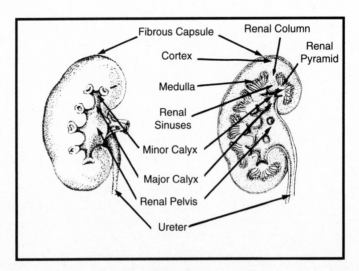

Fig. 6-3. The structure of a kidney. (From Bontrager KL: *Textbook of radiographic positioning and related anatomy,* ed 3, St Louis 1993, Mosby.)

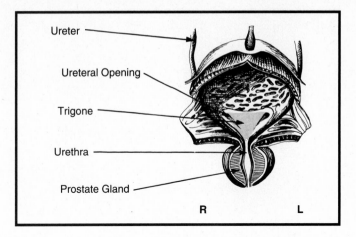

Fig. 6-4. An anterior, cut-away view of the bladder. (From Bontrager KL: *Textbook of radiographic positioning and related anatomy,* ed 3, St Louis 1993, Mosby.)

IMAGING CONSIDERATIONS
Intravenous Urography

Many different examinations exist to study the various aspects of the urinary system. The most common of these is the intravenous urogram (intravenous pyelogram or IVP), which remains the usual starting point for the diagnosis of urinary tract dysfunction. The indications for performing an intravenous urogram include suspected urinary tract obstruction, abnormal urinary sediment (especially hematuria), systemic hypertension, or frequently in men with symptoms of prostatism. While little or no serious adverse effects typically accompany the injection of urographic contrast agents, about 1 of 40,000 patients actually dies as a result of an allergic reaction to the contrast agents. The use of nonionic, low osmolar contrast agents significantly reduces moderate reactions, and may reduce the mortality figure associated with ionic agents.

A plain abdominal radiograph, often termed a *scout* or *preliminary* film, is the usual beginning for most intravenous urograms (Fig. 6-5,*A*, p. 246). Its primary purpose is to determine if adequate bowel preparation has been accomplished, and to visualize calculi of the kidneys, ureters, and bladder that may otherwise be hidden by the presence of contrast media. The radiologist also examines areas unrelated to the urinary tract, as they may hold clues to the diagnosis. The kidneys are frequently radiographically visible on this film because of the perirenal fat capsule that surrounds them. The kidneys are generally well fixed to the abdominal wall and are seen to move with respiratory effort. In addition, a male's kidneys are generally larger than those of the female.

Many intravenous urogram routines allow for a radiograph to be taken within 1 minute after contrast media injection. This is termed a *nephrogram* (phase) radiograph and may be used to demonstrate the contrast agent in the nephrons before it reaches the renal calyces. Ready visualization of the renal parenchyma allows for an inspection of the renal outline. Indentations and/or bulges may indicate the presence of disease. The neph-

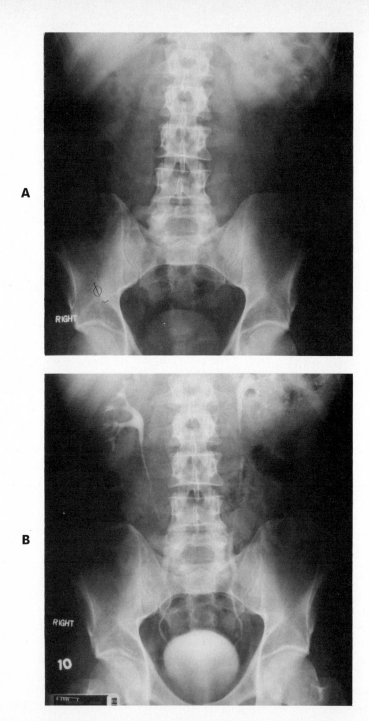

Fig. 6-5, *A.* "Scout film" of the abdomen taken in preparation for an intravenous urogram readily demonstrates renal and psoas shadows in this 39-year-old male. *B.* With other films interspersed, this 10-minute followup IVP film demonstrates good renal function with normal renal contours and collecting system. (Courtesy of Riverside Methodist Hospitals, Columbus, Ohio.)

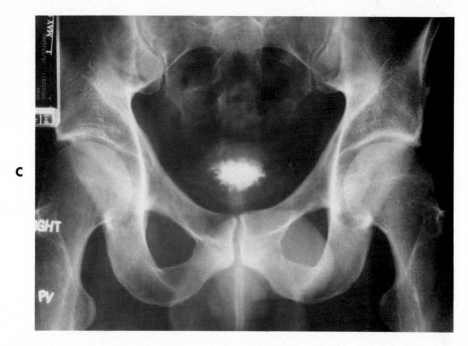

Fig. 6-5, *C.* Post-void film taken as part of this IVP series demonstrates good bladder function, completing a normal intravenous urogram. (Courtesy of Riverside Methodist Hospitals, Columbus, Ohio.)

rogram radiograph is also used to check for normal kidney position, which may be altered by congenital malposition or the presence of a retroperitoneal mass.

While the number and type of radiographs taken may vary from one institution to another, a series of collecting system sequence films are the final part of an intravenous urogram (Fig. 6-5,*B*). The renal pelvis, calyces, ureters, and bladder are examined for any abnormalities. The calyces should be evenly distributed and reasonably symmetrical. Usually, they present as "buttercup-shaped" projections surrounding the renal papillae. Calyceal dilatation may be demonstrated as a result of acute or chronic urinary tract obstruction, postobstructive uropathy, or reflux. Dilatation secondary to destruction of the renal pyramids is less common.

Due to the peristaltic activity of ureters, only part of their length in a collecting system sequence may be demonstrated. Sometimes nonopaque ureteral calculi cause filling defects and an obstructive dilatation of the ureter. The majority of all urinary tract calculi are found at the vesicoureteral junction. Any pronounced deviation of the ureter suggests the presence of a retroperitoneal mass. Various filling defects may be demonstrated in the contrast agent-filled ureter during an intravenous pyelogram, including tumors, blood clots, and nonopaque calculi. Common bladder defects visualized during an intravenous urogram include urinary catheter balloons and extrinsic deformities such as uterine or sigmoid colon tumors. A "post-void" film usually completes an intravenous urogram procedure, and allows assessment of the bladder function (Fig. 6-5,*C*).

Other Studies

Once the intravenous urogram is complete, the physician may order one of several additional tests designed to look at a select aspect of the urinary tract. Nephrotomography, for example, may be used as an adjunct study, using tomograms of the kidneys taken at suitable intervals. The indications for this may be small renal masses and better visualization of the renal parenchyma.

With retrograde pyelography, a catheter is placed into the ureteric orifice at cystoscopy to allow injection of contrast medium to outline the renal collecting system. Indications for this study may include hematuria of unknown cause, hydronephrosis, and in cases of a nonfunctioning kidney, where further information about the obstruction is desired. Percutaneous translumbar pyelography involves posterolateral insertion of a needle or catheter into the renal pelvis using medical sonography, fluoroscopy, or sometimes a combination of both modalities. The catheter may be left in place to provide drainage of an obstructed kidney or to allow retrieval of the calculus with a basket catheter. Sometimes the procedure is used to relieve obstruction in patients in which immediate surgery is not possible.

Extracorporeal shock wave lithotripsy (ESWL) is a method used to locate and treat renal calculi. After location of the stone is attained radiographically, fluoroscopy aids in alignment of a high-frequency shock wave directed at the stone of a patient. If the treatment is successful, the stone disintegrates into fragments that can be voided by the patient, often sparing a surgical procedure and a much more lengthy recovery period (Fig. 6-6).

Renal angiography is usually indicated to further evaluate a renal mass suspected of being malignant, but it also allows an assessment of renal artery stenosis, a cause of hypertension. With this procedure, a catheter is introduced into the femoral artery, with injection of contrast media into or above the renal arteries.

The most common examination for studying the lower urinary tract is the cystogram. This involves insertion of a catheter into the urethra and retrograde filling of the bladder with contrast material (Fig. 6-7, p. 252). A frequent indication for this procedure is to identify vesicoureteral reflux. In the normal bladder, increased pressure as the bladder fills effectively shuts down any chance of reflux. Bladder infection, however, can render the ureteral "valve" incompetent, refluxing infection into the kidney. Cystography is also used to study congenital bladder anomalies, tumors, diverticula, or calculi.

Voiding (micturition) cystography is sometimes used as a follow-up to a cystogram to allow study of the urethra upon voiding. Urethrography may be accomplished antegrade, as with a voiding cystourethrogram, or retrograde when a cystogram is not necessary. Its usual intent is to allow study of a urethral stricture.

For imaging other than radiographic or fluoroscopic, both ultrasound and CT play large roles. Ultrasound is useful in diagnosis of kidney stones, calcifications, hydronephrosis, abscesses, renal masses and cysts, and to assess renal atrophy. CT is particularly important in determining the nature of renal masses, either solid or cystic, and allowing for accurate biopsy. It is also useful in looking for sites of obstruction, assessing renal infection or trauma, and in staging of tumors of the lymph nodes or bladder. Nuclear medicine has a role in assessing the physiology associated with urine flow and in evaluating renal artery stenosis. As in the abdomen, the role of MRI is still being defined as respiratory motion problems are present.

Text continued on p. 252.

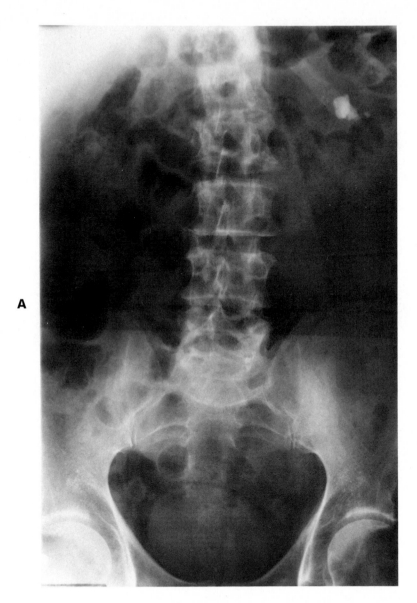

Fig. 6-6, *A.* ''Scout film'' taken before lithotripsy demonstrates a large, solid renal stone in the right kidney. (Courtesy of The Ohio Kidney Stone Center, Columbus, Ohio.)

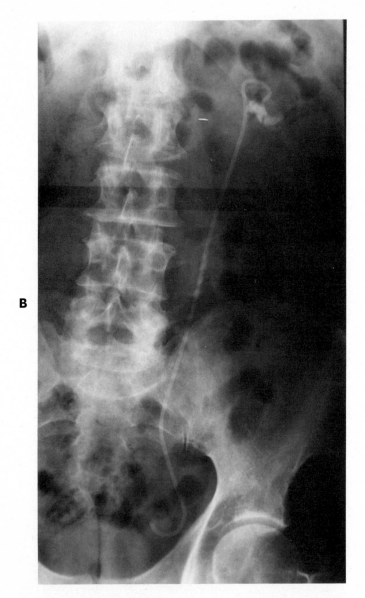

B

Fig. 6-6, *B.* Two months following lithotripsy, the stone is clearly seen to be fragmented and beginning to descend the right ureter. A stent has been placed in the right ureter to aid in draining urine. (Courtesy of The Ohio Kidney Stone Center, Columbus, Ohio.)

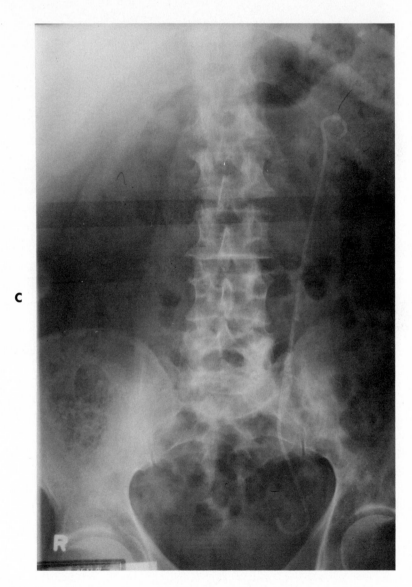

Fig. 6-6, *C.* A film taken 2 months later demonstrates further movement of stone fragments down the ureter. The stent is still in place. (Courtesy of The Ohio Kidney Stone Center, Columbus, Ohio.)

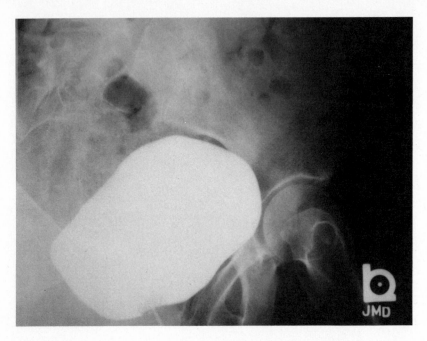

Fig. 6-7. Normal cystogram without reflux as seen in this oblique projection of the bladder in this 56-year-old female. (Courtesy of Riverside Methodist Hospitals, Columbus, Ohio.)

Urinary Tubes/Catheters

When certain types of pathology such as tumors or stone formation inhibit the normal flow of urine through the urinary system, several types of tubes may be used to allow drainage of the urine. A *nephrostomy tube* connects the renal pelvis to the outside of the body (Fig. 6-8). It is inserted percutaneously through the renal cortex and medulla into the renal pelvis to allow the urine to drain outside of the body directly from the renal pelvis. Special care must be taken when dealing with this type of patient because these patients are readily prone to infections because of the direct opening into the urinary system.

Ureteral stents may also be placed in cases of ureteral obstruction. Unlike nephrostomy tubes, ureteral stents do not connect the urinary system to the outside of the patient's body (see Fig. 6-6, *B*). Ureteral stents are placed surgically or via cystoscopy with the upper portion of the stent lying in the renal pelvis and the lower portion lying within the urinary bladder. The stent allows for patency of the diseased ureter, allowing the urine to flow normally. These stents are radiographically visible on plain abdominal radiographs.

Urinary catheterization is performed to obtain urine specimens, relieve urinary retention, monitor renal function, and in cases of urinary incontinence. A *Foley catheter* is the most common indwelling urinary catheter and is placed within the urinary bladder

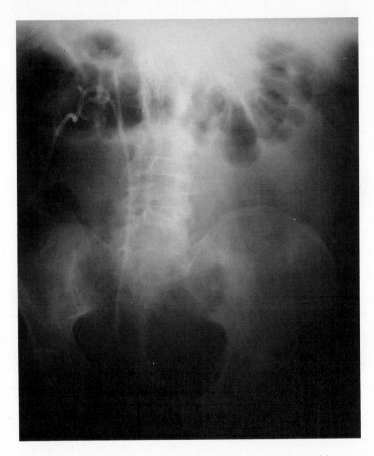

Fig. 6-8. A nephrostomy catheter is visible on the right, along with a stent catheter between the right renal pelvis and urinary bladder in this abdominal view of a 79-year-old male. A Greenfield filter is also seen in the inferior vena cava. (Courtesy of Riverside Methodist Hospitals, Columbus, Ohio.)

using sterile technique. Once the catheter is placed through the urethra and urinary sphincter, a small balloon is inflated to help the catheter remain in place within the urinary bladder. This catheter is generally connected to a bag that collects the urine as it flows through the catheter to the outside of the body. Care must be taken to ensure the catheter is not displaced during a radiographic procedure and the urine collection bag must remain lower than the patient's bladder at all times to prevent the reflux of urine back into the bladder, which could result in a urinary tract infection. A Foley catheter must be placed in an individual before performing cystography or cystourethrography to allow the installation of contrast material into the bladder. Again, the importance of proper sterile technique cannot be overemphasized.

CONGENITAL/HEREDITARY DISEASES

Anomalies of the kidneys and ureters are caused by errors in development. They can be classified as anomalies of number, size and form, fusion, and position. About 10% of all persons have some sort of congenital malformation of the urinary system. At least half of those with kidney anomalies have malformations elsewhere in the urinary system or other systems.

Number and Size Anomalies of the Kidney

Renal agenesis is a relatively rare anomaly that demonstrates as the absence of the kidney on one side with an unusually large kidney on the other side (Fig. 6-9), which is known as compensatory hypertrophy. The left kidney is more frequently missing, and the condition is more common in males than in females. The single kidney is normal and it is more subject to trauma because of its enlarged size. Protection against disease in an individual with only one kidney is very important.

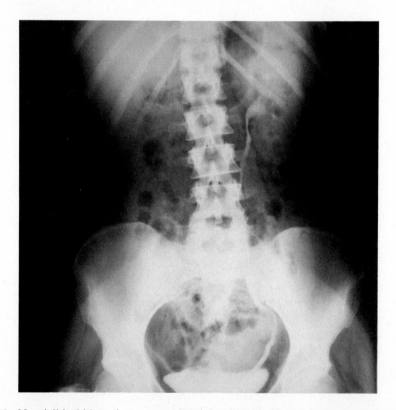

Fig. 6-9. No visible kidney is seen on the right side on this intravenous urogram. Angiography confirmed lack of a renal artery, and cystoscopy demonstrated no ureteric orifice; all are consistent with renal agenesis on the right. (Courtesy of Riverside Methodist Hospitals, Columbus, Ohio.)

A *supernumerary kidney* is also relatively rare and consists of the presence of a third, small, rudimentary kidney. It has no parenchymal attachment to a kidney, and usually drains from an independent renal pelvis into the ureter on that side. It often becomes symptomatic as a result of infection.

Hypoplasia is a rare anomaly of kidney size involving a kidney that is developed less than normal (Fig. 6-10). Usually hypoplasia is associated with hyperplasia of the other kidney. It requires renal arteriography to differentiate congenital hypoplasia from a kidney that is atrophic due to acquired vascular disease. The clinical significance of hypoplasia depends on the volume of functioning kidney. *Hyperplasia* is the opposite condition; it involves an overdeveloped kidney. Again, this is often associated with renal agenesis or hypoplasia of the other kidney.

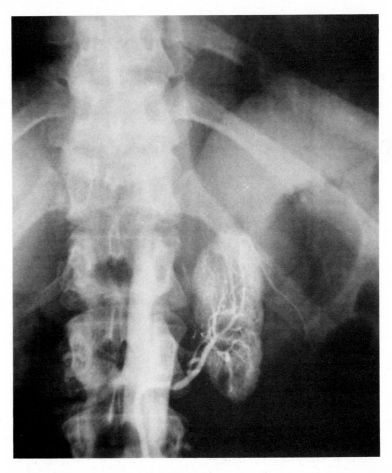

Fig. 6-10. Normal vasculature of this small kidney demonstrates renal hypoplasia (Courtesy of Riverside Methodist Hospitals, Columbus, Ohio.)

Fusion Anomalies of the Kidney

Fusion anomalies of the kidneys are often distinguishable on plain radiographs. *Horseshoe kidney* describes a condition in which the lower poles of the kidneys are joined across midline by a band of soft tissues, causing a rotation anomaly on one or both sides. The ureters exit the kidneys anteriorly instead of medially, and the lower pole calyces point medially rather than laterally with this condition (Figs. 6-11 and 6-12). Kidney function is generally unimpaired with this condition. *Crossed ectopy* exists when one kidney lies across the midline and is fused to the other kidney (Fig. 6-13, p. 258). Both kidneys demonstrate various anomalies of position, shape, fusion, and rotation with crossed ectopy. The crossed kidney generally lies inferior to the uncrossed one. Its drainage may be impaired by malposition of its ureter.

Position Anomalies of the Kidney

Anomalies of position are relatively common. *Malrotation* consists of incomplete or excessive rotation of the kidneys (Fig. 6-14, p. 258) as they ascend from the pelvis in utero. This is generally of little clinical significance unless an obstruction is created. An *ectopic kidney* is one that is out of its normal position, usually lower than normal. Such kidneys are often in a pelvic (Fig. 6-15, p. 259) or sacral location. Most are asymptomatic throughout life. In some lean and athletic persons, the kidney is mobile and may drop toward the pelvis in an erect position. Nephroptosis (prolapse) can be distinguished from a pelvic kidney by the length of the ureter; if the ureter is short, it is a congenital pelvic kidney.

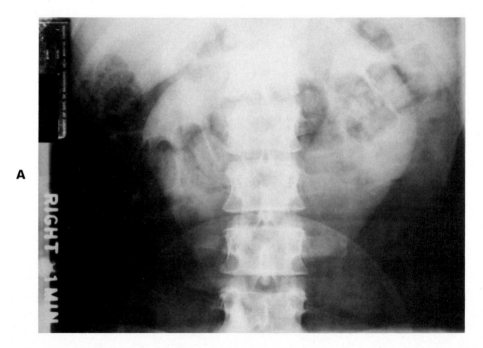

Fig. 6-11, *A.* Nephrogram phase of an intravenous urogram demonstrates fusing of the lower poles, as consistent with horseshoe kidney. (Courtesy of Riverside Methodist Hospitals, Columbus, Ohio.)

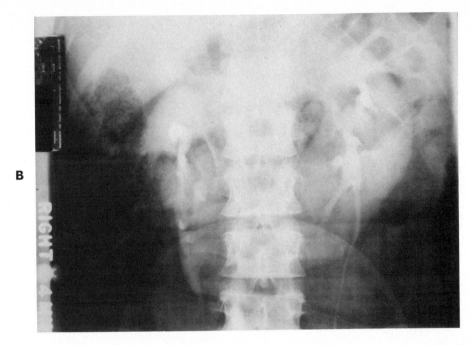

Fig. 6-11, *B.* Further excretion in the intravenous urogram demonstrates emptying of the malrotated kidneys via separate ureters. (Courtesy of Riverside Methodist Hospitals, Columbus, Ohio.)

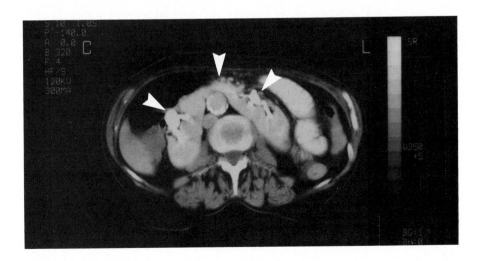

Fig. 6-12. Horseshoe kidney with apparent obstruction as seen on this CT of a 72-year-old female. (Courtesy of Riverside Methodist Hospitals, Columbus, Ohio.)

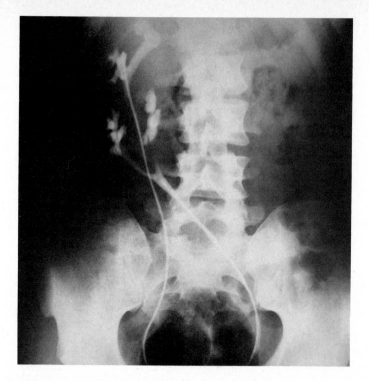

Fig. 6-13. Retrograde pyelogram demonstrates the left ureter crossing midline to connect with the lower pelvis of an anomalous right kidney, as consistent with crossed fused renal ectopy. (Courtesy of Riverside Methodist Hospitals, Columbus, Ohio.)

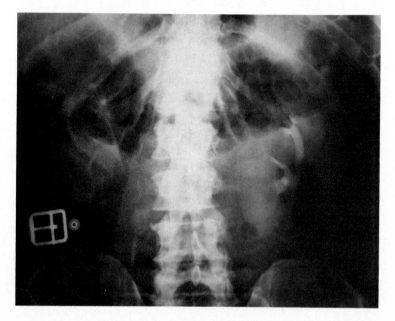

Fig. 6-14. Intravenous urography demonstrates that the left kidney's collecting system is along the lateral margin, consistent with malrotation. A restraining band is in place to slow renal excretion. (Courtesy of Riverside Methodist Hospitals, Columbus, Ohio.)

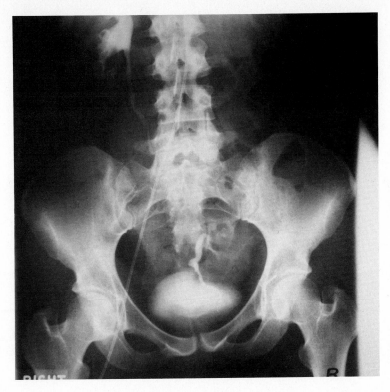

Fig. 6-15. An ectopic kidney, indicated by a urogram film taken at the end of an angiogram, demonstrates the left kidney with a shortened ureter in the left pelvis. (Courtesy of Riverside Methodist Hospitals, Columbus, Ohio.)

Renal Pelvis and Ureter Anomalies

Renal pelvis and ureter anomalies are frequent. They may be unilateral or bilateral, and they have a tendency to be asymmetric. Such anomalies may occur as double renal pelvis, double ureter (Fig. 6-16, p. 260), or a combination of both (Fig. 6-17, p. 260). The problem with these and other upper tract anomalies is that they may impair renal drainage, predisposing the patient to infection and calculi formation.

Lower Tract Anomalies

Simple *ureteroceles* are cystlike dilatations of a ureter near its opening into the bladder (Fig. 6-18, p. 261). These usually result from congenital stenosis of the ureteral orifice. Radiographically, a ureterocele presents as a filling defect in the bladder with a characteristic "cobra head" appearance. When a ureterocele appears with ureteral duplication, it often causes substantial obstruction and kidney infection. Treatment in this situation involves surgical removal to allow for increased flow of urine into the bladder.

Ureteral diverticula are probably a congenital anomaly and may actually represent a dilated, branched ureteric remnant. The appearance of these is the same as any other

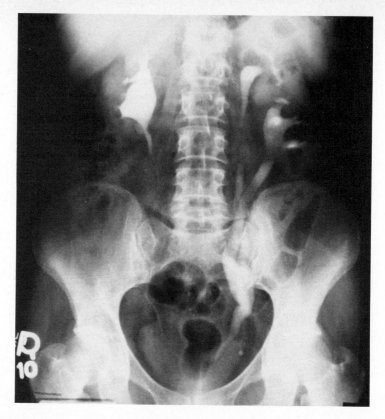

Fig. 6-16. Congenital double ureter is clearly seen on the left side. (Courtesy of Riverside Methodist Hospitals, Columbus, Ohio.)

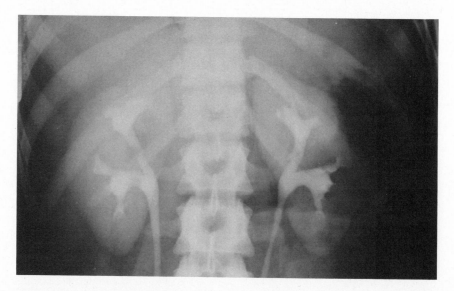

Fig. 6-17. Normal variation of the pelvicalyceal junction is seen in both kidneys. (Courtesy of the American College of Radiology, Reston, Virginia.)

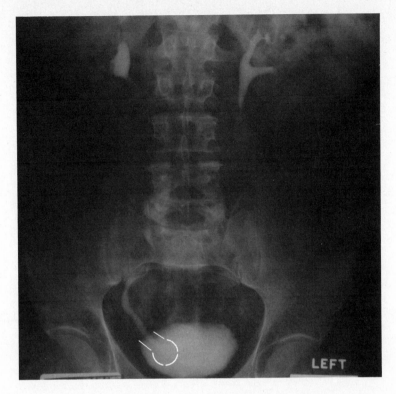

Fig. 6-18. A simple ureterocele seen as an opacified mass continuous with the terminal right ureter. (Courtesy of the American College of Radiology, Reston, Virginia.)

diverticula and is best demonstrated by retrograde urography. *Bladder diverticula* (Fig.6-19, p. 262) may occur as a congenital anomaly or be caused by chronic bladder obstruction and resultant infection. They usually occur in middle-aged men, with treatment aimed at eliminating the cause of obstruction and relief of infection.

    Urethral valves are mucosal folds that protrude into the posterior urethra as a congenital condition. These can cause significant obstruction to urine flow (Fig. 6-20, p. 262). Such ''valves'' occur in males and are usually discovered during infancy or early childhood.

Polycystic Kidney Disease

    Polycystic kidney disease is a familial kidney disorder that, though congenital in origin, usually presents in adults in their thirties. Innumerable tiny cysts that are present at birth gradually enlarge as the patient ages. This enlargement compresses and eventually destroys normal tissues. The late presentation of the condition occurs because the cysts are initially very small and do not cause problems until tissue destruction becomes significant. Radiographic indications of polycystic kidney disease show bilateral enlargement of the kidneys with poorly visualized outlines (due to the presence of cysts) and calyceal stretching and distortion (Figs. 6-21 and 6-22, p. 263). The diagnosis of multiple cysts is readily confirmed by ultrasound.

Text continued on p. 264.

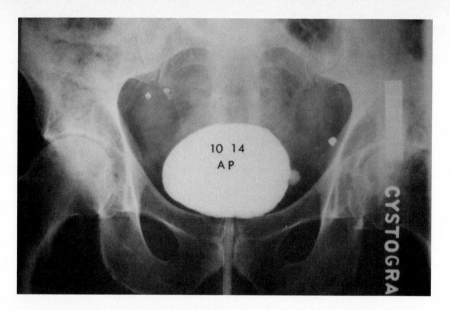

Fig. 6-19. Bladder diverticula seen on the bladder's left margin in this cystogram. (Courtesy of Riverside Methodist Hospitals, Columbus, Ohio.)

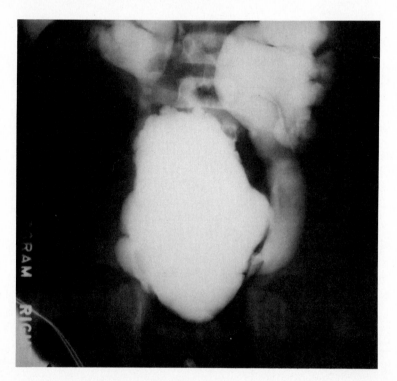

Fig. 6-20. Large, trabeculated bladder and large tortuous ureters and renal pelves seen on this cystogram of a 15-year-old boy, consistent with bladder outflow obstruction due to congenital posterior urethral valves. (Courtesy of the American College of Radiology, Reston, Virginia.)

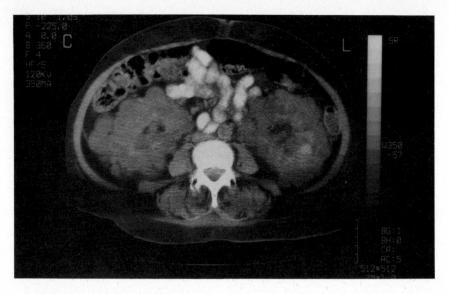

Fig. 6-21. Polycystic kidney disease as seen in both kidneys on this CT study of a 66-year-old male. (Courtesy of Riverside Methodist Hospitals, Columbus, Ohio.)

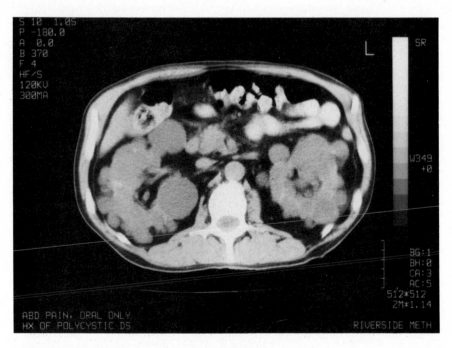

Fig. 6-22. Polycystic kidney disease seen as multiple masses in the kidneys in this CT of a 64-year-old male. (Courtesy of Riverside Methodist Hospitals, Columbus, Ohio.)

INFLAMMATORY DISEASES
Pyelonephritis

Acute pyelonephritis is a bacterial infection of the calyces and renal pelvis and thought to represent the most common renal disease. Any stagnation or obstruction to urine flow in any part of the urinary tract predisposes the patient to kidney infection. The bacteria involved likely reach the kidney via the blood stream. The condition is more common among women than men due to their increased incidence of reflux from the bladder. Acute pyelonephritis can occur during pregnancy as the increased size of the uterus acts to compress the ureter and decrease urine clearance of bacteria.

Patients presenting with acute pyelonephritis have fever, flank pain, and general malaise. Urinalysis demonstrates *pyuria,* the presence of pus created by the dumping of pus from abscesses formed in the kidneys into the collecting tubules. The diagnosis of the condition is usually made by laboratory results, as radiographic indications are not well demonstrated. In most cases an intravenous urogram is normal even during an acute attack. The calyces may be blunted and collecting structures may be less well visualized because of interstitial edema. Treatment consists of administering antibiotics to eliminate the infectious bacteria.

Chronic reflux of infected urine from the bladder into the renal pyramids can result in *chronic pyelonephritis.* This condition is often bilateral and leads to destruction and

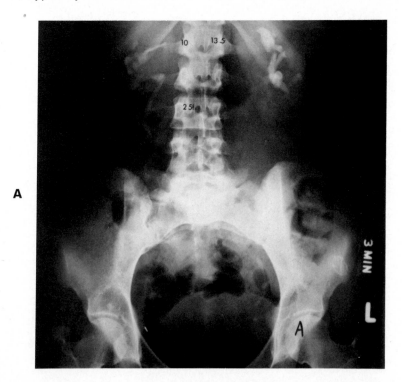

Fig. 6-23, *A.* Right kidney is small and has a scarred surface as seen on this intravenous urogram on a 25-year-old female with recurrent urinary tract infections. (Courtesy of the American College of Radiology, Reston, Virginia.)

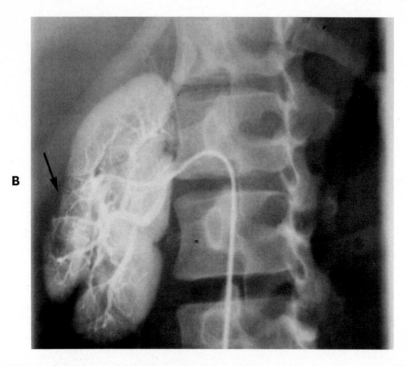

Fig. 6-23, B. Selective renal angiography demonstrates a thinned cortex caused by scarring and bunching of the renal vessels, as consistent with chronic pyelonephritis. (Courtesy of the American College of Radiology, Reston, Virginia.)

scarring of the renal tissue, with marked dilatation of the calyces. The eventual result is an overall reduction in kidney size, readily seen on intravenous urography (Fig. 6-23, A). The renal pyramids will also appear shrunken, giving the calyces a ''clubbed'' appearance. *Scars* may also be seen and appear as indentations of the renal cortex as seen on the kidney outline in the nephrogram phase (Fig. 6-23, B). This disease process may begin in childhood with a congenital anomaly of the ureterovesical junction that allows a chronic reflux of urine. It may also occur with obstruction or neurogenic bladder. Hypertension may result from chronic pyelonephritis. Treatment of pyelonephritis in a chronic stage centers on control of hypertension, removal of any cause for obstruction, and use of antibiotics to control infection.

Acute Glomerulonephritis

An antigen-antibody reaction in the glomeruli causes an inflammatory reaction of the renal parenchyma known as *acute glomerulonephritis*. Often this immunologic reaction occurs following streptococcal infection of the upper respiratory tract or the middle ear. It differs from acute pyelonephritis, which primarily affects the interstitial tissue rather than the nephrons. The condition occurs mainly in children following streptococcal infection, with most cases recovering completely. The diagnosis is again best made with laboratory

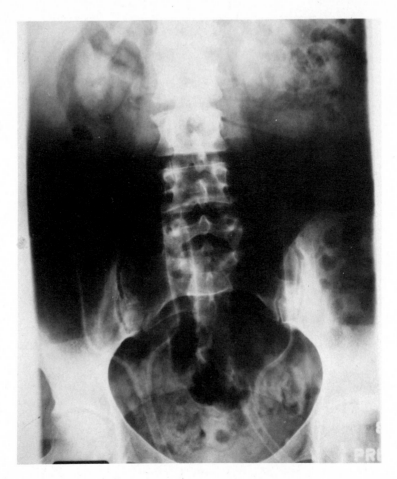

Fig. 6-24. Bilateral small kidneys, lack of contrast in the bladder, and a patient history of attacks of acute glomerulonephritis indicate chronic glomerulonephritis in this 28-year-old patient. (Courtesy of the American College of Radiology, Reston, Virginia.)

results. Radiographically, the kidneys appear larger, particularly during the nephrogram phase of an intravenous urogram, because of edematous accumulation. Treatment may include diuretic therapy to lessen edema and its resultant pressure on the glomeruli. Also, antibiotic therapy and bed rest may be used. Renal dialysis may be used for severe, chronic cases (Fig. 6-24).

Cystitis

Cystitis, inflammation of the bladder, is a fairly common infection, generally caused by bacteria, and may be either acute or chronic. Cystitis is more prevalent in women than in men because their short urethra permits easier access of bacteria into the bladder. The bladder lining's natural resistance to inflammation, however, serves as a protective mech-

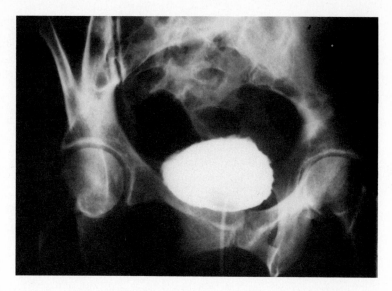

Fig. 6-25. Mildly trabeculated bladder as seen in this 34-year-old female with a small capacity bladder. (Courtesy of Riverside Methodist Hospitals, Columbus, Ohio.)

anism. Inflammation and congestion of the bladder mucosa cause the patient to experience burning pain on urination or the desire to urinate frequently. Although cystitis is not serious, the infection can cause further problems by spreading into the upper urinary passages, including the renal pelvis and kidney.

Vesicoureteral reflux, the backward flow of urine out of the bladder and into the ureters, may be seen in cases of cystitis. It can also result from a *neurogenic bladder,* a bladder dysfunction caused by interference with the nerve impulses concerned with urination. Cystography may demonstrate the presence of reflux as well as a roughening of the normally smooth bladder wall, a radiographic appearance referred to as *bladder trabeculae* (Fig. 6-25). Treatment of cystitis includes antibiotic therapy and an abundance of fluids. Prevention of pyelonephritis is paramount.

DEGENERATIVE/METABOLIC DISEASE
Nephrosclerosis

Nephrosclerosis is intimal thickening of predominately the small vessels of the kidney. It may occur as part of the normal aging process as well as in younger patients in association with hypertension and diabetes. Reduced blood flow caused by arteriosclerosis of the renal vasculature causes atrophy of the renal parenchyma. Local infarction may occur, demonstrating as an irregularity of the cortical margin, usually an indentation. The collecting system of the affected kidney is usually normal, but the kidney itself is decreased in size. Other conditions that cause the kidneys to appear smaller than normal include hypoplasia, atrophy following obstruction, and ischemia from large vessel obstruction. Treatment of nephrosclerosis consists of managing the associated hypertension and administration of diuretic agents and proper dietary restrictions (e.g., low sodium diet).

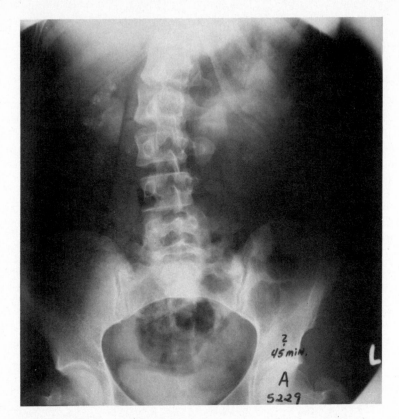

Fig. 6-26. Multiple small calcifications demonstrated in the renal pyramids of both kidneys caused by nephrocalcinosis secondary to hyperparathyroidism. (Courtesy of the American College of Radiology, Reston, Virginia.)

Nephrocalcinosis

Disturbances of calcium metabolism (e.g., hyperparathyroidism) may result in *nephrocalcinosis,* a condition characterized by tiny deposits of calcium dispersed throughout the renal parenchyma (Fig. 6-26). These deposits are readily seen on an intravenous urogram and even plain films of the abdomen. Calcium may also be deposited throughout the parenchyma as a result of tissue damaged by some other disease process or injury. In the case of a metabolic cause, treatment of the specific metabolic condition indirectly treats nephrocalcinosis. Treatment designed to lower serum calcium levels is also important.

Renal Failure

Renal failure represents the end result of a chronic process that gradually results in lost kidney function. The kidney's normal regulatory and excretory functions become impaired because of loss of glomerular filtration and subsequent deterioration of the renal

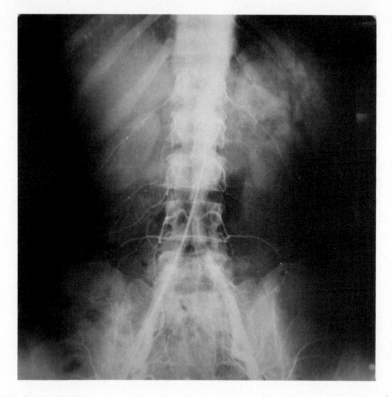

Fig. 6-27. Renal failure caused by chronic glomerulonephritis, indicated by bilaterally small kidneys with small outlines, no evidence of obstruction, and arterial changes associated with "end stage" kidneys. (Courtesy of the American College of Radiology, Reston, Virginia.)

parenchyma (Fig. 6-27). *Uremia* is characteristic of renal failure and consists of retention of urea in the blood. While not toxic in itself, urea is normally excreted by the kidneys. Its blood level correlates with the retention of other waste products and is thus a measure of the severity of renal failure.

The gradual deterioration of renal function brings with it a host of changes in other body systems. The affected patient will experience moderate anemia, hypertension, heart dysrhythmias, congestive heart failure, and other problems related to the body's severe imbalance of electrolytes and acid-base balance. Treatment consists of dialysis and possible transplantation.

Calcifications

With the exception of the gallbladder, more calculi are found in the urinary tract than anywhere else in the body. *Renal calculi* are stones that develop from urine, a supersaturated solution containing many crystalline materials, especially calcium and its salts. If

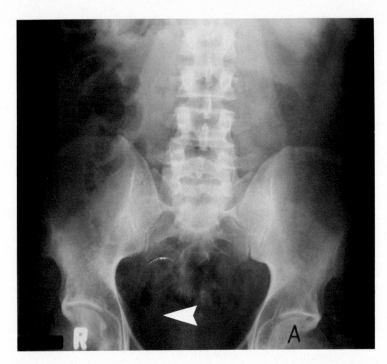

Fig. 6-28. A 3 mm, slightly calcified density is seen at the level of the right ischial spine on this plain film for an intravenous urogram. Subsequent films show distention of the collecting system to this point, as consistent with an opaque calculus at the ureterovesicular junction. (Courtesy of the American College of Radiology, Reston, Virginia.)

the body's normal equilibrium is upset, these products may precipitate out of the solution. Factors that can cause this precipitation include metabolic disorders such as hyperparathyroidism, excessive intake of calcium, and a metabolic rate that causes high urine concentration. Chronic urinary tract infections are also related to stone formation.

Males develop calculi more often than females, especially after the age of 30. Nearly all urinary tract calculi are calcified to some extent, appearing partially or totally opaque (Fig. 6-28). About 5% of stones do not calcify (Fig. 6-29). These are generally made of pure uric acid and present a more difficult diagnosis to the physician since they are one of several filling defects, including blood clots and tumors. Most stones are formed in the calyces or renal pelvis. A *staghorn calculus* is a large calculus that assumes the shape of the pelvicalyceal junction (Fig. 6-30). Beside intravenous urography, ultrasound is readily capable of demonstrating stones (Fig. 6-31, p. 272).

Stones tend to be asymptomatic until they begin to descend or cause an obstruction. The most common site for a calculus to lodge and create an obstruction is at the ureterovesical junction (Fig. 6-32, p. 272). Obstructions can also occur at the junction of the ureter and bladder and in the ureter at the pelvic brim. Movement of stones or acute obstruction results in severe, agonizing pain known as *renal colic*. It refers along the

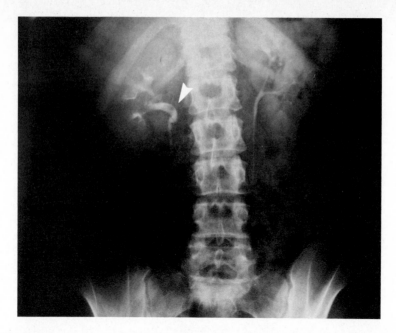

Fig. 6-29. Smooth, oval, noncalcified filling defect is seen in the right renal pelvis, as suggestive of a radiolucent uric acid stone in this 40-year-old woman with hematuria. (Courtesy of the American College of Radiology, Reston, Virginia.)

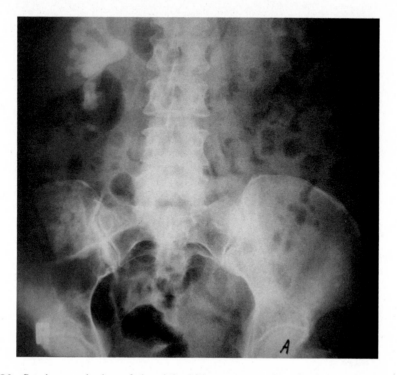

Fig. 6-30. Staghorn calculus of the right kidney as seen in a patient with a history of chronic pyuria. (Courtesy of the American College of Radiology, Reston, Virginia.)

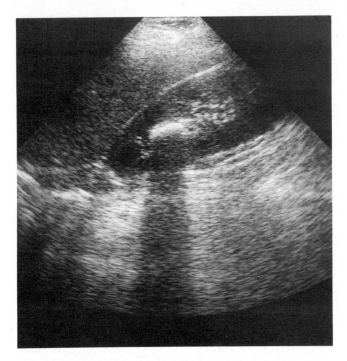

Fig. 6-31. Large calculi seen in the kidney on this ultrasound of a young female. Note the absence of sound transmission beyond the stone as indicated by the dark pathway beneath it. (Courtesy of Riverside Methodist Hospitals, Columbus, Ohio.)

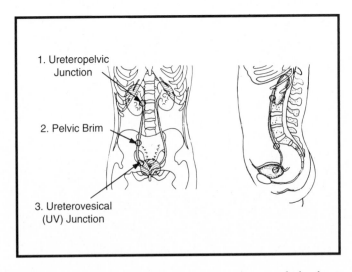

Fig. 6-32. The three usual points where kidney stones become lodged. (From Bontrager KL: *Textbook of radiographic positioning and related anatomy,* ed 3, St Louis 1993, Mosby.)

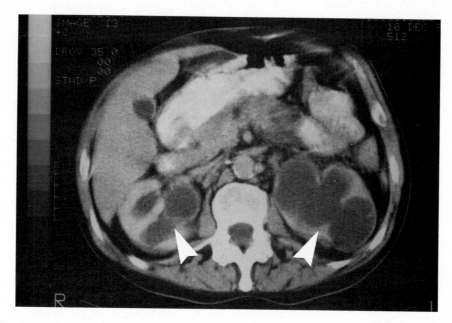

Fig. 6-33. Gross bilateral hydronephrosis as caused by pyelonephritis in this 64-year-old male. (Courtesy of Riverside Methodist Hospitals, Columbus, Ohio.)

course of the ureter toward the genital and loin regions and is highlighted by paroxysmal attacks, between which a constant low-grade pain is felt in the groin. The physician is generally able to distinguish between biliary and renal colic because biliary colic usually causes referred pain to the subscapular area or epigastrium, while renal colic causes referred pain as described.

Hydronephrosis is an obstructive disease of the urinary system that causes a dilatation of the renal pelvis and calyces with urine (Fig. 6-33). The resultant increase in intrarenal pressure causes ischemia, parenchymal atrophy, and loss of renal function. Although the most common cause of hydronephrosis is a calculus, it can also occur as a congenital defect or blockage of the system by a tumor, stricture, blood clot, or inflammation. Patients with hydronephrosis often complain of pain in their flanks, and their urine demonstrates blood or pus. The long-term changes of hydronephrosis are reversible if the cause of obstruction is relieved early in the process. A CT scan (Fig. 6-34, p. 274), an intravenous urogram, or a retrograde pyelogram readily demonstrates the marked dilatation characteristic of the condition. Treatment of obstructive disease includes antibiotics for the presence of any infection, and either lithotripsy of the stone or surgical excision of the cause of obstruction, or waiting until the stone passes.

Beside the kidneys, other sites of calcification in the urinary tract include the wall of the bladder and the prostate gland in the male. Calcification of the bladder wall is relatively rare and is usually due to calcium deposition on the surface of a bladder tumor. Prostatic calcification appears as numerous flecks of calcium of varying size below the bladder. It does not, however, correlate with either prostatic hypertrophy or carcinoma and usually is of no real significance.

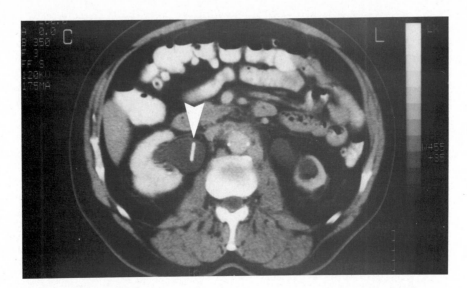

Fig. 6-34. Hydronephrosis of both kidneys as seen on this CT film, particularly in the right kidney where a stent is placed (*arrow*) to drain excess fluid to the bladder. (Courtesy of Riverside Methodist Hospitals, Columbus, Ohio.)

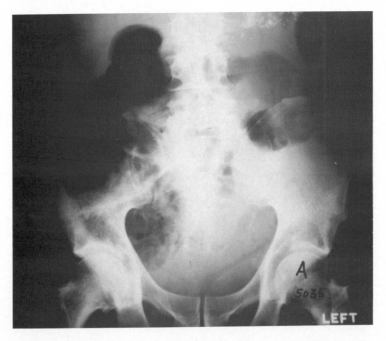

Fig. 6-35. Pancreatic calcification as indicated by the masses of calcium in the left upper quadrant that conform neatly to the shape of the pancreas. (Courtesy of the American College of Radiology, Reston, Virginia.)

Urinary tract calcifications are sometimes difficult to distinguish from other abnormal calcifications, such as gallstones, vascular calcifications, and calcified costal cartilages. To be in the kidney, the calcification must remain within the outline of the kidney on both frontal and oblique projections. In the case of gallstones, oblique projections of the abdomen help demonstrate if the calculus in question is anterior to the kidney. The pancreas may also demonstrate calcification that usually conforms to its shape (Fig. 6-35).

NEOPLASTIC DISEASES

Masses can cause filling defects in the urinary tract, becoming visible when they stretch and displace the collecting system. Almost all solitary masses are either malignant tumors or simple cysts.

Profuse hematuria resulting from a blood clot will also cause a filling defect. The diagnosis of such depends on the radiologist being aware of the history of hematuria. The distinction between a blood clot and a tumor is difficult for the physician. However, blood clots tend to have a smooth outline and show change on repeat examinations following treatment.

Renal Cysts

Renal cysts are an acquired abnormality common in adults. It is estimated that probably more than half of the population of age 50 have a renal cyst. They are usually asymptomatic and not an impairment to renal function, but they may cause symptoms from rupture, hemorrhage, infection, or obstruction. Their pathogenesis is unknown, but obstruction of nephrons by an acquired disease may have a relationship. They are commonly found in a lower pole of the kidney (Fig. 6-36, p. 276–277) and are readily demonstrated by CT (Fig. 6-37, p. 278) and diagnostic medical sonography.

Radiographically, cysts show calyceal spreading, but they can be distinguished from tumors by nephrotomography, in which a cyst shows an absence of a nephrogram phase following contrast media injection. By contrast, tumors, the majority of which have vascularity, may show irregular opacification during the nephrogram phase. Treatment, as needed, consists of aspiration of the cyst contents (Fig. 6-38, p. 278). Most cysts are asymptomatic and no treatment is needed.

Renal Carcinoma

The most common malignant tumor of the kidney is *adenocarcinoma* (hypernephroma). It occurs twice as frequently in males as in females, with an increased incidence after the age of 40 years. Its etiology is unknown, but chronic inflammation as from obstruction, cigarette smoking, and other agents is thought to contribute to the development of renal carcinoma. The affected patient often first presents for an intravenous urogram with hematuria.

Radiographically, the space-occupying lesion is shown to distort, stretch, and displace the kidney's collecting system (Fig. 6-39, *A*, p. 279). CT is also useful in demonstrating renal carcinoma and its metastases. Abnormal vascularity is readily seen on angiography (Fig. 6-39, *B*, p. 279), sometimes surrounding an avascular necrotic center. CT provides a good method to follow the progress of renal carcinoma (Fig. 6-40, p. 280).

Text continued on p. 280.

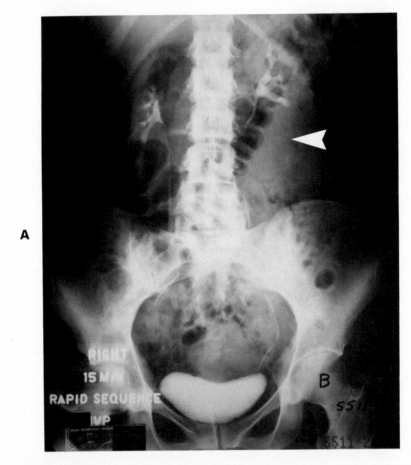

Fig. 6-36, *A.* Lower pole of the left kidney is grossly enlarged on this 15-minute film taken as part of an intravenous urogram, suggestive of a space-occupying lesion. (Courtesy of the American College of Radiology, Reston, Virginia.)

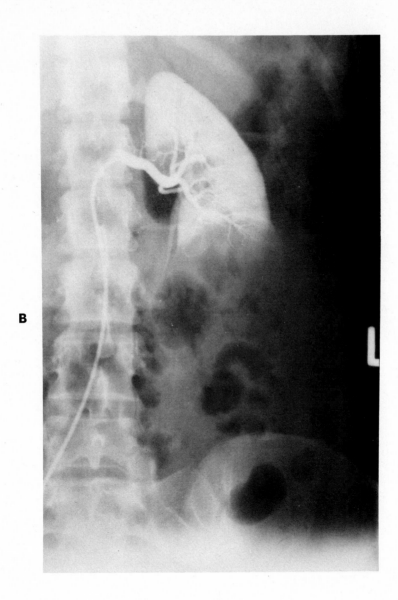

Fig. 6-36, *B.* Selective arteriography of the left kidney demonstrates an avascular mass, with vessels near it normal except for displacement. The diagnosis was simple renal cyst. (Courtesy of the American College of Radiology, Reston, Virginia.)

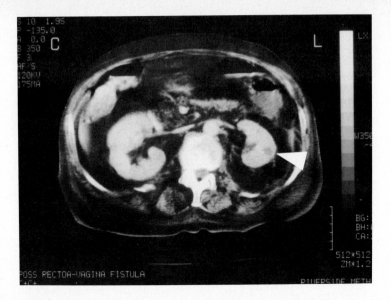

Fig. 6-37. Small renal cysts are seen on the relatively atrophic left kidney in this abdominal CT scan of a 73-year-old female. (Courtesy of Riverside Methodist Hospitals, Columbus, Ohio.)

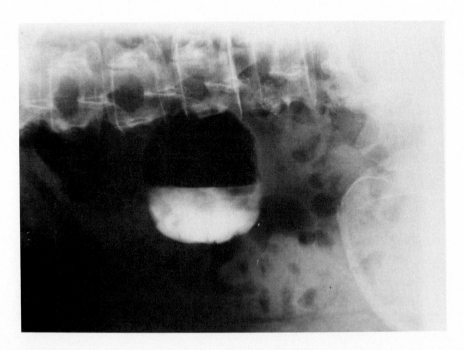

Fig. 6-38. An air-fluid level reveals removal of much of the contents of a renal cyst via a needle aspiration. (Courtesy of Riverside Methodist Hospitals, Columbus, Ohio.)

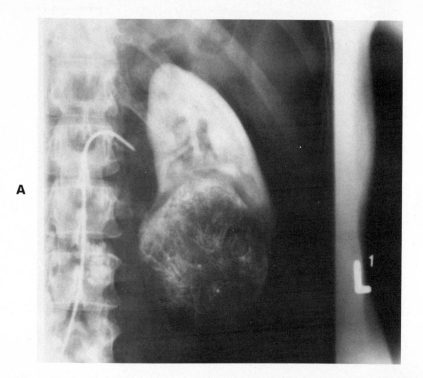

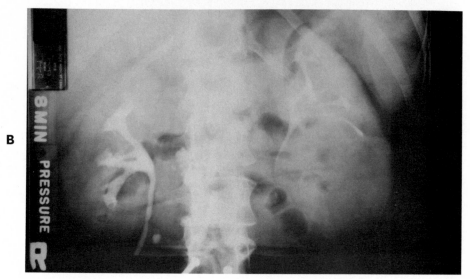

Fig. 6-39, *A.* Urography demonstrates displacement of the left lower pole calyces in this 54-year-old female with hematuria. *B.* Arteriography of the same patient demonstrates a large vascularized mass of the left lower pole, with grossly abnormal vasculature, indicative of renal cell carcinoma. (Courtesy of Riverside Methodist Hospitals, Columbus, Ohio.)

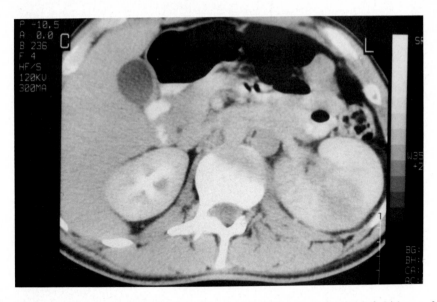

Fig. 6-40. CT demonstration of a large metastatic lesion seen in the left kidney of this 25-year-old male with renal adenocarcinoma. (Courtesy of Riverside Methodist Hospitals, Columbus, Ohio.)

If caught early, surgical excision of the kidney provides a good cure rate. The tendency of adenocarcinoma to metastasize early from the kidneys, however, poses a serious threat. The most common sites of metastasis are the lungs, brain, liver, and bone.

Nephroblastoma (Wilms' tumor)

Nephroblastoma is a malignant renal tumor found in children. It almost invariably develops before 5 years of age, with equal incidence between sexes. Children with nephroblastoma often present with a large, palpable abdominal mass that displaces the kidneys. On urography, the kidneys appear quite enlarged with marked calyceal spreading—an indication nearly diagnostic of the condition when seen in children (Fig. 6-41). Left untreated, the tumor will show widespread metastases to the lungs, liver, adrenal glands, and bone. Early surgical excision results in a very high cure rate, particularly when combined with radiation therapy and chemotherapy.

Bladder Carcinoma

Cancer of the bladder is usually seen three times as often in men as in women, particularly after 50 years of age. Its etiology is clearly related to cigarette smoking and certain industrial chemicals, and a link to excessive coffee drinking is being investigated. Hematuria is the chief symptom. Cystoscopy, often following an intravenous urogram, is the

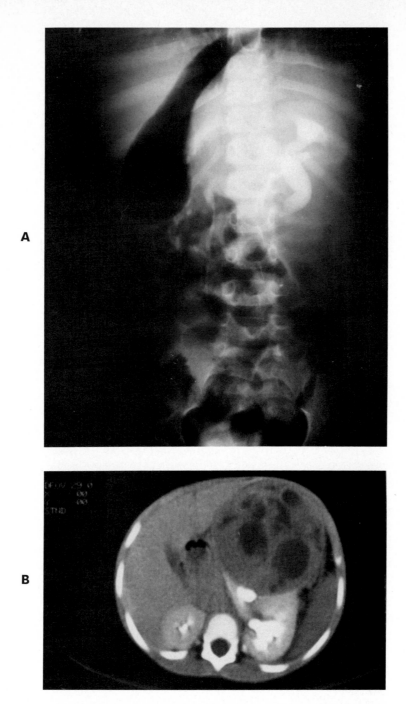

Fig. 6-41, *A.* An intravenous urogram on a 4-year-old female demonstrates an enlarged left kidney with distortion of the collecting system, and significant displacement of the stomach by the large mass. *B.* A CT image demonstrates a huge, noncalcified mass arising from the left kidney, as seen in nephroblastoma. (Courtesy of the American College of Radiology, Reston, Virginia.)

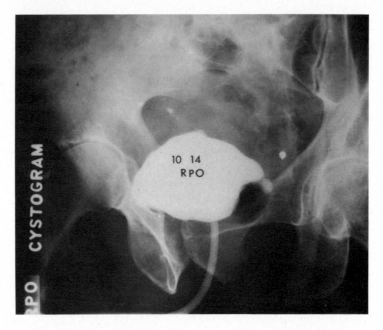

Fig. 6-42. Transitional cell carcinoma of the bladder, seen as a space-occupying lesion on this RPO of the bladder on a cystogram of a 67-year-old male. (Courtesy of the American College of Radiology, Reston, Virginia.)

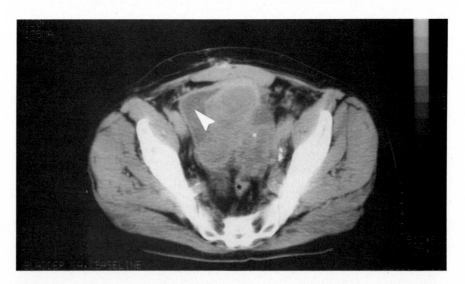

Fig. 6-43. Large bladder carcinoma in this 65-year-old male as seen on CT. (Courtesy of Riverside Methodist Hospitals, Columbus, Ohio.)

method of choice for investigation of bladder carcinoma. The tumor usually projects inward into the bladder and may be seen on a urogram as a filling defect of the bladder (Figs. 6-42 and 6-43).

Treatment consists of resection or a total cystectomy, depending on the amount of involvement and extent of metastasis, if any. Radiation therapy of the region follows. In the case of total cystectomy, the distal ureters are generally attached into a loop of the ileum. Distant metastases are usually late developing with bladder carcinoma.

▼ QUESTIONS

1. A malignant tumor of the kidney occurring in young children is:

  a. adenocarcinoma
  c. fibroadenoma
  b. hypernephroma
  d. nephroblastoma

2. Which of the following statements are true about the anatomy and function of the urinary system?
  1. The amount of urine formed in a typical day is about 1 to 1.5 liters.
  2. Urine is formed and excreted in the nephron, the microscopic unit of the kidney.
  3. The left kidney lies lower than the right because of the spleen's presence above.

  a. 1, 2
  c. 2, 3
  b. 1, 3
  d. 1, 2, 3

3. Which of the following statements are true of intravenous urography?
  1. Demonstration of contrast filling of only a partial ureter is always pathologic.
  2. Low osmolar contrast agents reduce the rate of mild and moderate reactions.
  3. Presence of renal colic is an indication for performing intravenous urography.

  a. 1, 2
  c. 2, 3
  b. 1, 3
  d. 1, 2, 3

4. Horseshoe kidney is an anomaly of:

  a. fusion
  c. position
  b. number
  d. size

5. Which of the following statements are true of urinary system anomalies?
  1. Crossed ectopy exists when one kidney lies across midline, fused to the other.
  2. Nephroptosis and a pelvic kidney are conditions identical to each other.
  3. Ureteroceles are ureteral dilatations occurring near the ureter's termination.

  a. 1, 2
  c. 2, 3
  b. 1, 3
  d. 1, 2, 3

6. Vesicoureteral reflux refers to the backward flow of urine into the:

  a. bladder
  d. urethra
  b. major calyx
  e. any of the above
  c. ureters

7. The "cobra head" is a radiographic appearance associated with:

  a. cystitis
  c. pyelonephritis
  b. nephrosclerosis
  d. ureteroceles

8. Which of the following conditions can make the kidneys appear smaller than normal?
   a. atrophy following obstruction
   b. chronic pyelonephritis
   c. hypoplasia
   d. nephrocalcinosis
   e. all of the above
   f. all but one of the above

9. The most common renal disease overall is:
   a. cystitis
   b. glomerulonephritis
   c. nephrocalcinosis
   d. pyelonephritis

10. Medical treatment designed to lower serum calcium levels would be important in management of:
    a. cystitis
    b. nephrocalcinosis
    c. nephrosclerosis
    d. polycystic kidney disease

11. Gradual and chronic deterioriation of the renal parenchyma eventually results in:
    a. glomerulonephritis
    b. polycystic kidney disease
    c. renal calculi
    d. renal failure

12. Renal failure is characterized by the abnormal retention of _____ in the blood.
    a. bilirubin
    b. calcium
    c. pus
    d. urea

13. Which of the following statements are true of renal calculi?
    1. Precipitation of solutes out of urine is the pathogenesis of renal calculi.
    2. Renal colic causes referred pain into the subscapular area or epigastrium.
    3. Stones tend to be asymptomatic until they move or cause an obstruction.
       a. 1, 2
       b. 1, 3
       c. 2, 3
       d. 1, 2, 3

14. Significant dilatation of the renal pelvis and calyces as a result of an obstruction from a stone is characteristic of:
    a. hypernephrosis
    b. renal failure
    c. nephroblastoma
    d. vesicoureteral reflux

15. Which of the following statements are true of neoplastic diseases of the urinary system?
    1. Chronic inflammation from obstruction can result in adenocarcinoma.
    2. Wilms' tumor is generally associated with elderly patients in renal failure.
    3. Early excision of nephroblastoma has shown a very high cure rate.
       a. 1, 2
       b. 1, 3
       c. 2, 3
       d. 1, 2, 3

16. The normal incidence of persons having some sort of urinary tract congenital anomaly is:
    a. 10%
    b. 25%
    c. 50%
    d. nearly 100%

17. An obese patient where visualization of renal parenchyma may be difficult might have a:

    a. cystogram   **c.** renal angiogram

    b. nephrotomogram   **d.** retrograde pyelogram

18. Which of the following studies would be useful in evaluating hypertension?

    a. cystogram   **c.** intravenous urogram

    b. high-infusion intravenous uro-   **d.** renal angiogram
        gram

19. Hyperplasia of one kidney is often associated with _____ of the other kidney.

    a. crossed ectopy   **c.** malrotation

    b. hypoplasia   **d.** renal diverticula

20. Polycystic kidney disease is what type of disorder?

    a. congenital   **c.** inflammatory

    b. degenerative   **d.** metabolic

7

The Reproductive System

▼

Upon completion of Chapter 7, the reader should be able to:

- Discuss the basic anatomic structures associated with the male and female reproductive systems.
- Describe the limitation of general radiography in the diagnosis and treatment of reproductive disorders.
- Briefly explain the role of diagnostic medical sonography in the diagnosis and treatment of reproductive system disorders.
- Compare and contrast breast imaging modalities, including diagnostic versus screening mammography, localization techniques, and sonography.
- Differentiate between the major congenital anomalies of the female reproductive system.
- Describe the various neoplastic diseases of both the female and male reproductive systems in terms of etiology, incidence, signs/symptoms, treatment, and prognosis.
- Differentiate between common disorders during pregnancy and explain the role of diagnostic medical sonography in the management of the gravid female.

THE FEMALE REPRODUCTIVE SYSTEM

ANATOMY AND PHYSIOLOGY REVIEW

The female reproductive system comprises one pair of ovaries, which are the primary sex organs, and the secondary sex organs, which include one pair of uterine tubes, the uterus, the vagina, and two breasts. (Fig. 7-1). This system functions in the production of the female reproductive cell (the ovum) and hormones and provides a cavity for the development of the zygote.

The uterus is a pear-shaped organ located within the pelvic cavity and can be divided into the upper portion, termed the *body* and the lower, neck portion, termed the *cervix*. Anatomically it is flexed so that the cervix and lower portion of the body lie anterior to the rectum, posterior to the urinary bladder, with the upper portion of the body normally lying superior to the bladder. The walls of the uterus include an inner, endometrial layer; a middle, muscular, myometrial layer; and an outer layer termed the *parietal peritoneum*. In actuality, the parietal peritoneum drapes over the upper three-fourths of the body but does not enclose the lower one-fourth of the body or the cervix. The actual cavity within the uterus is fairly small and can be well visualized via hysterosalpingography. It is divided into the internal os leading to the cervical canal and into the external os, which opens into the vagina. The uterus is held in place within the pelvic cavity via eight ligaments.

The uterine tubes extend from the upper, outer edges of the uterus and expand distally into the infundibula located close to, but not attached to, the ovaries. These tubes serve as a passageway for the mature ova and are the normal site of fertilization. In a normal pregnancy, the fertilized ovum will continue to travel through the uterine tube and implant into the endometrium of the uterus.

The ovaries are the primary reproductive glands and are responsible for ovulation and secretion of estrogen and progesterone. Each ovary contains numerous graafian follicles

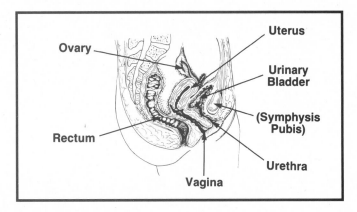

Fig. 7-1. Female pelvic organs. (From Bontrager KL: *Textbook of radiographic positioning and related anatomy,* ed 3, St Louis, 1993, Mosby.)

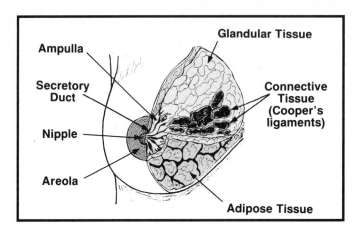

Fig. 7-2. Breast, anterior. (From Bontrager KL: *Textbook of radiographic positioning and related anatomy,* ed 3, St Louis, 1993, Mosby.)

enclosing ova. Following puberty, several graafian follicles and ova grow and develop each month. Normally only one follicle matures, migrates to the surface of the ovary, and degenerates, thus expelling a mature ovum. This is termed *ovulation.*

The breasts are also secondary sex organs, with the breast parenchyma differing according to age and parity. Females in their twenties and thirties, especially nulliparous women, have dense, fibroglandular parenchyma that may hide breast masses on both physical and mammographic examination. However, as age and parity increase, the breast typically becomes more fatty, enhancing the radiographic visibility of possible masses.

Anatomically, the breasts are attached via connective tissue to the pectoral muscles and consist of several lobes separated by connective tissue, much like the spokes of a wheel. The lobes are further divided into lobules clustered around small ducts. These small ducts join to form larger ducts, which terminate at the nipple (Fig. 7-2). The breasts function as an accessory reproductive gland to secrete milk for the newborn infant. During pregnancy, changes in the estrogen and progesterone levels prepare the breasts for lactation and approximately 3 days after delivery, a lactogenic hormone stimulates the secretion of milk.

IMAGING CONSIDERATIONS

Radiographic studies of the female reproductive system include investigation of gravid and nongravid females. The hysterosalpingogram is a common examination of the nongravid female, and is performed by injecting an opaque medium into the uterine cavity. This examination may be performed in cases of suspected infertility and to diagnose congenital anomalies. A common finding in cases of infertility is nonpatent uterine tubes. Radiography may also be used to locate intrauterine devices (IUDs) used for contraception (Fig. 7-3).

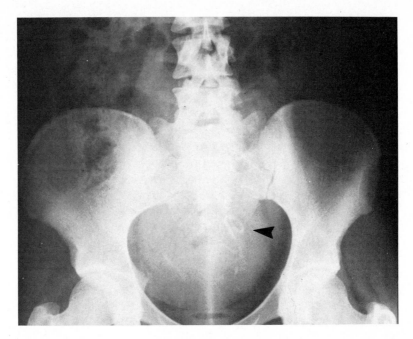

Fig. 7-3. Abdominal radiograph of a young female demonstrates proper placement of the IUD within the uterus. (Courtesy of Riverside Methodist Hospitals, Columbus, Ohio.)

Although rarely used today, pelvimetry is used to measure the dimensions of the bony pelvis in a gravid female. A fetal age study provides rough approximation of fetal age by visualizing ossification patterns of the fetal bones. However, much of this same information can be obtained with the use of diagnostic medical sonography.

Ultrasound has replaced radiographic examinations of the female reproductive system because of its excellent accuracy and because it presents no radiation hazards to the fetus or mother. Not only is ultrasound applicable in pregnancy, it is also useful in normal gynecologic examinations to visualize reproductive organs, to locate lost IUDs, or to follow the progress of a regimen of fertility medication.

Traditional pelvic sonography requires a distended urinary bladder to serve as an "acoustic window" for good visualization of the pelvic organs. In addition, the fluid within the urinary bladder helps to displace bowel gas away from the area of interest. Recent sonographic advancements have led to the use of transvaginal transducers that also provide accurate clinical information. The most common indications for sonography in the nongravid female include evaluation of pelvic, uterine, and ovarian masses because ultrasound can give information about mass size, location, internal characteristics, and its effect on surrounding organs. Sonography is often used to locate and identify IUDs. Obstetrically, ultrasound is the method of choice in visualizing the position of the placenta, multiple gestations, ectopic pregnancies, and determining gestational age. It is used to assist and guide the physician during amniocentesis and is invaluable in assessing fetal abnormalities, such as anencephaly, hydrocephaly, congenital heart defects, polycystic kidney disease, urinary tract obstructions, and GI tract obstructions, as well as determining fetal death.

The use of mammography as a diagnostic procedure for symptomatic patients is well documented. Mammography provides important information about specific clinical problems such as a breast mass, pain, nipple discharge, and abnormalities of the skin and lymph nodes. With the advent of modern mammographic equipment and techniques, radiation exposure is minimal. It is not known for certain if very low doses of radiation cause breast cancers; however, there is no evidence to suggest significant risk to women over 35 years of age. If a risk does exist, it is believed to be so minimal it has never been observed, only inferred, scientifically. In the accuracy of detecting breast pathologies, clinical investigations have revealed no significant difference between film/screen mammography and xeromammography. However, the glandular radiation dose is higher with xeromammography than with modern film/screen mammography.

Whether mammography is a safe method of screening asymptomatic women remains controversial. The use of mammography for screening purposes is based on its ability to detect nonpalpable breast lesions at an early stage when they are too small to be identified by physical examination. Current literature suggests that mammography can detect some cancers 2 years before they are palpable and survival depends on tumor size and lymph node involvement. It is generally agreed that women 50 years of age and older should undergo regular mammographic screening because in this age range the breast tissue is less sensitive to radiation and the incidence of breast cancer increases with age. The benefits far outweigh associated risks from radiation exposure.

Mammography is also a valuable examination tool in the detection and evaluation of breast disease in individuals with augmentation prostheses. Although experience with augmentation mammoplasty patients is limited, current research indicates mammography can demonstrate both palpable and non-palpable breast lesions. To demonstrate the underlying breast parenchyma in these individuals, technologists are encouraged to use manual exposure techniques, as well as additional ''pinch'' and/or axillary projections. Pinch projections require pushing the prosthesis posteriorly against the chest wall so the anterior breast tissue can be compressed and radiographed.

Needle or guidewire localization is a specialized procedure to identify non-palpable, mammographically detected abnormalities of the breast. They help direct the surgeon to the lesion in question and allow excision of the suspect tissue for biopsy. Needle guidewire localizations cause minimal morbidity with complications including hematoma formation, intraoperative wire dislodgement, and wire breakage. The development and refinement of localization techniques have greatly increased the percentage of positive findings upon surgical biopsy and allow more accurate diagnosis and treatment of early-stage carcinoma of the breast. Fine needle and large-core biopsy techniques offer an alternative to surgical biopsy as an initial step in investigation of breast masses.

Diagnostic medical sonography is an excellent modality for differentiating cystic masses from solid masses within the breast. However, sonography has major limitations in the diagnosis of malignant breast disease because of the solid nature of most breast cancers. It is not indicated as an established screening procedure for solid breast lesions and cannot differentiate between a solid benign mass and malignant disease.

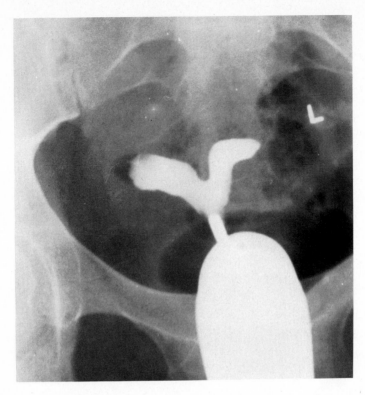

Fig. 7-4. Hysterosalpingogram demonstrates bicornuate uterus. (Courtesy of Riverside Methodist Hospitals, Columbus, Ohio.)

CONGENITAL ABNORMALITIES

Congenital anomalies of the female reproductive system occur in approximately 1% to 2% of women. The most common anomaly is the *bicornuate uterus*. This condition consists of paired uterine horns extending to the uterine tubes (Fig. 7-4). A *unicornuate uterus* occurs when the uterine cavity is elongated and has a single uterine tube emerging from it. *Uterus didelphys* is a rare congenital anomaly with complete duplication of the uterus, cervix, and vagina. Occasionally the normal uterus may lie in an abnormal position. If the uterus is more vertical than normal it is termed *retroflexed* and lies against the rectosigmoid region of the bowel. A uterus that lies more horizontal is termed *anteflexed* and it lies on top of the urinary bladder.

INFLAMMATORY DISEASE
Pelvic Inflammatory Disease

Pelvic inflammatory disease (PID) is a bacterial infection of the female genital system that is most often caused by gonococcus, staphylococcus, or streptococcus bacteria. PID may result from an unsterile abortion, following the insertion of an intrauterine contraceptive device (IUDs), or after introduction of a pathogen from other sources. This inflammation is generally bilateral and without treatment the infection will spread to the peritoneum, resulting in bacteremia. Tubo-ovarian abscess formation may also occur with PID, often resulting in sterility.

Common signs and symptoms of PID include pelvic and abdominal pain, dysmenorrhea, nausea and vomiting, elevated temperature, and leukocytosis. The most common treatment of PID is antibiotic therapy, but healing often results in scarring and obstruction of the uterine tubes, which predisposes the individual to ectopic pregnancy because of the narrowing of the uterine tubes. PID is a common indication for sonographic evaluation in a nongravid female. Severe cases with abscess formation may also require surgical intervention.

Mastitis

Inflammation of the breast or *mastitis* is most often caused by *S. aureus* bacteria. This bacterial infection usually occurs in the breasts of lactating females through cracks in the skin surrounding the nipple. Common signs and symptoms of mastitis include pain, redness, and swelling of the affected breast, elevated temperature, and, in severe cases, abscess formation. Mastitis is treated medically with antibiotic therapy and heat application to the affected breast. Mammography plays a very limited role in the diagnosis and treatment of mastitis.

NEOPLASTIC DISEASES
Ovarian Cystic Masses

Single cystic ovarian masses are fairly common in females within the reproductive age group. They include *follicular cysts* and *corpus luteum cysts*. The formation of follicular and corpus luteum cysts occurs as a part of the normal menstrual cycle; however, these cysts may occasionally increase in size and cause pelvic discomfort or abnormal pressure on the urinary bladder. Changes in the size of follicular and corpus luteum cysts occur quickly and vary with the menstrual cycle. Treatment is generally not necessary because they often disappear completely without medical intervention.

Multiple cystic masses may indicate *endometriosis,* a disease caused by the presence of endometrial tissue or glands in abnormal locations within the pelvis. External endometriosis commonly involves the ovaries, uterine ligaments, the rectovaginal septum, and the pelvic peritoneum; however, it may also attach to the rectal wall, the ureters, and/or the urinary bladder. The etiology of endometriosis is unknown, but it seems to respond to normal hormonal stimuli and is clinically significant in females between the ages of 20 to 40 years. The external endometrial tissue contains normal functioning endometrium, which continues to bleed cyclically. These blood-filled cysts are often visible upon ultrasonic examination. Long standing endometriosis results in the development of fibrosis, adhesions, scarring, and eventually sterility. Common signs and symptoms include pelvic and low back pain, dysmenorrhea, and infertility. Although ultrasound is useful in the diagnosis of endometriosis, a positive diagnosis is generally made via laparoscopy. Mild cases of endometriosis may be treated with hormone therapy, while severe cases generally require surgical intervention.

Polycystic ovaries consist of enlarged ovaries containing multiple small cysts. The ovaries are bilaterally enlarged and have a smooth exterior surface with the multiple cysts lying just below the outer surface. Polycystic ovaries are often associated with Stein-

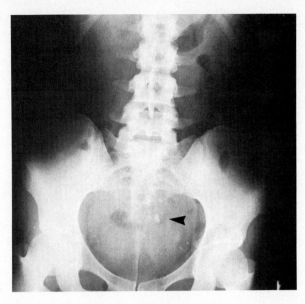

Fig. 7-5. Abdominal radiograph of a young female demonstrates a radiographically visible tooth within a cystic teratoma. (Courtesy of Riverside Methodist Hospitals, Columbus, Ohio.)

Leventhal syndrome, a fairly rare disease. Females with Stein-Leventhal syndrome rarely ovulate because of an endocrine abnormality that inhibits maturation and release of the ovarian follicle. In addition, these individuals may experience amenorrhea and sterility.

Benign *cystic teratomas* of the ovary, often called *dermoid cysts,* account for approximately 15% of ovarian tumors and are the most common type of germ cell tumor containing mature tissue. These masses arise from an unfertilized ova that undergoes neoplastic change. Cystic teratomas are composed of tissue derived from the ectoderm, endoderm, and mesoderm, and they often contain hair, thyroid tissue, keratin, sebaceous secretions, and occasionally teeth (Fig. 7-5). The treatment for cystic teratomas is surgical removal of the mass.

Cystadenocarcinoma

Cystadenocarcinoma is a malignant neoplasm of the ovary (Fig. 7-6, p. 294) occurring in females over the age of 40 years. Although it is less common than other female genital carcinomas, cystadenocarcinoma is the most lethal and has a very poor prognosis. The etiology of this neoplasm is unknown. Sonographic evaluation demonstrates a rough, irregular ovarian surface with the tumor often containing both cystic and solid areas. Serous tumors are frequently bilateral; mucinous tumors are more likely to be unilateral. The signs and symptoms of cystadenocarcinoma are very vague, including urinary bladder or rectal pressure. In many cases the disease is completely asymptomatic, delaying diagnosis and treatment, thus reducing the chance for cure. Serous cystadenocarcinomas have a 10-year survival rate of 13% and mucinous cystadenocarcinomas have a 10-year

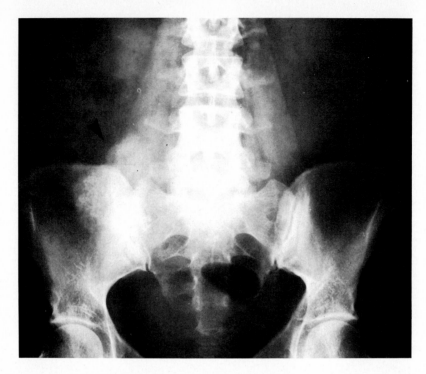

Fig. 7-6. Abdominal radiograph of a 47-year-old female diagnosed with a cystadenocar-cinoma. Note the calcifications within the lesion that make it radiographically visible. (Courtesy of Riverside Methodist Hospitals, Columbus, Ohio.)

survival rate of approximately 34%. These tumors often spread to other pelvic organs, the small intestines, the omentum, the stomach, and the liver, frequently presenting with associated ascites and pleural effusions. Common treatment of cystadenocarcinoma includes surgery in combination with chemotherapy or radiation therapy.

Carcinoma of the Cervix

Cervical carcinoma or *dysplasia* is a common malignancy of the female genital system caused by an abnormal growth pattern of epithelial cells around the neck of the uterus. Cervical intra-epithelial neoplasias (CIN) are classified or staged as mild (I), moderate (II), or severe (III), and are generally diagnosed by a Pap smear and confirmed by surgical biopsy. Research indicates that a history of multiple sexual partners and/or prior sexually transmitted infections predisposes females to this disease. Symptoms commonly associated with cervical dysplasia include abnormal bleeding, especially postcoitally. The treatment of cervical dysplasia varies according to the classification. Pap smears allow early detection of this disease, thus improving the chance of cure and survival. The 5-year survival rate ranges from 90% for Stage I dysplasias to less than 15% for advanced disease. The primary treatment is radiation therapy, however, surgical intervention may also be necessary.

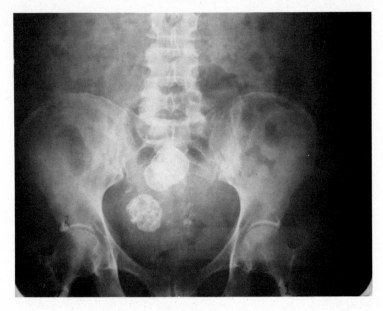

Fig. 7-7. Abdominal radiograph of a 50-year-old female demonstrates leiomyomas of the uterus with radiographically visible calcifications. (Courtesy of the American College of Radiology, Reston, Virginia.)

Uterine Masses

Leiomyomas (Uterine fibroids). *Leiomyomas* are benign, solid masses of the uterus that develop from an overgrowth of the uterine smooth muscle tissue. They are present in approximately 25% of all females over the age of 30 years and are the most common benign tumors of the female genital system. The etiology of this neoplasm is unknown; however, they tend to grow under the influence of estrogen, may enlarge during pregnancy, and stop growing at menopause. Following menopause leiomyomas are replaced largely by fibrous scar tissue, leading to the misnomer ''uterine fibroids.'' In addition, they often contain radiographically visible calcifications (Fig. 7-7). The tumors vary in size, number, and location; they are frequently asymptomatic until they grow large enough to place pressure on surrounding structures; and they are usually detected upon pelvic examination. Sonographically, they appear as sharply circumscribed, encapsulated lesions and may contain cystic areas. Malignant transformation is rare and treatment depends on patient symptoms, ranging from no treatment to surgical removal of the uterus.

Adenocarcinoma of the Endometrium. *Adenocarcinoma of the endometrium* is often termed *carcinoma of the uterus*. It is histopathologically different from cervical carcinoma and is one of the most common cancers of the female reproductive system, second only to breast cancer. The incidence of adenocarcinoma of the endometrium has remained fairly static, occurring mainly in postmenopausal women and increasing in incidence with age. The development of this neoplasm has strong ties to hormonal changes within the female and is more common in nulliparous women. Adenocarcinoma of the endometrium is believed to be preceded by adenomatous hyperplasia. It then passes through an in situ stage before reaching its final invasive stage, often completely filling the uterine cavity. The cancer is graded according to cellular differentiation and staged according to the extent of the disease. The most frequent symptom is irregular or post-menopausal bleeding. Treatment varies with the stage of the disease. Stage 0 is curable via hysterectomy and Stages I and II are usually treated with a combination of surgery and radiation therapy with a 5-year survival rate of 80%.

Breast Masses

Fibroadenoma. A *fibroadenoma* is the most common benign breast tumor. It consists of a well-defined mass that does not invade surrounding tissue. The neoplasm is formed by an overgrowth of fibrous and glandular tissue and is commonly located in the upper, outer quadrant of the breast. Fibroadenomas occur most frequently in females between the ages of 15 to 35 years, appear to be estrogen dependent, and may grow rapidly during pregnancy. These lesions are often painless and can usually be moved about within the breast. Mammography, in conjunction with physical breast examination and sometimes ultrasound, plays a vital role in the detection of fibroadenomas (Figs. 7-8 and 7-9). Surgical removal of the lesion is curative.

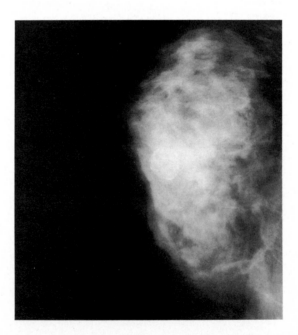

Fig. 7-8. Fibroadenoma of the breast with a well-circumscribed border in a 49-year-old female. (Courtesy of Riverside Methodist Hospitals, Columbus, Ohio.)

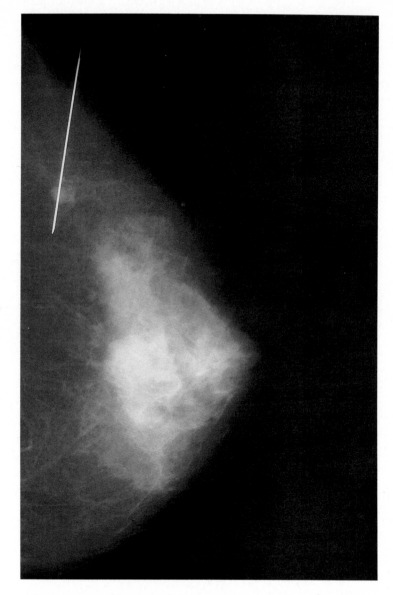

Fig. 7-9. Needle localization of fibroadenoma of the breast pinpoints to the location of the mass for surgical biopsy. (Courtesy of Riverside Methodist Hospitals, Columbus, Ohio.)

Fibrocystic Breasts. An overgrowth of fibrous tissue and/or cystic hyperplasia results in *fibrocystic breasts*. This is the most common disorder of the female breast and occurs in some degree in approximately 50% of premenopausal females. This condition may be unilateral, however, it is most frequently bilateral, with various sized cysts located throughout the breasts (Fig. 7-10). The severity of this disorder varies greatly and it is believed to result from fluctuations in the hormone levels during the menstrual cycle. The most common sign/symptom associated with fibrocystic breasts is a mass or masses that increase in size and tenderness immediately preceding the onset of the menstrual period. Ultrasound is extremely useful as a follow-up to mammography in differentiating solid masses from cystic masses in females with fibrocystic breasts (Fig. 7-11). Large cysts are commonly aspirated for cytologic evaluation of the fluid. If the aspiration is unsuccessful, surgical biopsy is often performed. Although controversy exists about the correlation of fibrocystic breasts and an increased incidence of breast cancer, it is well known that a fibrocystic condition may mask a coexistent cancer.

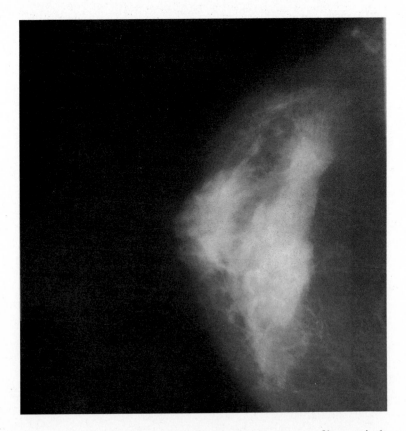

Fig. 7-10. Mammogram of a 35-year-old female demonstrates a fibrocystic breast pattern. (Courtesy of Riverside Methodist Hospitals, Columbus, Ohio.)

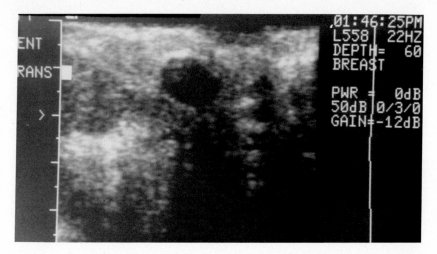

Fig. 7-11. Sonogram demonstrating a large cystic lesion within the breast of a 35-year-old female with a fibrocystic breast pattern. Notice the well-circumscribed borders of the cyst. (Courtesy of Riverside Methodist Hospitals, Columbus, Ohio.)

Carcinoma of the Breast. *Breast carcinoma* is a very common malignancy among females in the United States and accounts for approximately 27% of all female cancers. It also has the highest mortality rate of all female cancers with approximately 18% of all annual female cancer deaths in the United States attributed to breast cancer. Current literature suggests that one of every nine women in the United States will develop breast cancer during her lifetime, with an increased incidence in females between the ages of 30 to 50 years. The incidence continues to rise throughout the postmenopausal years because of changes in estrogen levels. Approximately 50% of all lesions occur in the upper, outer quadrant of the breast. Although the exact etiology of breast cancer is unknown, it is believed to be a multifactorial disorder. Heredity, endocrine influence, dietary habits, oncogenic factors (such as viruses), and environmental factors (such as chemical carcinogens) appear to play a role in the development of this disease. In terms of endocrine influence, current research suggests the amount of biologically available estrogen and progesterone is a key factor in the development of breast cancer. A strong family history of certain cancers also places a female at increased risk in developing breast cancer.

Scirrhous, infiltrating, papillary, and *medullary breast cancers* generally begin as slow growing, relatively painless masses, but as they grow, they may infiltrate the suspensory ligaments, causing them to shorten and retract the overlying skin. Physical signs of breast cancer include nipple retraction and distorted breast contour. The neoplasm may infiltrate and block lymphatic vessels, causing edema in the overlying skin and enlargement of the axillary and/or supraclavicular lymph nodes. The skin edema may cause the normal cutaneous hair follicles to appear as multiple small depressions on the skin surface, known as a *peau d'orange* appearance. As the tumor progresses it may attach to surrounding fascia and may ulcerate the surrounding skin.

Mammography plays a very important role in the diagnosis and management of breast cancer. The tumors commonly appear radiographically as dense, irregular, stellate masses that infiltrate surrounding tissue (Fig. 7-12). Many of these neoplasms contain numerous calcifications that are radiographically visible (Fig. 7-13). Needle localization of mammographically detected, nonpalpable cancerous breast lesions is reliable in directing the surgeon to the lesion in question and allows excision of the suspect tissue. The tissue specimen is radiographed and forwarded to a pathologist for histologic evaluation. Statistics demonstrate that this method of localization causes minimal morbidity and the development and refinement of mammographic localization has greatly increased the percentage of positive findings upon surgical biopsy. This invasive technique allows more accurate diagnosis and treatment of early stage carcinoma of the breast. If the tumor can be removed before the lesion is palpable the survival rate is greatly increased.

Treatment of breast carcinoma depends on the extent of the disease. Once the carcinoma is confirmed by surgical biopsy, an axillary lymph node resection is performed to

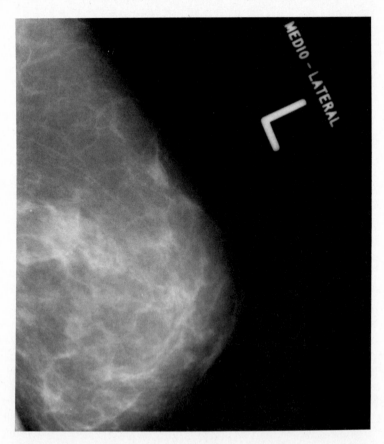

Fig. 7-12. Mammogram of the left breast of a 63-year-old female demonstrating a stellate mass commonly associated with carcinoma of the breast. Notice the irregular borders of the mass. (Courtesy of Riverside Methodist Hospitals, Columbus, Ohio.)

assist in the staging of the disease. Much controversy exists in terms of determining the best approach to management and treatment of breast cancers. In the past 40 years, the 5-year survival rate for breast cancer has remained virtually unchanged. Currently, two surgical options are recommended for Stage I and Stage II breast cancers: 1. modified radial mastectomy, or 2. breast-conserving surgery followed by radiation therapy. Both methods require axillary lymph node resection; randomized clinical trials have not demonstrated a significant difference in the survival rate between these two surgical options.

Though indications for chemotherapy are continuously under review, most experts agree patients should be referred to a medical oncologist following surgery. Treatment with an established combination of chemotherapeutic drugs is considered standard care for premenopausal females with lymph node involvement. Breast carcinomas are also classified by a hormone receptor test. Many tumors require hormones for continued growth, and these carcinomas may undergo temporary regression if hormonal balances are altered.

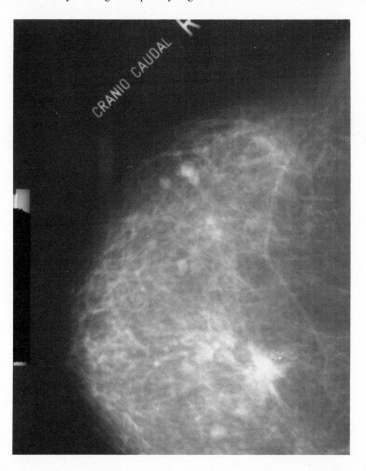

Fig. 7-13. Mammogram of the right breast in an elderly female demonstrating a stellate mass containing microcalcifications commonly associated with carcinoma of the breast. (Courtesy of Riverside Methodist Hospitals, Columbus, Ohio.)

DISORDERS DURING PREGNANCY

Diagnostic medical sonography is often used in the diagnosis of multiple and ectopic pregnancies. Ultrasonic examination is also indicated if the pregnant uterus is too small or too large for the calculated delivery date.

Amniotic Fluid

Amniotic fluid is produced by various physiologic functions within the mother and the fetus. The amount of amniotic fluid present varies with the stage of pregnancy. *Oligohydramnios* occurs when too little amniotic fluid is present and *polyhydramnios* occurs with an excess of amniotic fluid. The normal fetus swallows several hundred milliliters of fluid per day. This fluid is absorbed by the fetal intestines with a portion excreted via the fetal urinary system and a portion transferred across the placenta into the mother's circulatory system. The major source of amniotic fluid arises from the fetus urinating fluid once the kidneys are developed. Therefore oligohydramnios often results from poor fetal kidney function or blockage of the ureters. If a fetus is unable to swallow, polyhydramnios may occur. Two causes of this disorder are anencephaly or a high gastrointestinal obstruction.

Ectopic Pregnancy

Ectopic pregnancy refers to the development of an embryo outside the uterine cavity and occurs in approximately 1% of all pregnancies. The most common site for an ectopic pregnancy is the uterine tube, but it may also occur in the ovary, cervix, or abdominal cavity. In the case of a tubal pregnancy, the uterine tube distends to accommodate the growing embryo, causing the blood vessels to rupture. This may produce serious internal hemorrhage and can be life threatening. If a tubal pregnancy goes untreated, the embryo will only develop and survive for 2 to 6 weeks.

Common signs/symptoms associated with ectopic pregnancy are the same as early pregnancy, but distention of the tube causes abdominal pain and tenderness. If internal hemorrhage occurs, loss of blood can cause fainting and shock. Ectopic pregnancies are more common in females who have had pelvic inflammatory disease and/or have a partial obstruction of the uterine tube. The etiology of tubal pregnancies is obstruction of the normal passageway for the ovum. Although ultrasound is useful in assessing ectopic pregnancies, diagnosis is confirmed via laparoscopy. The treatment involves the surgical removal of the embryo and the affected uterine tube.

Placenta Disorders

Placenta previa is a condition in which the placenta develops in the lower half of the uterus and encroaches on and partially or completely covers the internal cervical os. In cases of placenta previa, the mother experiences bleeding during the later stages of pregnancy because of the partial separation of the placenta from the uterine wall. Hemorrhage can occur, and this condition can be life threatening to both the mother and child. Ultrasound is a good method of determining placenta location in cases of suspected previa and useful in the management of the pregnancy. Normal delivery cannot occur in patients with placenta previa so a caesarean section is normally performed.

Occasionally a normally implanted placenta may prematurely separate from the uterus. This condition is termed *abruptio placentae* and may also be life-threatening.

THE MALE REPRODUCTIVE SYSTEM

ANATOMY AND PHYSIOLOGY REVIEW

The male reproductive system is composed of glands, ducts, and supporting structures. The glands of the male reproductive system include a pair of testes, a pair of seminal vesicles, a pair of bulbourethral glands, and one prostate gland. The testes are enclosed by a white, fibrous covering within the scrotum. They are responsible for the production of sperm and hormone secretion, mainly testosterone. The prostate gland lies just inferior to the bladder, and the urethra actually passes through this gland (Fig. 7-14 and 7-15). The prostate gland is responsible for secreting the majority of the seminal fluid.

The ducts that connect the glands include a pair of epididymides, a pair of vas deferens, a pair of ejaculatory ducts, and one urethra. The testes are divided into lobules that contain seminiferous tubules, which converge into larger ducts and emerge at the head of the epididymis. The epididymides lie superior and lateral to the testes and serve as a passageway for sperm. They are also responsible for secreting a portion of the seminal fluid. The vas deferens extend from the epididymides and pass through the inguinal canal into the pelvic cavity. They pass superior to the bladder and continue down the posterior surface of the bladder to join the ducts emerging from the seminal vesicles. This junction forms the ejaculatory ducts. These ducts eventually empty into the urethra, which is responsible for delivering the seminal fluid to the exterior of the body.

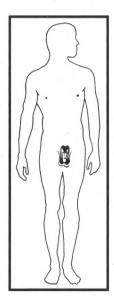
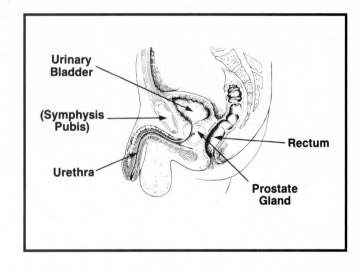

Fig. 7-14, left. The male reproductive system. (From Bontrager KL: *Textbook of radiographic positioning and related Anatomy,* ed 2, St Louis, 1993, Mosby.)

Fig. 7-15, right. The male urinary bladder, anterior cut away. (From Bontrager KL: *Textbook of radiographic positioning and related Anatomy,* ed 3, St Louis, 1993, Mosby.)

IMAGING CONSIDERATIONS

Radiographic investigation of the male reproductive system is limited mainly to urethrograms, intravenous urography, and CT. However, ultrasound is commonly used to evaluate testicular masses, an enlarged scrotum, and to help differentiate between epididymitis and orchiditis or testicular torsion. Prostatic ultrasound via a rectal probe is used to evaluate nodules and guide the physician during biopsies of the prostate.

NEOPLASTIC DISEASES
Prostatic Hyperplasia

Prostatic hyperplasia is a common benign enlargement of the prostate gland caused by the development of discrete nodules within the organ. The etiology of prostatic hyperplasia is unknown, but it is believed to be caused by hormonal changes associated with aging, thus generally affecting males 50 years of age and older. The benign nodules most frequently occur in the median lobe and central portions of the lateral lobes of the prostate gland. Due to this location, the nodules often compress the portion of the urethra passing through the prostate gland, thus interfering with urination.

Symptoms associated with this disorder include difficulty in starting, stopping, and maintaining a flow of urine and the inability to completely empty the bladder. Once the flow of urine is inhibited, urinary tract infections may occur, and in some cases urinary tract obstructions may result from an overgrowth of the prostate gland. The most common treatment of prostatic hyperplasia is partial excision of the prostate gland. A transurethral resection of the prostate (TURP) is performed by passing an endoscope through the urethra to core out the gland. Prostatic enlargement may be demonstrated on an intravenous urographic examination as a filling defect at the base of the bladder. Hyperplastic changes are also readily visible on CT of the pelvic area (Fig. 7-16). There is no con-

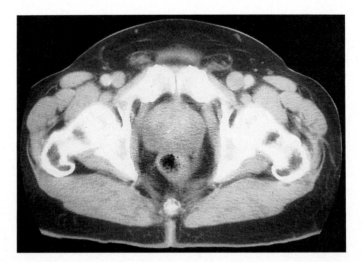

Fig. 7-16. Pelvic CT of a 68-year-old male demonstrating prostatic hyperplasia. Notice the indentation into the urinary bladder. (Courtesy of Riverside Methodist Hospitals, Columbus, Ohio.)

clusive evidence to suggest that development of prostatic hyperplasia increases an individual's chance of developing prostatic carcinoma.

Many males over the age of 50 years develop small, multiple calcifications within the prostate. These are termed *prostatic calculi* and may be radiographically visible on plain abdominal or pelvic images. The development of these calculi is of no clinical significance.

Carcinoma of the Prostate

Adenocarcinoma of the prostate is a common cancer in males. It most frequently affects elderly men with the incidence increasing with age. The etiology of prostate cancer is unknown, but it generally affects the outer group of prostate glands and occurs more frequently in the posterior lobe of the prostate. This disease is most frequently diagnosed by physical examination and an elevation of acid phosphatase levels in the blood. Common signs and symptoms associated with prostate cancer include urinary tract obstructions, a hard, enlarged prostate upon rectal palpatation, and low back pain, often caused by metastatic spread to the pelvis and lumbar spine.

Some types of prostate cancer are fairly dormant, but others are very aggressive and yield a higher mortality rate. If it is diagnosed in an early stage, the initial treatment is surgical removal of the tumor. This neoplasm is very testosterone dependent, so the testes are often removed. In some instances, female hormones may be administered to control the growth of the tumor.

Prostate cancer is staged A to D and graded I to III, depending on the extent of the disease. It is the third leading cause of cancer deaths in males and has a 5-year survival rate of approximately 33%. Skeletal metastases occur in approximately 75% of all cases and manifest on plain radiographs as sclerotic lesions within the bone (Fig. 7-17).

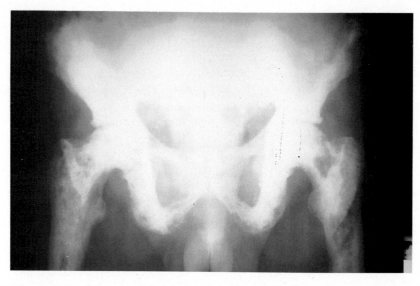

Fig. 7-17. Skeletal metastatic disease of the pelvis and spine secondary to prostate cancer. (Courtesy of Riverside Methodist Hospitals, Columbus, Ohio.)

Testicular Masses

Malignant testicular tumors comprise approximately 1% of all male cancers with a peak incidence around the age of 30 years and a second smaller peak around the age of 75 years. The etiology of malignant tumors of the testes is unknown, but research has shown a strong hereditary association. The most common signs include enlargement and/or palpable hardness of the testis. As with other cancers, testicular tumors are staged I to III depending on the size and extent of the disease. All types of malignant testicular neoplasms are treated with surgical resection. Chemotherapy and/or radiation therapy may also be used in conjunction with surgery depending on the type and staging of the disease. There are four types of malignant germ cell tumors: *seminomas, embryonal carcinomas, teratomas,* and *choriocarcinomas.*

Seminomas arise from the seminiferous tubules and account for approximately 40% of malignant testicular tumors. Seminomas grow rapidly but tend to remain localized for a fairly long time before metastasizing. These neoplasms have an excellent prognosis because of their extreme radiosensitivity. If treated with radiation therapy, seminomas carry a 10-year survival rate of approximately 90%.

Teratomas arise from primitive germ cells and account for approximately 25% of the malignant testicular masses. These neoplasms are composed of various cell types such as connective tissue, muscle, and thyroid glandular tissue. Teratomas are associated with a poorer prognosis than seminomas and carry a 10-year survival rate of approximately 50% to 75%.

Embryonal carcinomas make up approximately 20% of malignant testicular tumors. They are smaller in size than seminomas; however, they are very invasive and metastasize fairly quickly. Embryonal carcinomas carry a 10-year survival rate of approximately 35%.

Choriocarcinomas compose the smallest portion of malignant testicular tumors, accounting for only 1% of malignant neoplasms of the testes. However, choriocarcinomas are very small and aggressive neoplasms. They are often nonpalpable and metastasize very early. Choriocarcinomas carry the worst prognosis, with a 10-year survival rate of approximately 10%.

Benign masses of the testes may be associated with *epididymo-orchitis.* Other common benign masses include *hydroceles* and *spermatoceles.* Ultrasound may be used to differentiate between benign hydroceles/spermatoceles and solid, malignant neoplasms.

▼ QUESTIONS

1. The neck portion of the uterus is termed the:
    a. body
    b. cervix
    c. fundus
    d. internal os

2. The innermost layer of the uterine walls is termed the:
    a. endometrium
    b. myometrium
    c. parietal peritoneum

3. The primary sex organs of the female reproductive system include the:
    a. breasts
    b. ovaries
    c. uterus
    d. all of the above

4. Imaging studies performed on a nongravid female include:
    a. hysterosalpingography
    b. IUD localization examinations
    c. pelvic sonography
    d. all of the above

5. Regular, yearly mammographic screening should occur in females ____ years of age or older.
    a. 20
    b. 30
    c. 40
    d. 50

6. The congenital disorder resulting in a complete duplication of the uterus, cervix, and vagina is:
    a. bicornuate uterus
    b. retroflexed uterus
    c. unicornuate uterus
    d. uterus didelphys

7. Pelvic inflammatory disease may be caused by which of the following?
    1. gonococcus   2. staphylococcus   3. streptococcus
    a. 1, 2
    b. 1, 3
    c. 2, 3
    d. 1, 2, 3

8. The formation of which of the following cystic ovarian masses may occur as a part of the normal menstrual cycle?
    1. corpus luteum cysts
    2. cystadenomas
    3. follicular cysts
    a. 1, 2
    b. 1, 3
    c. 2, 3
    d. 1, 2, 3

9. All of the following may result in sterility EXCEPT:
    a. cystic teratoma
    b. endometriosis
    c. polycystic ovaries
    d. PID

10. A malignant neoplasm of the ovary is a:
    a. cystoadenocarcinoma
    b. cystadenoma
    c. leiomyoma
    d. fibroadenoma

11. Diagnosis of which type of neoplastic disease is often made via a Pap smear and confirmed by surgical biopsy?
    a. adenocarcinoma of the endometrium
    b. cervical carcinoma
    c. leiomyoma of the uterus

12. The majority of breast masses occur in which anatomical region of the breast?
    a. lower, inner quadrant
    b. lower, outer quadrant
    c. upper, inner quadrant
    d. upper, outer quadrant

13. Factors influencing the development of breast cancer include:
    a. nulliparity
    b. family history of breast cancer
    c. viruses
    d. all of the above

14. Physical signs of breast cancer include:
    a. nipple discharge
    b. peau d'orange appearance
    c. massive weight loss
    d. all of the above

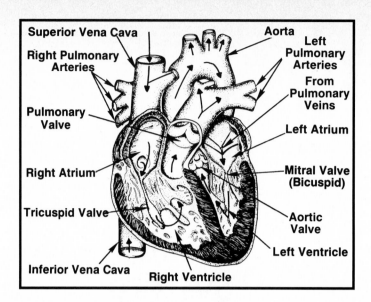

Fig. 8.1. Blood flow through the heart. (From Bontrager KL: *Textbook of radiographic positioning and related anatomy,* ed 3, St Louis, 1993, Mosby).

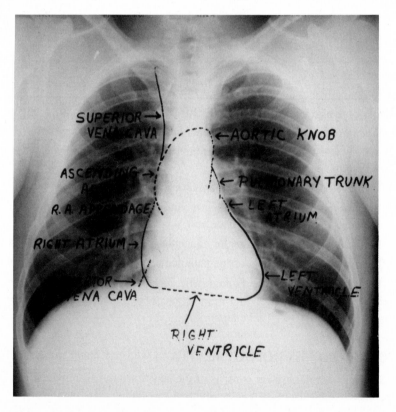

Fig. 8-2. PA chest radiograph with heart chambers and great vessels outlined. (Courtesy of The American College of Radiology, Reston, Virginia.)

4. Imaging studies performed on a nongravid female include:
    a. hysterosalpingography   **c.** pelvic sonography
    b. IUD localization examinations   **d.** all of the above

5. Regular, yearly mammographic screening should occur in females ____ years of age or older.
    a. 20   **c.** 40
    b. 30   **d.** 50

6. The congenital disorder resulting in a complete duplication of the uterus, cervix, and vagina is:
    a. bicornuate uterus   **c.** unicornuate uterus
    b. retroflexed uterus   **d.** uterus didelphys

7. Pelvic inflammatory disease may be caused by which of the following?
    1. gonococcus   2. staphylococcus   3. streptococcus
    a. 1, 2   **c.** 2, 3
    b. 1, 3   **d.** 1, 2, 3

8. The formation of which of the following cystic ovarian masses may occur as a part of the normal menstrual cycle?
    1. corpus luteum cysts
    2. cystadenomas
    3. follicular cysts
    a. 1, 2   **c.** 2, 3
    b. 1, 3   **d.** 1, 2, 3

9. All of the following may result in sterility EXCEPT:
    a. cystic teratoma   **c.** polycystic ovaries
    b. endometriosis   **d.** PID

10. A malignant neoplasm of the ovary is a:
    a. cystoadenocarcinoma   **c.** leiomyoma
    b. cystadenoma   **d.** fibroadenoma

11. Diagnosis of which type of neoplastic disease is often made via a Pap smear and confirmed by surgical biopsy?
    a. adenocarcinoma of the endometrium
    b. cervical carcinoma
    c. leiomyoma of the uterus

12. The majority of breast masses occur in which anatomical region of the breast?
    a. lower, inner quadrant   **c.** upper, inner quadrant
    b. lower, outer quadrant   **d.** upper, outer quadrant

13. Factors influencing the development of breast cancer include:
    a. nulliparity   **c.** viruses
    b. family history of breast cancer   **d.** all of the above

14. Physical signs of breast cancer include:
    a. nipple discharge   **c.** massive weight loss
    b. peau d'orange appearance   **d.** all of the above

15. The presence of an excess amount of amniotic fluid is termed:
    a. abruptio placentae   c. placenta previa
    b. oligohydramnios   d. polyhydramnios

16. The most common site for an ectopic pregnancy is in the:
    a. abdominal cavity   c. ovary
    b. cervix   d. uterine tube

17. The testes are responsible for secreting which of the following hormones?
    a. estrogen   c. testosterone
    b. progesterone

18. Benign hyperplasia of the prostate most commonly affects which lobes of the prostate?
    1. median lobe   2. lateral lobes   3. posterior lobe
    a. 1, 2   c. 2, 3
    b. 1, 3   d. 1, 2, 3

19. The prostate gland is located ____ to the urinary bladder.
    a. anterior   c. posterior
    b. inferior   d. superior

20. Prostatic calculi are a strong indication of adenocarcinoma of the prostate.
    a. true   b. false

21. Prostatic hyperplasia most frequently occurs in males:
    a. under the age of 30 years
    b. between the ages of 30 to 50 years
    c. over the age of 50 years

22. The most common sites for skeletal metastases of adenocarcinoma of the prostate are the:
    1. lumbar spine   2. pelvis   3. ribs
    a. 1, 2   c. 2, 3
    b. 1, 3   d. 1, 2, 3

23. Benign tumors of the testes include:
    1. hydroceles   2. seminomas   3. spermatoceles
    a. 1, 2   c. 2, 3
    b. 1, 3   d. 1, 2, 3

24. Malignant tumors of the testes arising from primitive germ cells are termed:
    a. choriocarcinomas   c. seminomas
    b. embryonal carcinomas   d. teratomas

25. Which type of malignant neoplasm of the testes is associated with the best prognosis?
    a. choriocarcinoma   c. seminoma
    b. embryonal carcinoma   d. teratoma

8

The Cardiovascular System

▼
Upon completion of Chapter 8, the reader should be able to:

- Describe the anatomical components of the cardiovascular system.
- Explain the appearance of the various portions of the heart on conventional chest radiographs.
- Describe each segment of the cardiac cycle.
- Discuss the role of other imaging modalities in the diagnosis, treatment, and management of cardiovascular disorders.
- Differentiate between the major congenital anomalies of the cardiovascular system.
- Identify the pathogenesis of the pathologies cited and typical treatments for them.
- Describe, in general, the radiographic appearance of each of the given pathologies.

ANATOMY AND PHYSIOLOGY REVIEW

The cardiovascular system consists of the heart, arteries, capillaries, and veins and may be further divided into two subsystems of circulation. The pulmonary circulation transports blood between the heart and lungs, whereas the systemic circulation transports blood between the heart and the rest of the body.

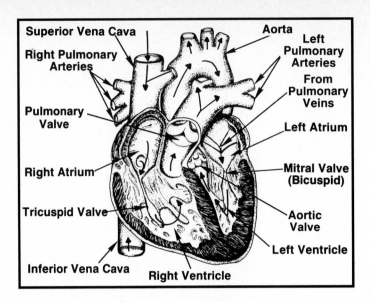

Fig. 8.1. Blood flow through the heart. (From Bontrager KL: *Textbook of radiographic positioning and related anatomy,* ed 3, St Louis, 1993, Mosby).

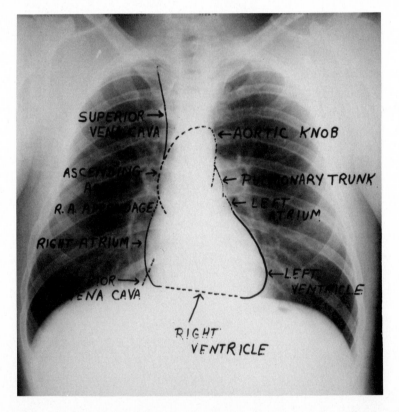

Fig. 8-2. PA chest radiograph with heart chambers and great vessels outlined. (Courtesy of The American College of Radiology, Reston, Virginia.)

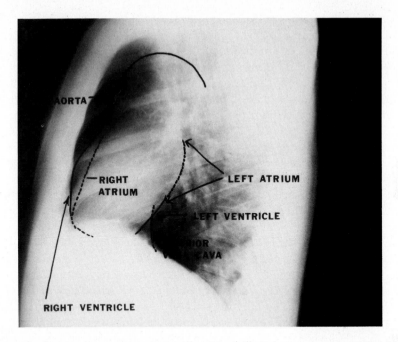

Fig. 8-3. Lateral chest radiograph with heart chambers and great vessels outlined. (Courtesy of The American College of Radiology, Reston, Virginia.)

The Heart

The *heart* acts as a pump to propel the blood throughout the body via the circulatory vessels. It lies in the anterior chest within the mediastinum and is clearly visible on a chest radiograph. The interior of the heart is divided into two upper chambers, termed the *right* and *left atria,* and two lower chambers termed the *right* and *left ventricles* (Fig. 8-1). It is important to note that the heart lies in an oblique plane within the mediastinum; therefore a conventional posteroanterior (PA) chest radiograph does not clearly demonstrate all chambers of the heart.

A frontal projection of the chest shows a cardiac silhouette; the right side is composed of mainly the right atrium and the left side is composed mainly of the left ventricle. The right ventricle lies midline within the cardiac shadow and is located anterior to the right atrium and left ventricle. The left atrium is located midline and is the posterior-most aspect of the heart (Fig. 8-2). Therefore, it is necessary to obtain a lateral projection of the chest to best demonstrate the right ventricle and left atrium. On a lateral projection of the chest, the right ventricle constitutes the anterior portion of the cardiac silhouette, and the left atrium and left ventricle constitute the posterior portion of the cardiac shadow (Fig. 8-3).

The heart contains three tissue layers. The innermost layer, termed the *endocardium,* is smooth. The valves located within and between the various chambers are also composed of endocardium. Although the valve tissue is relatively thin, in a normal heart it is able to prevent the backflow and passage of blood when the valve is closed. The middle layer is muscular and is termed the *myocardium*. This is the thickest layer of heart tissue and the muscle receives blood supply from the right and left coronary arteries that arise directly from the aorta, just superior to the aortic valve. Maximum blood flow through the coronary arteries occurs during diastole, while the heart is relaxed. The outermost layer is a protective covering termed the *epicardium*. The entire heart is enclosed within a pericardial sac, which contains a small amount of fluid to lubricate the heart as it contracts and relaxes, thus reducing friction between the heart and other mediastinal structures.

In the normal heart, the right atrium receives deoxygenated blood from the body via the superior and inferior vena cavae. The deoxygenated blood passes through the right atrioventricular or tricuspid valve into the right ventricle. The right ventricle contracts, thus propelling the blood to the lungs through the pulmonary valve and pulmonary trunk, which bifurcates into the right and left main pulmonary arteries, respectively. Approximately 60% of the deoxygenated blood enters the right lung, and approximately 40% enters the left lung.

The exchange of gases occurs at the capillary/alveolar level, and the now oxygenated blood is returned to the left atrium via the four pulmonary veins. The oxygenated blood flows from the left atrium to the left ventricle via the left atrioventricular or bicuspid valve. The left ventricle is responsible for pumping the oxygenated blood throughout the systemic circulatory system; therefore the left ventricle has a thicker layer of myocardium and contracts with greater force than does the right ventricle. The oxygenated blood flows through the aortic valve into the aorta when the left ventricle contracts.

The Cardiac Cycle

The contraction of the myocardium is termed *systole* and the subsequent relaxation is termed *diastole*. The pacemaker of the heart is the sinoatrial (SA) node, which is located in the upper portion of the right atrium near the superior vena cava. An electrical current is transmitted through the myocardium, resulting in a heartbeat.

Electrocardiography graphically displays this electrical activity. The elements of an electrocardiogram include the P wave, PR interval, QRS complex, T wave, and QT duration (Fig. 8-4). The P wave is the graphic display of the spread of the electrical impulse from the atria. The PR interval shows the amount of time required for the electrical impulse to travel from the SA node to the ventricular muscle fibers. The spread of the electrical impulse through the ventricles is displayed by the QRS complex, and the period in which the ventricles recover from the spent electrical impulse is graphically displayed by the T wave. The QT duration represents the total time from ventricular depolarization (QRS) to ventricular repolarization (T).

Circulatory Vessels

Arteries are blood vessels that carry blood away from the heart and they are composed of three layers. The outermost layer is termed the *adventitia*, the middle layer is the *media*, and the innermost layer is the *intima*. The internal, tubular structure of the vessel is termed the *lumen*. *Veins* are blood vessels that carry blood to the heart. They are composed of the same three layers; however, venous walls are thinner than arterial walls and veins contain valves at set intervals to help with blood return to the heart. *Capillaries* are microscopic vessels that connect the arteries and veins (Fig. 8-5). They are responsible for the exchange of substances necessary for nutrient and waste transport.

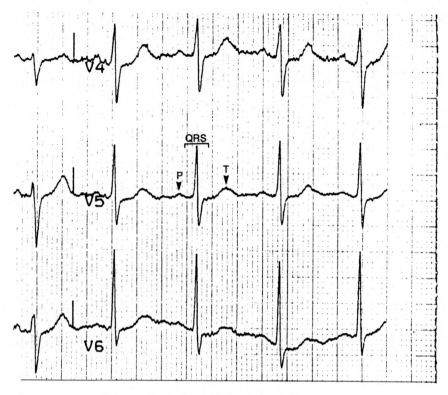

Fig. 8-4. Electrocardiograph demonstrating the P wave, PR interval, QRS wave, and T wave. (Courtesy of Riverside Methodist Hospitals, Columbus, Ohio.)

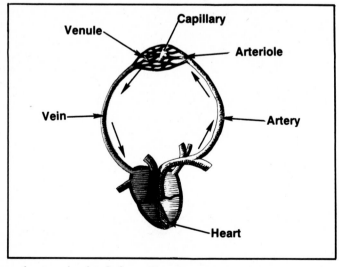

Fig. 8-5. General systemic circulation. (From Bontrager KL: *Textbook of radiographic positioning and related anatomy,* ed 3, St Louis, 1993, Mosby.)

IMAGING CONSIDERATIONS

Radiography is important in the diagnosis and management of cardiovascular disease. Conventional chest radiographs provide information concerning heart shape and size. However, the technologist must be aware that many factors may affect the cardiac image. Some factors can be controlled by the technologist, whereas others cannot.

Controllable Factors

Factors that the technologist can control include patient posture, degree of inspiration, correct positioning, geometric factors, and exposure technique selection. Whenever possible, chest radiographs should be taken with the patient in an erect position. If a patient is semi-recumbent or recumbent, the heart appears to be enlarged because the abdominal organs push the diaphragm and heart up into the thoracic cavity. It is important to identify cases in which the patient is not erect to aid the physician in diagnosis and interpretation.

Chest radiographs obtained without a good inspiration also distort heart shape and size (Figs. 8-6 and 8-7). Remember that at least 10 posterior ribs should be visible within

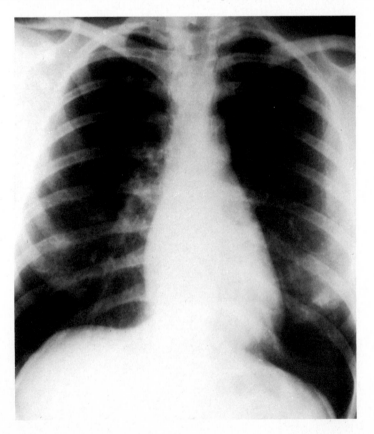

Fig. 8-6. PA chest radiograph with good inspiration. (Courtesy of the American College of Radiology, Reston, Virginia.)

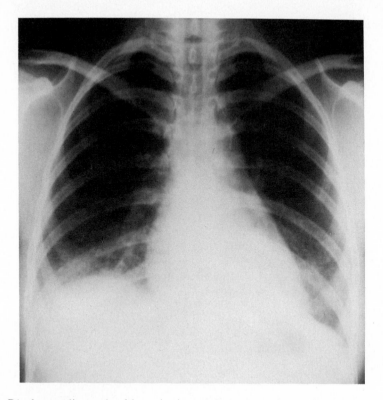

Fig. 8-7. PA chest radiograph with expiration on the same patient as in Fig. 8-6, notice the enlargement of the cardiac shadow on this radiograph. (Courtesy of the American College of Radiology, Reston, Virginia.)

the lung fields on a good inspiratory chest radiograph. The sternoclavicular joints should be an equal distance from the spine and the scapulae should be rolled out of the lung fields on a well-positioned PA chest radiograph. When positioning for a lateral chest, the arms and shoulders should be placed above the patient's head to ensure that they are above the apices.

Geometric factors affecting heart shape and size include source-to-image receptor distance (SID) and object-to-image receptor distance (OID). Conventional chest radiographs are generally obtained using a 72-inch SID to decrease magnification of the heart to an approximate factor of 10%. Again, it is important to document variations in SID to aid in the proper diagnosis of heart disorders. Because the heart is located fairly anterior in the mediastinum, it is preferable to obtain PA chest images whenever possible. This places the heart closest to the image receptor, allowing for the smallest OID. Positioning the patient for a PA projection also helps decrease magnification of the cardiac silhouette. A third geometric factor that is frequently overlooked is the anode-heel effect. Technologists can use this phenomenon to their advantage by placing the anode over the apical region and the cathode toward the base of the lungs, thus distributing the radiographic density more evenly throughout the chest radiograph.

Adequate penetration of the mediastinal structure is also critical in chest radiography and requires the use of a relatively high kilovoltage. A minimum of 100 kilovolts peak (kVp) should be used. Compensating filters, such as trough filters, may also be used to ensure adequate penetration of the mediastinum while maintaining optimum visualization of the vascular markings within the lung fields. Vascular markings within the chest help the physician assess ventricular function. The pulmonary vessels also provide information about pulmonary artery pressure. Dilatation of these vessels often indicates problems with the right ventricle. Exposure times of less than 1/60 of a second or less should be used whenever possible to decrease involuntary cardiac motion. It has been documented that heart motion may increase the size of the cardiac shadow.

In most institutions, chest radiography is the most commonly performed procedure, and technologists all too often underestimate the importance of these basic radiographic principles. Well-positioned diagnostic chest radiographs are crucial in the diagnosis and treatment of cardiovascular disorders. In a normal adult the transverse diameter of the cardiac shadow should be less than half the transverse diameter of the thorax on a PA erect chest radiograph. An enlarged heart is termed *cardiomegaly* (Fig. 8-8), which is indicative of many cardiovascular disorders.

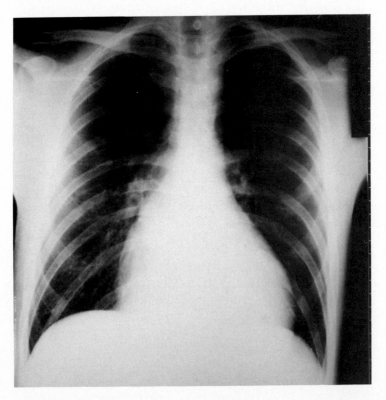

Fig. 8-8. PA chest radiograph of a 53-year-old male with aortic insufficiency resulting in cardiomegaly. (Courtesy of The American College of Radiology, Reston, Virginia.)

Uncontrollable Factors

Factors affecting cardiac shape and size that are not under the technologist's control include patient body habitus, bony thorax abnormalities, and pathologic conditions, such as a pneumothorax or pulmonary emphysema. Bony abnormalities of special concern include scoliosis and pectus excavatum. Individuals with pectus excavatum present with a funnel-shaped depression of the sternum. The abnormal placement of the xiphoid causes displacement of the heart to the left and distortion of the cardiac shadow.

Other Imaging Modalities

At times it may be necessary to fill the esophagus with barium sulfate to better demonstrate the borders of the heart (Figs. 8-9 and 8-10). When positioning for a cardiac series, a 45-degree right anterior oblique position is adequate to project the heart shadow into the left lung field free from the other mediastinal structures. However, it is necessary to use

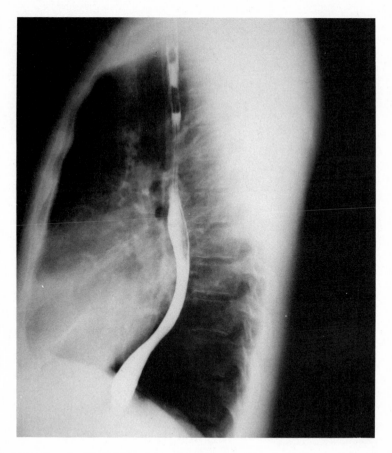

Fig. 8-9. Lateral projection of the chest with barium sulfate outlining the left atrium of the heart. (Courtesy of Riverside Methodist Hospitals, Columbus, Ohio.)

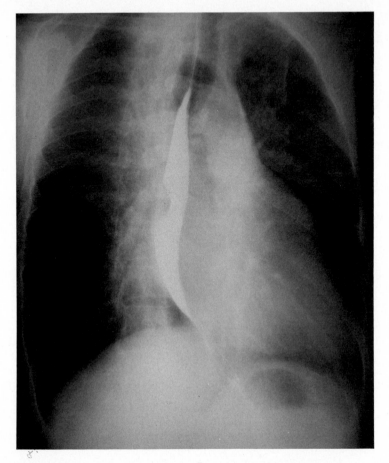

Fig. 8-10. Right anterior oblique position of the chest with barium sulfate outlining the left atrium of the heart. (Courtesy of Riverside Methodist Hospitals, Columbus, Ohio.)

approximately a 60-degree left anterior oblique position to project the heart into the right lung field so that it is not superimposed on other mediastinal structures.

Fluoroscopy may be used to visualize cardiac calcifications and chamber motion. In general, however, cardiac fluoroscopy is of limited value in the diagnosis of heart disease. Echocardiography is a noninvasive allied procedure that can provide detailed information concerning heart anatomy and function and vessel patency.

Echocardiography provides a good examination of the left atrium, left ventricle, and the aortic root and allows evaluation of left ventricular function. Cardiac sonography is also used to measure the thickness of the ventricular walls and provides an accurate assessment of cardiac motion and valve function. In addition, it is an excellent modality for visualizing the ascending and abdominal aorta in cases of suspected aneurysm.

Nuclear medicine procedures used in the assessment of cardiovascular disease include myocardial perfusion scans, gated cardiac blood pool scans, and radionuclide angiocardiography. Myocardial perfusion scans with thallium 20 are the most widely used procedure in nuclear cardiology. It is especially useful in detecting regions of myocardial ischemia and scarring. Gated cardiac blood pool scans are used to evaluate left ventricular function; radionuclide angiocardiography is mainly used in the management of congenital heart defects in pediatric patients. In addition, positron emission tomography (PET) is emerging as a promising method of demonstrating myocardial viability and metabolic imaging.

Angiography is still the most commonly performed procedure for cardiovascular disease. It may be performed to provide diagnostic information or for therapeutic purposes such as percutaneous transluminal angioplasty or thrombolysis.

CONGENITAL/HEREDITARY DISEASES

Because fetal circulation and blood-gas exchange occur within the placenta, certain characteristics are present in the fetal circulatory system that should normally disappear at birth. These characteristics include an opening in the septum between the atria, termed the *foramen ovale,* which allows the blood to bypass the pulmonary circulatory system, and a small vessel termed the *ductus arteriosus,* which connects the pulmonary artery and the descending aorta. If these anatomical structures persist, a variety of congenital anomalies can develop in the newborn infant. The incidence of congenital cardiovascular anomalies is approximately 8 per 1000 live births.

Etiology of congenital heart disease includes heritable disorders, chromosomal aberrations (such as Down's syndrome), and environmental factors (such as drugs, infection, radiation, and maternal disease). In addition, individuals presenting with congenital anomalies of the heart are at an increased risk of developing endocardial infections. Approximately one third of all infants born with congenital anomalies of the heart, die within the first month of life. Therefore immediate diagnosis and treatment are vital. Radiography and diagnostic medical sonography play a critical role in the diagnosis and treatment of congenital anomalies, along with the diagnosis of heart murmurs by physical examination and abnormal heart rates demonstrated by electrocardiography.

Patent Ductus Arteriosus

If the ductus arteriosus does not close at birth, *patent ductus arteriosus* results (Fig. 8-11, p. 320). Chest radiographs of the infant will demonstrate cardiomegaly and increased pulmonary vascular congestion. This condition is more common in premature infants, especially in cases of respiratory distress syndrome.

Because the left ventricle contracts with more force than the right ventricle, the arterial blood within the aorta is shunted into the pulmonary trunk via the open ductus arteriosus. This increases the volume of blood propelled into the lungs, thus increasing pulmonary vascular congestion and the volume of blood returning to the left atrium. Infants with this condition generally display cyanotic features resulting from the shunting. Echocardiography is the imaging method of choice when evaluating the severity of this anomaly.

Coarctation of the Aorta

Although the ductus arteriosus may close normally at birth, a narrowing of the aorta may occur at the junction site. This anomaly is termed *coarctation of the aorta.* It occurs

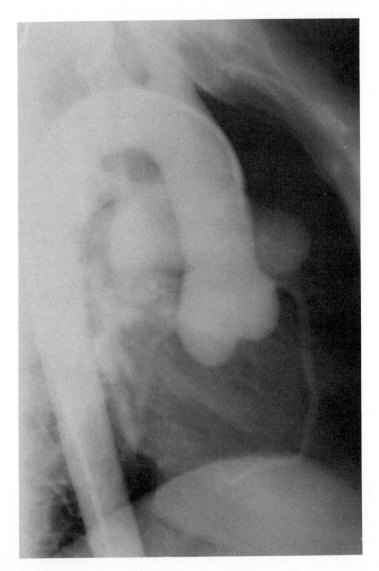

Fig. 8-11. Aortogram demonstrating patent ductus arteriosus. Notice filling of the pulmonary vessels as well as the aorta. (Courtesy of Riverside Methodist Hospitals, Columbus, Ohio.)

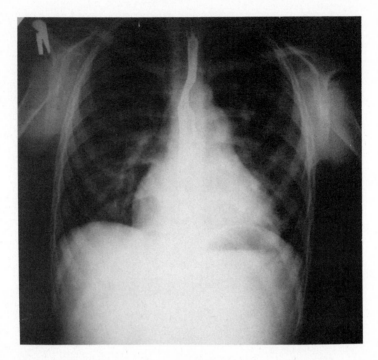

Fig. 8-12. Chest radiograph depicting ventricular septal defect. Notice the enlargement of the right heart border. (Courtesy of Children's Hospital, Columbus, Ohio.)

anatomically inferior to the vessels responsible for circulation to the head, neck, and upper extremities, so circulation to these anatomic regions is not affected. However, blood flow to the abdomen and lower extremities is compromised and the femoral pulse is very weak in most individuals possessing this anomaly. Radiographically, two bulges of the aorta will be demonstrated in the aortic arch region, one superior to and one inferior to the stenosis. Coarctation of the aorta may be successfully treated surgically by removing the narrowed region of the aorta and reattaching the normal aorta superior and inferior to the coarctation.

Septal Defects

A defect in either the ventricular or atrial septum allows the blood to be shunted between the two chambers (Fig. 8-12). The blood is generally shunted from the left to the right chamber because of increased pressure in the left side of the heart. This shunting of the blood results in an enlargement of the right side of the heart and increased pulmonary vascularitis.

If the foramen ovale does not close at birth, an opening remains between the right and left atria. In most cases this does not require surgical intervention. The most serious septal defects would occur between the ventricular chambers because the pressure is greater in the left ventricle. Surgical intervention depends on the size of the defect and the risk of developing bacterial endocarditis at the site of the defect.

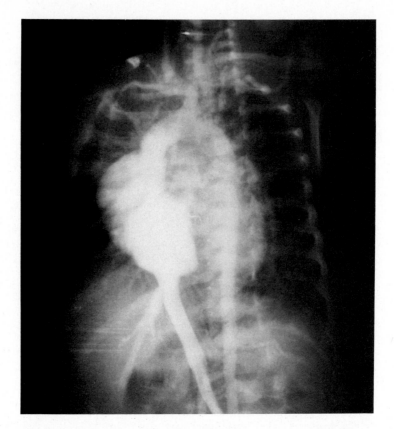

Fig. 8-13. Angiogram demonstrating transposition of great vessels. Notice the "closed" system of the right side of the heart. The blood is returned via the vena cavae, and redistributed via the aorta, thus bypassing the lungs. (Courtesy of Children's Hospital, Columbus, Ohio.)

Transposition of Great Vessels

Transposition of great vessels is a serious congenital defect of the circulatory system that does not allow the pulmonary and systemic subsystems to communicate. This anomaly exists when the aorta arises from the right ventricle instead of the left ventricle and the pulmonary trunk arises from the left ventricle instead of the right ventricle (Fig. 8-13).

Deoxygenated blood returns to the right atrium, travels through the right ventricle, and is pumped through the aorta back into the systemic subsystem without becoming oxygenated. The oxygenated blood returns to the left atrium, travels through the right ventricle and is pumped through the pulmonary trunk back to the lungs for gas exchange to occur. Obviously, this anomaly is incompatible with life. Because immediate recognition and treatment of this defect is imperative, an emergency cardiac catheterization and balloon septostomy should be performed to enlarge the opening between the atria to increase mixing of venous and arterial blood and to decompress the left atrium. Surgical correction of this anomaly is indicated after the age of 6 months.

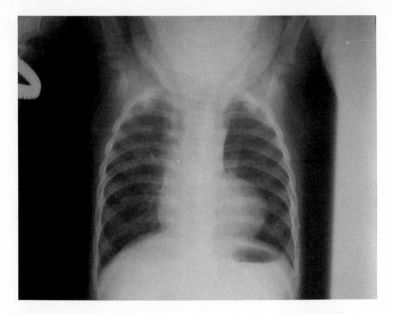

Fig. 8-14. Chest radiograph on an infant with tetralogy of Fallot. Notice the "boot-shaped" cardiac shadow. (Courtesy of Children's Hospital, Columbus, Ohio.)

Tetralogy of Fallot

Tetralogy of Fallot is a combination of four defects: pulmonary stenosis, ventricular septal defect, overriding aorta, and hypertrophy of the right ventricle. The narrowing of the pulmonary valve prevents passage of a sufficient volume of blood from the right ventricle to the lungs and results in the most common cause of cyanosis in infants with cardiovascular anomalies. Normally, the aorta should arise from the left ventricle, but in cases of tetralogy of Fallot, the aorta arises from a ventricular septal defect. In other words, it overrides the right ventricle, which in turn results in hypertrophy of the right ventricle. Enlargement of the right ventricle is demonstrated radiographically as a "boot-shaped" cardiac shadow caused by displacement of the heart apex (Fig. 8-14). Corrective surgery is usually performed after the age of 1 year.

VALVULAR DISEASE

The most common cause of chronic valve disease of the heart is rheumatic fever. This condition most frequently affects the bicuspid (mitral) and aortic valves and is more common in females than in males. Because of advances in pharmaceuticals, technology, and medical care, the incidence of rheumatic heart disease is on the decline. Rheumatic fever produces inflammatory changes within the connective tissues of the body, thus affecting the valves within the heart. This may result in stenosis, insufficiency, and/or incompetency. Individuals suffering from rheumatic heart disease present with a distinct heart murmur audible upon physical examination.

Valvular stenosis is caused by a scarring of valve cusps that eventually adhere to one

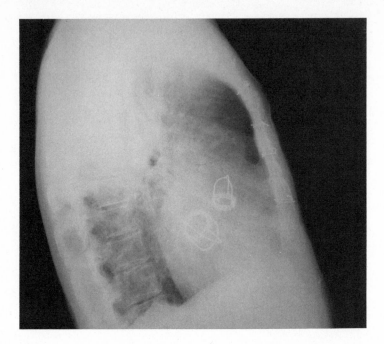

Fig. 8-15. Lateral chest radiograph demonstrating two prosthetic valve replacements clearly visible within the heart. (Courtesy of the American College of Radiology, Reston, Virginia.)

another. The results of valvular stenosis become apparent in adult life because it generally takes years for the scarring to affect valve function. Mitral valve stenosis inhibits blood flow from the left atrium into the left ventricle. This slows the blood flow through the lungs and the right side of the heart, resulting in an enlargement of the right side of the heart and the left atrium. Insufficiency and incompetency occur when the valves do not close properly and allow blood to reflux during systole. This complication often follows endocarditis and most commonly affects the mitral or aortic valve.

Radiographically the heart silhouette appears enlarged and the diseased valves may contain small calcifications. In severe cases, the diseased valves are replaced with prosthetic devices that are clearly visible on conventional chest radiographs (Fig. 8-15).

CONGESTIVE HEART DISEASE

Congestive heart failure occurs when the heart is unable to propel blood at a sufficient rate and volume. This results in congestion of the subcirculatory systems and does not allow a sufficient supply of blood to reach the tissues of the body. Congestive heart failure is most commonly caused by hypertension but may result from other disease processes that overburden the heart, such as valvular disease. Congestive heart failure may affect either side of the heart, and it may develop gradually or have a quick onset in combination with pulmonary edema. However, regardless of the original side affected, prolonged strain on

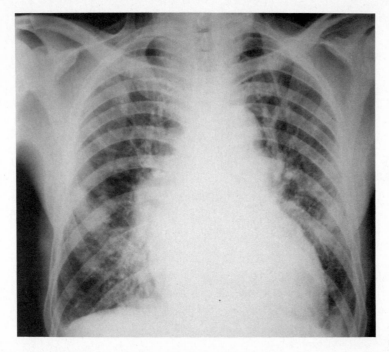

Fig. 8-16. Chest radiograph demonstrating left-sided congestive heart failure. Notice the engorgement of the pulmonary vessels and interstitial fluid accumulation within the lung tissue. (Courtesy of the American College of Radiology, Reston, Virginia.)

the heart eventually affects the entire organ. Signs and symptoms may vary with the extent and location of the disease. The treatment of congestive failure depends on the cause and severity of the disease and may include surgical intervention, especially in cases of valvular disease.

Left-Sided Failure

When the left ventricle of the heart cannot pump an amount of blood equal to the venous return in the right ventricle, the pulmonary subcirculatory system becomes overloaded. The fluid that accumulates in the capillaries of the lungs leaks into the interstitial tissues within the lungs. This results in pulmonary edema, which can be a life-threatening condition. Radiographically the heart is enlarged and the hilar region of the lungs are congested with increased vascular markings (Fig. 8-16). Upon physical examination, individuals with left-sided heart failure present with an increased heart rate because the heart tries to compensate for the deficiency. Individuals commonly complain of difficulty in breathing and/or shortness of breath upon exertion and respiratory distress severe enough to awaken them during the night. As the disease progresses, sleeping in a recumbent position becomes impossible. The most common causes of left-side failure are aortic and mitral valvular disease, hypertension, or coronary artery disease.

Right-Sided Failure

Right ventricular failure is not as common as left-sided failure and occurs when the right ventricle cannot pump as much blood as it receives from the right atrium. This causes the venous blood flow to slow down producing engorgement of the superior and inferior vena cavae and edema of the lower extremities. A common complaint from individuals with right-sided failure is swelling of their ankles. Radiographically, the right atrium and right ventricle appear enlarged. Common causes of true, right-sided failure are pulmonary valve stenosis, emphysema, or pulmonary hypertension secondary to pulmonary emboli.

DEGENERATIVE DISEASES
Atherosclerosis

Atherosclerosis is a degenerative condition affecting the major arteries of the body, often termed "*hardening of the arteries.*" It is the most prevalent disease in humans, occurring in epidemic proportions in the United States. The etiology of atherosclerosis is unknown, and researchers are not sure whether it is genetic in origin or whether it is an acquired, environmental disease. It affects sexes equally, however, it tends to affect males at an earlier age than females. Atherosclerosis may occur in any artery (Fig. 8-17), but it has a predilection for the aorta, coronary arteries, and cerebral arteries. Risk factors associated with this disorder include increased age, increased serum lipoproteins and cholesterol, hypertension, increased blood sugar levels, cigarette smoking, and a sedentary lifestyle. In addition, some other disease processes, such as diabetes mellitus, predispose individuals to atherosclerotic disease.

Three theories are currently being debated regarding the cause of the development of *atheroma formations* (fibro-fatty plaques) within the vessel. The most common theory suggests that the disease process first affects the intima or inner layer of the artery, which narrows the lumen, and secondarily affects the media or middle layer, causing a weakening in the vessel wall. As the disease progresses, the atheroma may calcify, hemorrhage, ulcerate, or include a superimposed thrombosis. These arterial changes often occur silently, and symptoms may not be present until atheroma formation occludes over two thirds of the vessel. In some cases, this slow narrowing allows enough time for the formation of collateral vessels to maintain blood supply distal to the stenotic site. If normal blood supply is decreased and/or stopped completely, *ischemia* occurs. Unfortunately the most common signs/symptoms associated with atherosclerotic disease result from ischemia of a vital organ such as the heart or brain, or a weakening of a vital artery resulting in an aneurysm. Atherosclerotic disease is the most common cause of coronary heart disease and cerebrovascular accidents.

Cardiovascular angiography is often used in the diagnosis and treatment of atherosclerosis through the use of percutaneous transluminal angioplasty. MRI and echocardiography are both noninvasive modalities that may also visualize blood flow without the use of contrast agents.

Coronary Artery Disease (CAD)

Coronary artery disease results from the deposition of atheromas in the arteries supplying blood to the heart muscle. As the plaques accumulate in the coronary arteries, blood supply to the heart muscle is decreased, resulting in ischemia and myocardial damage.

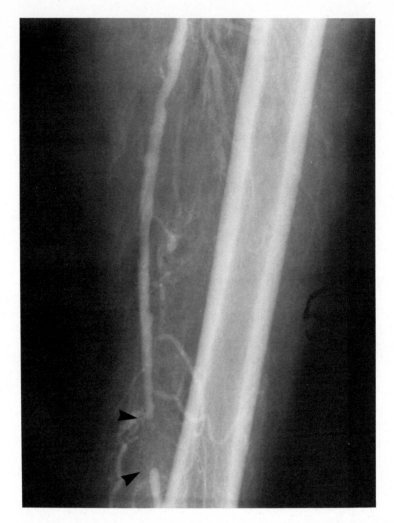

Fig. 8-17. Arteriogram on a 47-year-old male demonstrating an occluded femoral artery caused by atherosclerosis. (Courtesy of Riverside Methodist Hospitals, Columbus, Ohio.)

Major complications of coronary artery disease include angina pectoris (chest pain), myocardial infarction, and subsequent myocardial necrosis, if the patient survives the heart attack. Acute myocardial infarction causes approximately 35% of deaths in men in the United States between the ages of 35 and 50 years. It is the single most frequent cause of death in the United States with approximately 90% of the cases demonstrating significant widespread atherosclerotic disease of the coronary arteries upon autopsy.

Clinical signs/symptoms of myocardial infarction include a sudden onset of severe crushing chest pain that may radiate down the left arm or up into the neck. It may be accompanied by profuse sweating, shortness of breath, nausea, or vomiting. In some cases, it may be passed off as indigestion. Immediate medical attention is critical to the survival of individuals experiencing a myocardial infarction. Approximately 20% to 25% of these patients die before reaching the hospital. Early medical intervention significantly increases survival. Survival rates are approximately 85% for those first attack victims receiving medical attention within the first 30 minutes after the attack. The prognosis of coronary artery disease is variable, depending largely on the importance of the occluded vessel, the extent of damage to the heart muscle, and the amount of collateral circulation available. Angiography plays a major role in the diagnosis of stenotic and/or occluded heart vessels. In some cases, percutaneous transluminal angioplasty may be performed to open these vessels.

Medical treatments of coronary artery disease may include the use of antianginal drugs to improve circulation and decrease the amount of oxygen consumed by the myocardium. Other cases may be treated surgically with coronary artery bypass grafts, which involve bypassing the obstruction with a segment of the saphenous vein. A portion of the saphenous vein is removed from the patient's leg and one end is attached to the aorta above the level of the coronary arteries. The lower end of the graft is attached to the coronary artery, beyond the site of the occlusion.

Nuclear medicine studies such as thallium myocardial perfusion scans and gated examinations are important noninvasive methods of determining the presence and extent of coronary artery disease; these studies also assist in the clinical management of post-myocardial patients. In addition, echocardiography may be used to provide needed clinical information in the diagnosis, treatment, and management of coronary artery disease.

Cerebrovascular Accident

Atherosclerotic disease affecting the blood supply to the brain results in a *cerebrovascular accident (CVA)* or stroke. There are basically three causes for this disease: brain hemorrhage, infarction caused by thrombosis of a cerebral artery, or embolism to the brain from a thrombus elsewhere in the body.

Brain hemorrhage results from a weakening in the diseased vessel wall. The onset of this type of CVA is sudden and often lethal because it expands rapidly. Brain hemorrhages account for approximately 10% to 15% of all cerebrovascular accidents, with most bleeds occurring in the cerebrum and bleeding into the lateral ventricle. Most commonly they are preceded by an intense headache that is often accompanied by vomiting. Loss of consciousness follows within minutes and leads to total contralateral hemiplegia or death. The prognosis of this type of CVA is very poor; it has a 30-day survival rate of approximately 17%.

The most frequent type of CVA results from infarction and may be easily diagnosed with angiography. An infarct caused by thrombosis of a cerebral artery is termed an *atherothrombic brain infarction (ABI)*. These most commonly occur at the bifurcation of the common carotid artery (Fig. 8-18), within the carotid sinus, or at the termination of the internal carotid artery giving rise to the cerebral arteries. Symptoms associated with ABI develop slowly over a period of hours or days and include confusion, hemiplegia, and aphasia. This type of CVA may be preceded by a temporary episode of neurologic dysfunction termed a *transient ischemic attack (TIA)*, which includes hemiparesis, hemiparesthesia, or monocular blindness. These symptoms should clear within 24 hours.

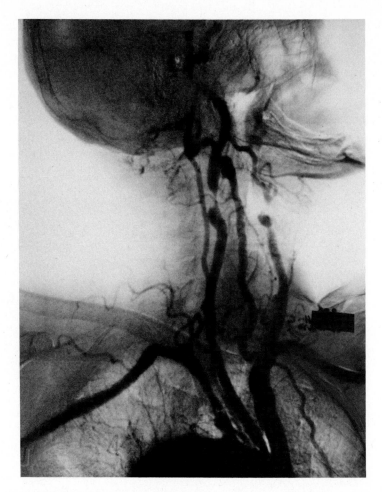

Fig. 8-18. A digital subtraction arteriogram demonstrating atherosclerotic disease of carotid artery. Notice that the carotid artery is almost completely occluded. (Courtesy of The American College of Radiology, Reston, Virginia.)

Infarction may also be caused by an embolism to the brain from a thrombus elsewhere in the body, most commonly from the left side of the heart. CVAs resulting from cerebral embolism have a sudden onset of symptoms without warning. The prognosis is much better for CVAs caused by infarct compared with those from hemorrhage. The 30-day survival rate associated with infarct is approximately 73%. Angiography, Doppler sonography, and CT all play a vital role in the diagnosis and management of CVAs.

ANEURYSMS

A localized ''ballooning'' or outpouching of a vessel wall is called an *aneurysm*. This results when the vessel wall has been weakened by atherosclerotic disease, trauma, infection, or congenital defects. Aneurysms are usually classified as saccular, fusiform, or dissecting. A *saccular aneurysm* is a localized bulge involving one side of the arterial wall (Fig. 8-19). If this bulging includes the entire circumference of the vessel wall, it is termed *fusiform*. A *dissecting aneurysm* results when the intima tears and allows blood to flow within the vessel wall, thus forming an intramural hematoma. Symptoms of a dissecting aneurysm often mock those of a heart attack. Angiography is often used in the diagnosis of aneurysms. CT and diagnostic medical sonography are often of value, especially in the case of a dissecting aneurysm.

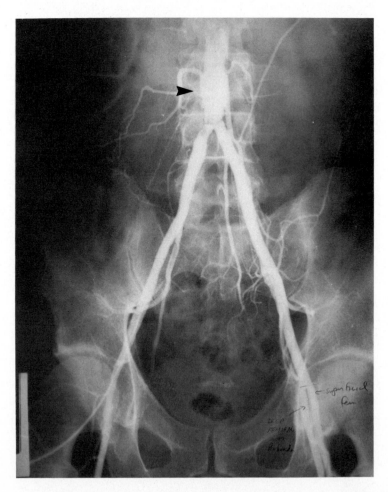

Fig. 8-19. Abdominal aortogram on a 53-year-old male demonstrating a saccular abdominal aneurysm and bilateral areas of stenosis at the bifurcation of the aorta into the common iliac arteries. (Courtesy of Riverside Methodist Hospitals, Columbus, Ohio.)

VENOUS THROMBOSIS

The formation of blood clots within a vein is called *venous thrombosis*. These clots commonly form in the veins of the lower extremities (Fig. 8-20) and result from a slowing of the blood return to the heart. The contraction of the leg muscles assists with venous blood return, therefore postoperative or bedfast patients are especially prone to this disorder. *Phlebitis,* an inflammation of the vein, is often associated with venous thrombosis. The medical term used to specify the combination of these disorders is *thrombophlebitis*.

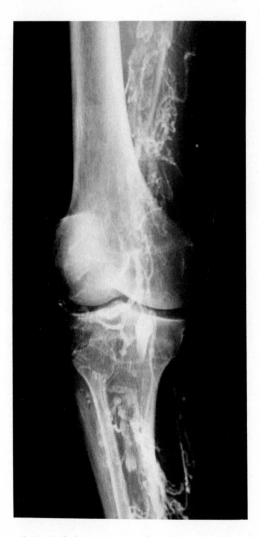

Fig. 8-20. Venogram of the left lower extremity demonstrating deep vein thrombosis. (Courtesy of Riverside Methodist Hospitals, Columbus, Ohio.)

Venography is often performed to provide information concerning the location and the extent of this disease. One major complication associated with deep vein thrombosis is a pulmonary embolism. Filters are often placed in the patient's inferior vena cava to prevent these clots from reaching the kidneys and chest. These filters may be inserted under fluoroscopic control and are clearly visible on plain radiographs of the abdomen (Fig. 8-21).

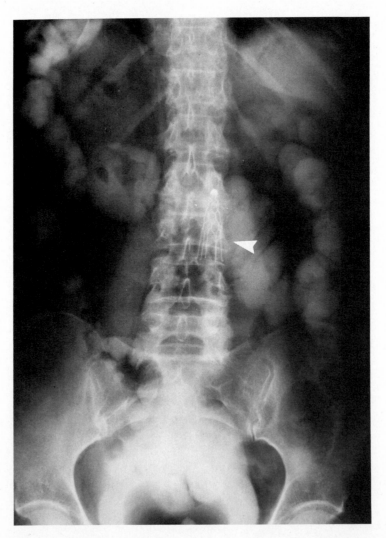

Fig. 8-21. Abdominal radiograph on an elderly female demonstrating the proper placement of a venal caval filter. (Courtesy of Riverside Methodist Hospitals, Columbus, Ohio.)

▼ QUESTIONS

1. The heart chamber located most anteriorly and comprising the anterior border of the cardiac shadow on a lateral chest radiograph is the:
   a. left atrium
   b. left ventricle
   c. right atrium
   d. right ventricle

2. Vessels responsible for carrying blood toward the heart are:
   a. arteries
   b. capillaries
   c. veins

3. The middle or muscular layer of the heart is termed the:
   a. endocardium
   b. epicardium
   c. myocardium
   d. pericardium

4. The bicuspid valve is also known as the:
   a. left atrioventricular valve
   b. right atrioventricular valve
   c. aortic valve
   d. pulmonary valve

5. Contraction of the myocardium is termed:
   a. diastole
   b. systole

6. Which one or more of the following factors affect heart size on a radiograph?
   a. patient posture
   b. SID
   c. scoliosis
   d. a, b
   e. a, b, c

7. How many posterior ribs should be visible on a good inspiration PA chest radiograph?
   a. 12
   b. 10
   c. 8
   d. 6

8. In a fetus, the ductus arteriosus connects which two structures?
   a. aorta and SVC
   b. aorta and pulmonary trunk
   c. right and left atria
   d. right and left ventricles

9. In cases of complete transposition of great vessels, the aorta arises from the:
   a. left atrium
   b. left ventricle
   c. right atrium
   d. right ventricle

10. Foramen ovale is an opening between the right and left:
    a. atria
    b. ventricles

11. Tetralogy of Fallot includes which one or more of the following defects?
    a. pulmonary stenosis
    b. ventricular septal defect
    c. hypertrophy of right ventricle
    d. a, c
    e. a, b, c

12. Which one or more valves are most commonly affected in cases of rheumatic heart disease?
    a. mitral
    b. pulmonary
    c. tricuspid
    d. all of the above

13. A narrowing of the scarred valve is termed:
    a. incompetency
    b. insufficiency
    c. stenosis

14. Valvular disease is more common in:
   a. females   **b.** males

15. A condition in which the left ventricle cannot pump an amount of blood equal to the venous return of the right ventricle is:
   a. coronary artery disease
   b. left-sided congestive heart failure
   c. right-sided congestive heart failure
   d. patent ductus arteriosus

16. Risk factors associated with atherosclerosis include:
   1. low blood sugar levels
   2. hypertension
   3. cigarette smoking
   a. 1, 2   **c.** 2, 3
   b. 1, 3   **d.** 1, 2, 3

17. A decrease in tissue blood supply is termed:
   a. atheroma   **c.** ischemia
   b. infarction   **d.** necrosis

18. The single most frequent cause of male deaths in the United States is:
   a. congestive heart failure   **c.** transposition of great vessels
   b. coronary artery disease   **d.** valvular disease

19. Clinical signs of a myocardial infarction include:
   1. shortness of breath
   2. crushing chest pain
   3. neck pain
   a. 1, 2   **c.** 2, 3
   b. 1, 3   **d.** 1, 2, 3

20. Coronary artery bypass grafts are performed using which type of vessels as the graft material?
   a. arteries   **c.** veins
   b. capillaries

21. The term *atherothrombic brain infarction* denotes:
   a. brain hemorrhage due to atherosclerosis
   b. infarction caused by thrombosis of a cerebral artery
   c. an embolism to the brain from a left heart thrombus

22. Symptoms associated with a cerebrovascular accident resulting from a cerebral embolism develop over a period of hours or days.
   a. true   **b.** false

23. Imaging procedures that may be used to demonstrate an abdominal aneurysm include:
   a. Angiography   **d.** a, b
   b. CT   **e.** a, b, c
   c. Diagnostic sonography

24. An aneurysm that results when the intima tears and allows blood to flow within the vessel wall is termed:

    a. dissecting   **c.** saccular

    b. fusiform

25. Inflammation of the vein is termed:

    a. phlebitis   **c.** venous thrombosis

    b. thrombophlebitis-

9

The Hemopoietic System

ANATOMY AND PHYSIOLOGY REVIEW

The hemopoietic system consists of blood, lymphatic tissue, bone marrow, and spleen. The circulating blood contains both plasma and blood cells with the plasma comprising approximately 55% of the total blood volume. The plasma is about 90% water and 10% solutes such as proteins, glucose, amino acids, and lipids. Three basic types of blood cells—erythrocytes, leukocytes, and thrombocytes (Table 9-1)—make up the remaining 45% of the total blood volume.

The *erythrocytes* or red blood cells are very small in relation to the other blood cells. They do not possess a nucleus and are shaped like biconcave disks. Erythrocytes are responsible for transporting oxygen and carbon dioxide to and from the various organs of the body. This is accomplished via the hemoglobin found in the erythrocytes, which

▼**Table 9-1**   Type of Blood Cell

Type	Formed by	Function	Life Span
Erythrocyte:	myeloid tissue within red bone marrow	transporting O_2 & CO_2	120 days
Leukocyte:	**Granular:** red bone marrow **Nongranular:** lymphatic tissue	body defense, immunity	**Granular:** 2 weeks **Nongranular:** years
Thrombocyte:	myeloid tissue within red bone marrow	blood clotting	10 days

allows oxygen or carbon dioxide molecules to attach to the cell for transport. Individuals with a hemoglobin level of less than 12 grams per 100 ml of blood are considered *anemic*. The total number of red blood cells is determined by a laboratory test termed *hematocrit*.

Erythrocytes are formed by specialized cells called *hemocytoblasts* that are located in the myeloid tissue found within red bone marrow. These cells live approximately 120 days and are phagocytosed by the *reticuloendothelial system*. The reticuloendothelial system consists of specialized cells in the liver, spleen, and bone marrow. During the phagocytosis, the iron within the hemoglobin is released and bilirubin is formed. The iron is used again in the development of new erythrocytes and the bilirubin is excreted in the bile.

Erythrocytes may contain various antigens that determine blood type. This is especially critical when performing blood transfusions because blood type incompatibility can have fatal results. Erythrocytes may contain no antigens, either the A or B antigen, or both the A and B antigen. The resulting blood types are "O" (no antigen), "A", "B", and "AB". If incompatible blood types are mixed (e.g., a type O patient receives type AB blood), the erythrocytes from the donor clump together in the serum of the recipient. Since the type O recipient does not possess the A or B antigen, antibodies are formed to fight against the foreign red blood cells. This is termed *agglutination*. Eventually the recipient destroys the donor erythrocytes with the rejection, possibly resulting in immediate shock. In some cases the reaction may be delayed, resulting in fever, pain, and ultimate renal failure as the kidneys try to excrete the by-products produced from the destruction of the erythrocytes. Cross-matching of blood types to eliminate the chance of a recipient receiving incompatible blood is essential. Type "O" blood is considered the universal donor, because it does not contain any antigens and can be given to anyone, regardless of blood type. Type "AB" is considered the universal recipient because it possesses both antigens and can receive any type of blood (Table 9-2). In addition, the Rh blood factor should also be considered. The *Rh factor* is termed such because it was first discovered in the blood of the rhesus monkey. Approximately 85% of the human population contains this factor and are classified as *Rh-positive*. Individuals not possessing the Rh factor are *Rh-negative*. The Rh factor becomes a problem in cases where an Rh-

▼**Table 9-2**   Cross-Matching of Blood Types

Recipient Blood Type	Acceptable Donor Type			
	A	B	AB	O†
A	yes	no	no	yes
B	no	yes	no	yes
AB*	yes	yes	yes	yes
O†	no	no	no	yes

*AB - Universal Recipient
†O - Universal Donor

positive father transmits the factor to a fetus carried by an Rh-negative mother. The first pregnancy generally progresses normally, but in subsequent pregnancies the mother builds anti-Rh antibodies that attack the fetal blood. This scenario can be avoided by Rh immunization of the mother before pregnancy.

Leukocytes or white blood cells may be classified as granular or nongranular. Granular leukocytes contain cytoplasmic granules and irregular nuclei. They are formed within the red bone marrow and include basophils, neutrophils, and eosinophils. The names of these cells correspond to the manner in which they respond to certain dyes for microscopic inspection. Nongranular leukocytes do not contain cytoplasmic granules and they possess regular nuclei. They are mainly formed in the lymphatic tissue of the spleen and include lymphocytes and monocytes. Leukocytes play an important role in the body's defense system. They are able to move out of capillaries into tissue to "attack" and phagocytose foreign substances. The life span varies of leukocytes depending on the type of cell. Granular leukocytes live for only about 2 weeks, whereas lymphocytes may live for years. Normal blood contains between 5000 to 9000 leukocytes per cubic milliliter. Changes in the number of leukocytes often indicate the presence of disease and are of clinical significance.

The lymphatic system is a subsystem of the circulatory system and comprises both lymphatic vessels and nodes. Lymphatic vessels contain a milky liquid substance termed *lymph*. The lymph nodes are small ovoid bodies attached in a chainlike pattern along the vessels. Major areas of lymph node chains include the neck, mediastinum, axillary, retroperitoneal, pelvic, and inguinal regions. These lymph nodes often become enlarged when the body is invaded by an infectious agent and in cases of neoplastic disease.

Mature *lymphocytes* are the most important cell in the development of immunity. T-lymphocytes are derived from the thymus gland and B-lymphocytes are derived from the bone marrow. These two types of lymphocytes work together with macrophages to ingest foreign substances and process the specific foreign antigens. Via a complex process, an antibody is formed capable of attacking the foreign antigen. An antibody is an immunoglobulin produced by plasma cells and can be categorized into one of five classifications: IgG, IgM, IgA, IgD, IgE. This is the systemic response that can have a negative effect on tissue grafts and organ transplants. The human body sees the transplant as foreign, therefore the lymphocytes and macrophages try to destroy the foreign antigens, resulting in rejection of the graft or organ.

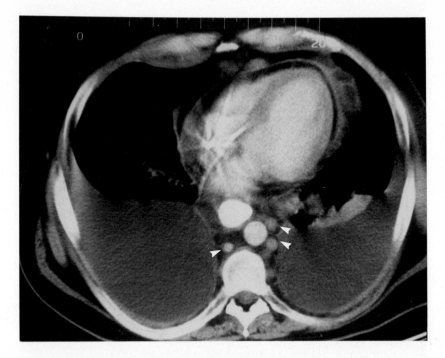

Fig. 9-1. CT of the lower chest/upper abdomen demonstrating enlargement of lymph nodes on a 27-year-old male with lymphoma. (Courtesy of The Ohio State University Hospitals, Columbus, Ohio.)

The third major type of blood cells are the *thrombocytes* or platelets. These cells are necessary for blood to clot properly and respond within seconds to initiate the coagulation process. The thrombocytes are also formed in the myeloid tissue within the red bone marrow and have a life span of approximately 10 days.

Although the risk of whole body radiation exposure is of little concern in diagnostic radiology, it is important for the radiographer to remember that exposure to X or gamma rays can have a harmful effect on the blood marrow and lymphoid tissue. It takes a whole body dose of approximately 50 to 75 rads to cause a detectable change in the blood cells. The most radiosensitive blood cells are the lymphocytes, followed by the leukocytes and thrombocytes.

IMAGING CONSIDERATIONS

Radiography plays a limited role in the diagnosis and treatment of hemopoietic disorders. Skeletal radiography may be used in cases of multiple myeloma and for some types of leukemia. Chest radiographs are helpful in identifying lymphatic changes within the mediastinum and various opportunistic infections associated with acquired immune deficiency syndrome (AIDS). Abdominal CT is also of great value in the assessment of lymph node enlargement (Fig. 9-1) and may be followed by lymphography to further determine the location and extent of neoplastic diseases of the lymphatic system. During lymphography initial radiographs or lymphangiogram films are taken immediately follow-

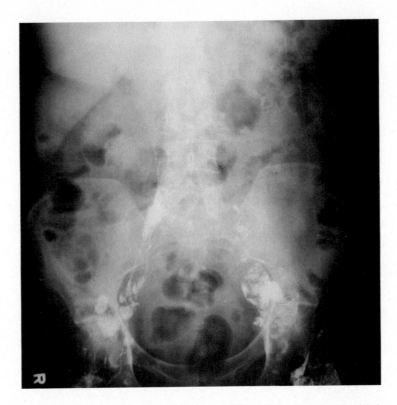

Fig. 9-2. 24-hour lymphadenogram on a 70-year-old female diagnosed with lymphosarcoma. (Courtesy of The Ohio State University Hospitals, Columbus, Ohio.)

ing the injection of contrast material to visualize the lymphatic vessels. The patient then returns in approximately 24 hours for additional radiographs, termed *lymphadenograms,* which visualize the lymph nodes (Fig. 9-2). MRI is a state of the art modality that is proving to be quite useful in imaging bone marrow and the diseases that affect the marrow. Although MRI produces a signal void in areas of compact bone, changes in the trabecular pattern are quite visible and useful in the diagnosis of many disorders (Fig. 9-3).

Many bloodborne pathogens may be transmitted to the health care worker. Therefore it is of utmost importance that radiographers always practice universal precautions in terms of blood and body fluids. Precautions must be taken when the radiographer may come into contact with blood or body fluids, and gloves should be worn whenever the possibility of contamination exists. Additional protective apparel may be necessary in cases in which large amounts of body fluids may be encountered. Needles should not be recapped; they should be placed in puncture-proof containers for hazardous waste disposal. Handwashing cannot be overemphasized, because it plays an important role in good infection control practices. It is the single most significant factor in infection control.

A

B

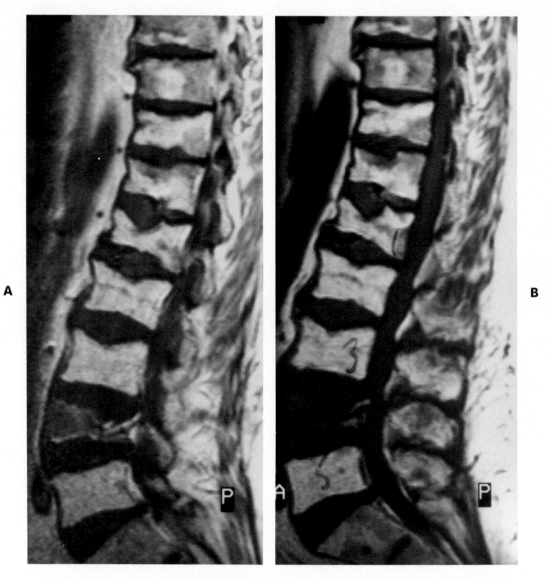

Fig. 9-3, *A.* A T2 weighted sagittal MRI view without gadolinium demonstrates an obvious L4 lesion. *B.* A T2 weighted sagittal MRI view with gadolinium demonstrates L4 destruction, consistent with multiple myeloma in this 55-year-old male. (Courtesy of Riverside Methodist Hospitals, Columbus, Ohio.)

ACQUIRED IMMUNE DEFICIENCY SYNDROME

Acquired immune deficiency syndrome (AIDS) was first recognized in 1981. It is caused by the *human immunodeficiency virus* (HIV) and acts to paralyze the normal immune mechanisms within the human body. This virus inhibits the body's response to the presence of a variety of diseases, thus one major sign of AIDS is the presence of unusual opportunistic infections such as *pneumocystis carinii, toxoplasma gondii, cryptococci, mycobacterium avium,* herpes, and Kaposi's sarcoma. Other signs/symptoms include generalized lymphadenopathy, malaise, fever, and weight loss. HIV may also affect the central nervous system resulting in apathy, memory loss, the inability to concentrate, and dementia.

AIDS is currently the greatest health crisis with no known cure and carries approximately a 90% mortality rate. HIV may lie dormant in an individual for years, however this does not happen in most patients. Emerging treatments are extending the life of individuals, hence the 90% mortality rate.

HIV most frequently affects homosexual and bisexual males and intravenous drug users. However, it can affect anyone, regardless of age or sexual persuasion. The virus is transmitted through sexual contact and exposure to infected blood and body fluids.

One of the most common life-threatening infections associated with AIDS is *pneu-*

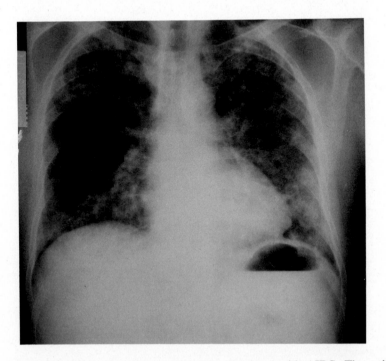

Fig. 9-4. Chest radiograph of a 53-year-old male diagnosed with AIDS. The radiograph demonstrates pneumocystis carinii pneumonia with diffuse bilateral airspace parenchymal infiltrative densities. (Courtesy of the American College of Radiology, Reston, Virginia.)

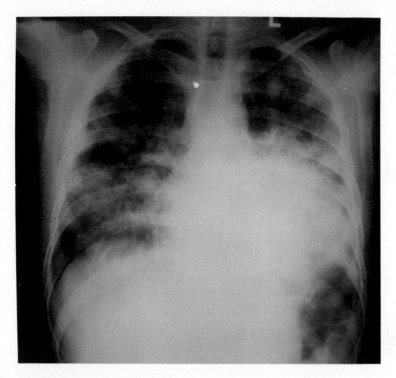

Fig. 9-5. Chest radiograph of a 27-year-old male with Kaposi sarcoma of the skin and pulmonary involvement showing nodular diffuse patchy parenchymal infiltration with nodular densities in the upper lobes. (Courtesy of the American College of Radiology, Reston, Virginia.)

mocystis carinii pneumonia often in combination with a cytomegalovirus. It occurs in over half of all AIDS patients. Chest radiographs (Fig. 9-4) reveal bilateral perihilar reticular-interstitial infiltrates that rapidly progress within 3 to 5 days to diffuse consolidation.

Kaposi's sarcoma is present in approximately 25% to 30% of AIDS patients and may affect the connective tissue in various sites within the body. It most often affects the skin, the lymph nodes, and gastrointestinal system. About 20% of patients with Kaposi's sarcoma also demonstrate pulmonary involvement. Radiographically the patients present with hilar adenopathy, nodular pulmonary infiltrates, and pleural effusion (Fig. 9-5).

NEOPLASTIC DISEASE
Multiple Myeloma

Multiple myeloma is a neoplastic disease of the plasma cells that results in cell proliferation. It is usually confined to the bone marrow and forms discrete tumors that weaken the affected bone. Multiple myeloma most frequently affects the pelvis, spine, ribs, and skull. The abnormal plasma cells produce large amounts of protein, specifically the immunoglobulins, which create a variety of problems in addition to skeletal involvement. This

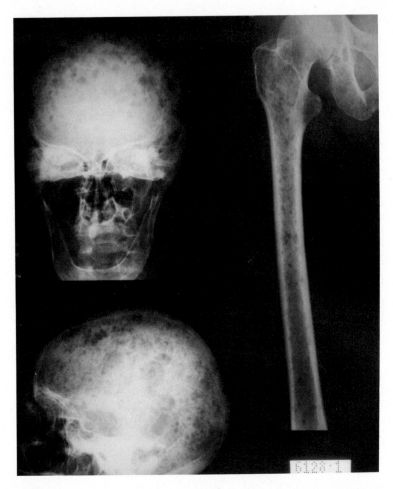

Fig. 9-6. Radiographs of a 65-year-old male with multiple myeloma demonstrating the presence of innumerable, discrete, lytic, well-circumscribed skeletal defects. (Courtesy of the American College of Radiology, Reston, Virginia.)

protein is excreted via the urine and disrupts normal renal function. The protein can be detected in both the blood and urine.

Signs/symptoms of multiple myeloma include progressive bone pain, anemia, fatigue, bleeding disorders, renal insufficiency/failure, hypercalcemia, and recurrent bacterial infections, especially pneumococcal pneumonia. Radiography plays a vital role in the diagnosis and treatment of multiple myeloma because skeletal radiographs will demonstrate diffuse osteoporosis with discrete osteolytic regions (Fig. 9-6). Chemotherapy and palliative radiation therapy may be prescribed, but the prognosis is poor because as the disease progresses it leads to multiple bone lesions, renal failure, and infections. The median survival of patients with multiple myeloma is approximately 2 to 3 years.

Leukemia

Leukemia is a term associated with neoplastic disease of leukocytes that results in an overproduction of white blood cells. This increase in leukocytes interferes with normal blood cell production and may lead to anemia, bleeding, and infection. Leukemias can infiltrate lymphatic tissue and organs such as the liver and spleen. The cause of leukemia is unknown, but certain risk factors such as exposure to irradiation and certain chemicals (especially benzene) seem to predispose individuals to developing this disorder.

Leukemias are classified according to cell type and cell maturity. Granulocytic or myelocytic leukemias develop from primitive or stem cells. Monocytic leukemias develop from precursor cells (the cells from which leukocytes are derived) and are the least common type of leukemia. Lymphocytic leukemias arise from lymphoid cells. Additionally, leukemias are classified as either acute or chronic. Acute leukemias have an abrupt onset and may present as a hemorrhagic episode. They generally are associated with primitive or poorly differentiated cells. Chronic leukemias progress at a relatively slow pace with nonspecific signs such as fatigue and weakness. They are associated with mature or well-differentiated cells. These terms are used in combination to describe the specific type of leukemia. Acute lymphocytic leukemia (ALL) predominantly affects children. Chronic lymphocytic leukemia (CLL) predominantly affects individuals over the age of 50 years. Chronic myelocytic leukemia (CML), also called chronic granulocytic leukemia (CGL), most often affects adults between the ages of 20 to 50 years. Acute myelocytic leukemia (AML) and acute monoblastic leukemia (AMOL) can affect anyone at any age. Leukemias, in general, account for approximately 33% of all cancer deaths in children under the age of 15 years.

In many cases, proper therapy can stop the pathologic process. Regardless of the type of leukemia, all forms require the destruction of cells by either radiation or antileukemic drug therapy that renders the patient severely immunosuppressed. In some cases bone marrow transplants may be attempted. Most patients with acute leukemias die within 6 months without treatment. More than 90% of acute lymphocytic leukemias carry a 5-year remission rate of 50% or better following treatment. Acute myelocytic and acute monoblastic leukemias result in 70% to 85% remission following treatment. In all cases, survival depends on complete remission. Chronic granulocytic leukemia, however, is progressive with an average survival of about 3 to 4 years following the onset of the disease and carries a 5-year survival rate of approximately 20%.

Radiography plays a limited role in the diagnosis and treatment of most leukemias. Diagnostic medical ultrasound and CT are of value in assessing lymphatic disease. Additionally, lymphography (Fig. 9-7, p. 345) may be helpful in staging the disease.

Hodgkin's Disease

Hodgkin's disease is another neoplastic disease affecting the lymphoid tissue and is a type of lymphoma. It has an unknown etiology, commonly affects individuals between the ages of 20 to 40 years, and tends to affect males slightly more often than females. Common signs and symptoms associated with Hodgkin's disease are general malaise, fever, anorexia, and enlarged lymph nodes. Mediastinal lymph nodes are often visible on a chest radiograph and definite diagnosis is made via biopsy of the lymphatic tissue. Specific cells termed *Reed-Sternberg cells* differentiate Hodgkin's lymphomas from other types of lymphatic disease. As with other neoplastic disorders, Hodgkin's disease is staged ac-

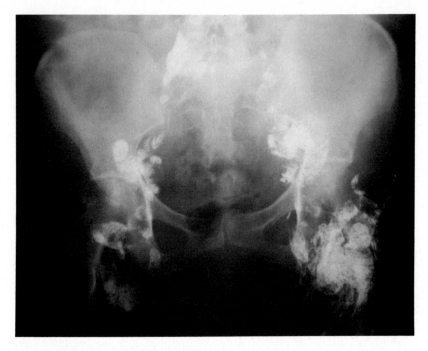

Fig. 9-7. Lymphogram of a 70-year-old female with lymphosarcoma. Notice the enlarged lymph nodes with partial obstruction of the left channels at the hip area and extravasation of contrast material. (Courtesy of The Ohio State University Hospitals, Columbus, Ohio.)

cording to the extent of the disease. Stage I denotes one anatomic node location versus Stage IV, which denotes extranodal spread to the bone marrow, the lungs, or the liver. There are four histoplastic types of Hodgkin's lymphomas with the prognosis varying with the type.

Hodgkin's disease is most commonly treated with a combination of radiation and chemotherapy. Stage I Hodgkin's lymphoma is associated with a 5-year survival rate of 90%. Stage IV Hodgkin's disease only boasts approximately a 20%, 5-year survival rate. The overall prognosis is associated with a 5-year survival rate of approximately 42%. Again, ultrasound, computed tomography, lymphography, and nuclear medicine studies are of value in staging the disease.

▼ QUESTIONS

1. The portion of the blood comprising the majority of blood volume is the:
   a. erythrocytes
   b. leukocytes
   c. plasma
   d. thrombocytes

2. Red blood cells are also termed:
   a. erythrocytes
   b. leukocytes
   c. platelets
   d. thrombocytes

3. Myeloid tissue may be found in:
   a. red bone marrow   **b.** yellow bone marrow

4. Bilirubin is formed during the destruction of:
   a. erythrocytes   **c.** plastocytes
   b. leukocytes   **d.** thrombocytes

5. Which type of blood is considered to be a "universal donor?"
   a. A   **c.** AB
   b. B   **d.** O

6. Granular leukocytes include:
   1. basophils
   2. eosinophils
   3. neutrophils
      a. 1,2   **c.** 2,3
      b. 1,3   **d.** 1,2,3

7. Which type of cells are most important in the development of immunity?
   a. erythrocytes   **c.** platelets
   b. lymphocytes   **d.** thrombocytes

8. Acquired immune deficiency is caused by what type of virus?
   a. AIDS   **c.** pneumococcal
   b. HIV   **d.** Kaposi

9. Which type of pneumonia is commonly associated with AIDS?
   a. pneumococcal   **c.** streptococcal
   b. pneumocystic carinii **d.** all of the above

10. Kaposi's sarcoma is frequently associated with AIDS, and it may affect the:
    a. gastrointestinal system   **c.** skin
    b. lymph nodes   **d.** all of the above

11. One neoplastic disease of the plasma is:
    a. Hodgkin's disease   **c.** lymphoma
    b. leukemia   **d.** multiple myeloma

12. Which type of leukemia predominately affects children?
    a. acute lymphocytic   **c.** chronic myelocytic
    b. chronic lymphocytic   **d.** acute myelocytic

13. Leukemias associated with mature or well-differentiated cells are classified as:
    a. acute   **b.** chronic

14. Reed-Sternberg cells are associated with what type of neoplastic disease?
    a. leukemia   —   **c.** multiple myeloma
    b. Hodgkin's disease   **d.** uremia

15. Hodgkin's disease affects what type of blood cells?
    a. erythrocytes   **c.** plastocytes
    b. lymphocytes   **d.** thrombocytes

10

$$\blacktriangledown$$
$$\blacktriangleleft$$
$$\blacktriangledown$$
$$\blacktriangledown$$
$$\blacktriangleleft$$
$$\blacktriangledown$$

The Central
Nervous System

▼

Upon completion of Chapter 10, the reader should be able to:

- Describe the anatomical components of the central nervous system (CNS) and their general function.
- Discuss the role of the various imaging modalities in evaluation of the CNS, particularly magnetic resonance imaging (MRI) and computed tomography (CT).
- Discuss common congenital anomalies of the CNS.
- Characterize a given condition as inflammatory, degenerative, or neoplastic.
- Identify the pathogenesis of the pathologies cited, and typical treatments for them.
- Describe, in general, the radiographic appearance of each of the given pathologies, as possible, or alternative means of imaging.

ANATOMY AND PHYSIOLOGY REVIEW

The central nervous system (CNS) comprises the brain and the spinal cord. It is composed of neurons (nerve cells) and neuroglia (the interstitial tissue). The CNS extends peripherally through nerves that carry motor messages through efferent nerves to the muscles and sensory messages from the skin and elsewhere back to the spinal cord and brain through afferent nerves. This chapter will concentrate on conditions involving the brain and spinal cord.

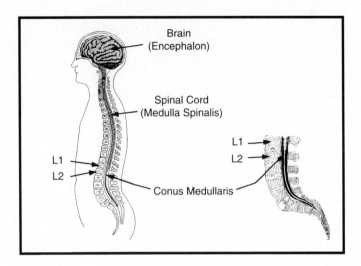

Fig. 10-1. Central nervous system. (From Bontrager KL: *Radiographic positioning and related anatomy,* ed 3, St Louis 1993, Mosby.)

The brain consists of the cerebrum (right and left hemispheres), cerebellum, diencephalon (including the hypothalamus), and the brain stem. The brain stem, composed of the midbrain, pons, and the medulla oblongata, serves to connect the cerebrum with the spinal cord. The innumerable motor and sensory nerves pass through the brain stem into the spinal cord. The spinal cord originates as an extension of the medulla oblongata at the foramen magnum in the base of the skull. It extends to approximately the level of the second or third lumbar vertebra to terminate with a cone-shaped area called the conus medullaris (Fig. 10-1). Spinal nerves beyond this point are referred to as the cauda equina.

Both the brain and the spinal cord are invested by the meninges, which consist of three distinct layers (Fig. 10-2, p.350). The dura mater is the outermost and is tough and fibrous in nature. It has three major extensions: the falx cerebri, which divides the cerebral hemispheres; the falx cerebelli, which similarly divides the cerebellar hemispheres; and the tentorium cerebelli, which separates the occipital lobe of the cerebrum from the cerebellum. The arachnoid is the middle layer of the meninges and has the appearance of cobwebs. The pia mater is innermost and adheres directly to the cortex of the brain and the spinal cord. The subarachnoid space, at its deepest at the base of the brain, is located between the arachnoid and the pia mater. It is filled with cerebrospinal fluid (CSF) to continuously bathe the brain and spinal cord with nutrients and to cushion it against shocks and blows. CSF is secreted by the choroid plexi, a network of capillaries located in the brain's ventricles.

The ventricles are four interconnected cavities within the brain. As noted, they house the choroid plexi that serves to secrete CSF. The right and left lateral ventricles are located in their respective cerebral hemispheres (Fig. 10-3, *A* and *B*, p. 350). They may

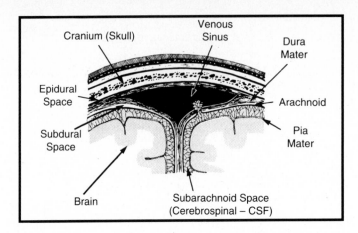

Fig. 10-2. Coronal perspective of meninges and meningeal spaces. (From Bontrager KL: *Radiographic positioning and related anatomy,* ed 3, St Louis 1993, Mosby.)

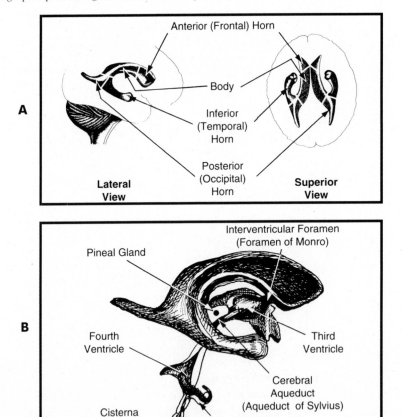

Fig. 10-3, *A.* Lateral and superior views of the lateral ventricles. *B.* A lateral view of the ventricular system. (From Bontrager KL: *Radiographic positioning and related anatomy,* ed 3, St Louis 1993, Mosby.)

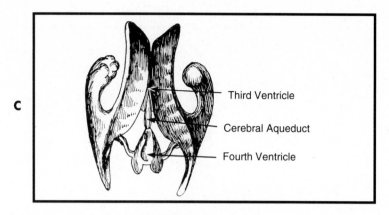

C

Third Ventricle

Cerebral Aqueduct

Fourth Ventricle

Fig. 10-3, C. A superior view of the ventricular system. (From Bontrager KL: *Radiographic positioning and related anatomy,* ed 3, St Louis 1993, Mosby.)

be further divided into anterior, posterior, and inferior horns, as well as a body and a trigone. CSF flows from the lateral ventricles into the third ventricle via interventricular foramina (of Monroe). The third and fourth ventricles are midline structures connected to each other by the cerebral aqueduct (Fig. 10-3, C). From there it flows through a median and two lateral foramina (Magendie and Lushka, respectively) into the subarachnoid space surrounding the brain and the spinal cord.

Most of the brain's blood is supplied anteriorly via the bilateral carotid arteries and posteriorly via the bilateral vertebral arteries. After entering the cranial vault through the foramen magnum, the vertebral arteries converge to form the basilar artery. The basilar artery and portions of the internal carotid arteries form the Circle of Willis (Fig. 10-4, p. 352) to distribute oxygenated, arterial blood through various branches to all parts of the brain. Venous blood is returned to large venous sinuses in the dura mater, which ultimately drain into the internal jugular veins (Fig. 10-5, p. 352).

The capillaries that connect the arteries and veins function somewhat differently in the brain than in other organs. Here, they serve to prevent the passage of unwanted substances into the brain through a special function called the *blood-brain barrier.* This is accomplished in a number of ways but especially as a result of these capillaries having a very tight junction that prevents macromolecules and fluids from leaking out into the brain parenchyma. This protects the brain by keeping toxins out, yet it allows removal of the waste products of brain metabolism. These specialized capillaries are found everywhere in the brain except for the pineal and pituitary glands and the choroid plexus. The significance of the blood-brain barrier in terms of imaging is that contrast media enhancement in the brain occurs only where the barrier breaks down from ischemia or neoplastic growth (with its new vascularity). Also, glucose readily passes over this barrier and is the primary agent used so far in positron emission tomography (PET) scanning.

While the intervertebral disks are not part of the CNS, they often impact on it when they rupture and impinge on adjacent spinal nerves. Disks serve to cushion movement of the vertebral column. They comprise a tough outer covering, known as the *annulus fibrosus,* and a pulpy center, called the *nucleus pulposus* (Fig. 10-6, p. 353).

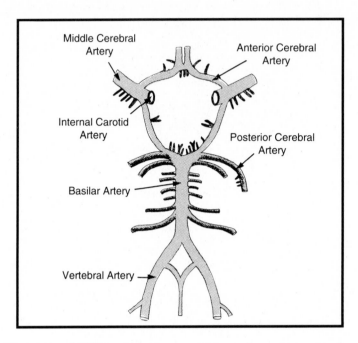

Fig. 10-4. The circle of Willis. (From Bontrager KL: *Radiographic positioning and related anatomy,* ed 3, St Louis 1993, Mosby.)

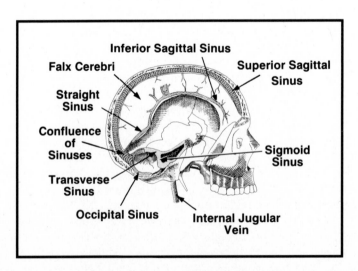

Fig. 10-5. Dura mater sinuses and venous drainage of the brain. (From Bontrager KL: *Radiographic positioning and related anatomy,* ed 3, St Louis 1993, Mosby.)

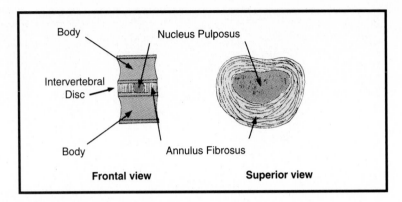

Fig. 10-6. An intervertebral disk. (From Bontrager KL: *Radiographic positioning and related anatomy,* ed 3, St Louis 1993, Mosby.)

IMAGING CONSIDERATIONS

Radiographic demonstration of the various cranial structures can provide information important in evaluation of the CNS. Its role, however, has largely been reduced to evaluation of cranial trauma because of the rapid ascent of MRI and continued refinements in CT. Other studies important in evaluation of the CNS include angiography, sonography, nuclear medicine, and PET scanning.

Beside the visualization of fractures caused by trauma as described in Chapter 2, plain skull films may also reveal normal variants. Blood vessels such as the middle meningeal artery commonly cause radiolucent impressions on the inner table of the cranial vault (Fig. 10-7, p. 354). Their linear progression and bilateral appearance help distinguish them from fractures. Visualization of an enlarged or deformed pituitary fossa can provide information concerning the presence of a pituitary tumor and/or increased intracranial pressure (Fig. 10-8, p. 354). A calcified pineal gland situated in the midline may be seen on about 60% of all plain skull films (Fig. 10-9, p. 355). Its displacement can indicate the presence of a pathologic lesion if it is greater than 2 to 3 mm. The choroid plexus (Fig. 10-10, p. 355), falx cerebri (Fig. 10-11, p. 356), and falx cerebelli, may also be calcified.

The role of plain films in evaluation of the spine was described in Chapter 2. A number of conditions that impact on the spinal cord can readily be demonstrated. The fluoroscopic procedure of myelography has been a staple of radiology for years, allowing for visualization of conditions (such as herniated disks) that impinge on the spinal cord. Its role, however, is greatly diminishing because of the significant specificity of MRI.

MRI has emerged as the modality of choice for a wide variety of conditions related to the CNS (Fig. 10-12, pp. 356–357). Its sensitivity is excellent in evaluation of all types of spinal disease, including tumors and disk disease. The ability of MRI to evaluate brain tumors and conditions such as stroke, cranial tumors, and infection surpasses that of CT. Evaluation of demyelinating disease such as multiple sclerosis is substantively enhanced by MRI. Although evolving rapidly in technology, it currently has only a small role in evaluation of trauma, mainly as limited to evaluation of spinal cord compression.

Text continued on p. 358.

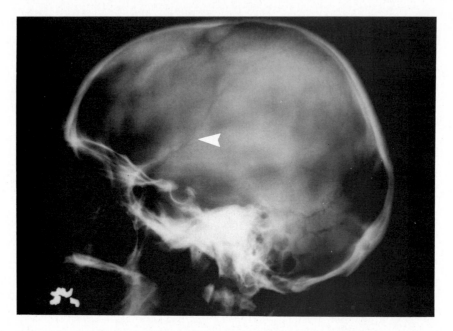

Fig. 10-7. Normal appearance of the middle meningeal artery as indicated on this lateral skull radiograph. (Courtesy of the American College of Radiology, Reston, Virginia.)

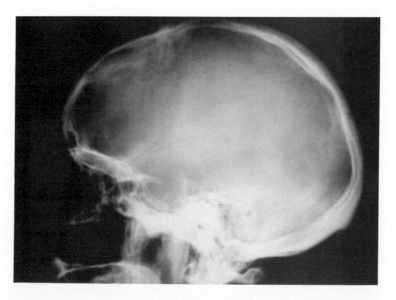

Fig. 10-8. An enlarged sella turcica on this lateral skull radiograph evidences a pituitary macroadenoma. (Courtesy of the American College of Radiology, Reston, Virginia.)

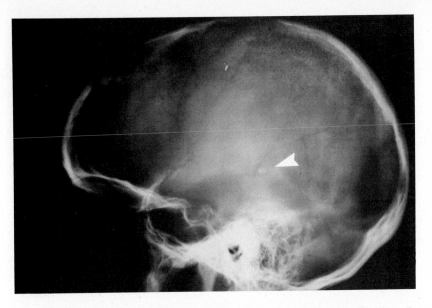

Fig. 10-9. Normal calcification of the pineal gland as seen on this lateral skull radiograph of a 44-year-old male. (Courtesy of the American College of Radiology, Reston, Virginia.)

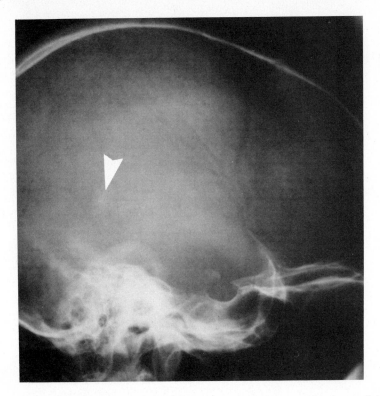

Fig. 10-10. Normal calcification of the choroid plexus in the posterior horn of the lateral ventricle as seen in this lateral skull radiograph of a 60-year-old female. (Courtesy of the American College of Radiology, Reston, Virginia.)

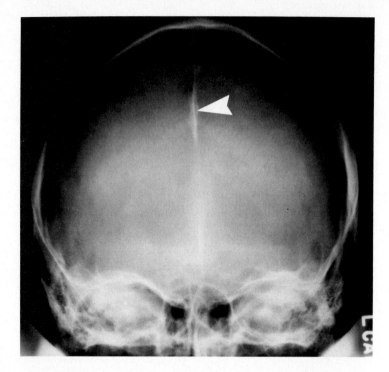

Fig. 10-11. Normal calcification of the falx cerebri as seen in this PA skull projection of a 59-year-old male. (Courtesy of the American College of Radiology, Reston, Virginia.)

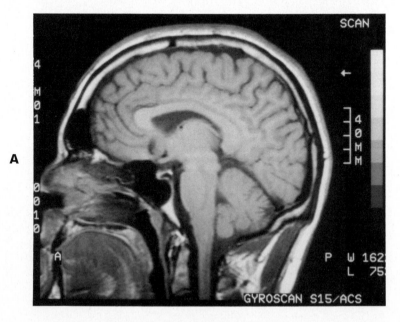

Fig. 10-12, *A.* Normal MRI of a young female with a history of seizures as seen in a sagittal, T1 weighted view without gadolinium contrast. (Courtesy of Riverside Methodist Hospitals, Columbus, Ohio.)

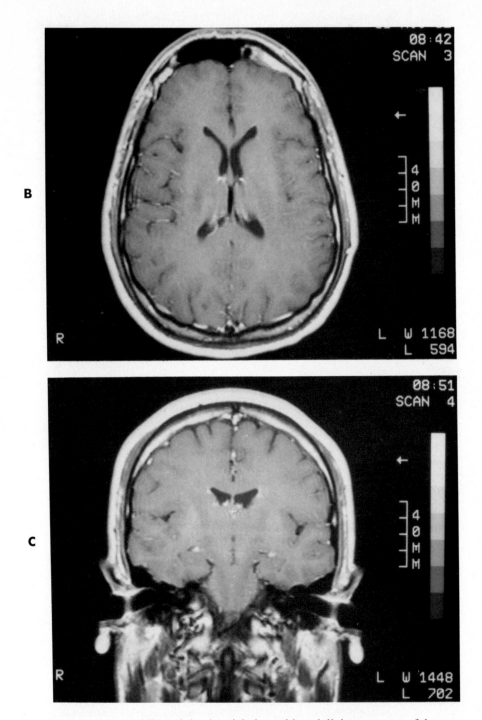

Fig. 10-12, *B.* A normal T1 weighted, axial view with gadolinium contrast of the same patient. *C.* A normal T1 weighted, coronal view with gadolinium contrast of the same patient. (Courtesy of Riverside Methodist Hospitals, Columbus, Ohio.)

CT continues to play a significant role in evaluation of the CNS. It is rapid, noninvasive, safe, and quite accurate. CT is particularly useful in evaluation of cerebral bleeding post-trauma because it readily reveals the extent of any hematoma present. Other related roles include any kind of routine anatomic evaluation as might be seen in assessment of shunt functioning or the sinuses (as discussed in Chapter 3). Postmyelographic CT of the spine is also fairly prevalent but is decreasing with the more widespread use of MRI. CT is also used to evaluate vertebral fractures as bony detail is not seen as well on MRI.

Other modalities used to evaluate the CNS include angiography, ultrasound, nuclear medicine, and PET scanning. As elsewhere in the body, angiography is used to study the vasculature. A variety of conditions involving cerebral circulation can have wide effects on the brain, as discussed in Chapter 9. Ultrasound is useful in evaluating the brain of neonates before closure of the fontanelles, because the fibrous tissue covering the fontanelles provides a ready "window" into the brain. It is also useful intraoperatively in evaluation of tumors and guidance for shunt placement (Fig. 10-13). New efforts are being made to apply ultrasound to assessment of blood flow through the intracranial parts of the carotid arteries. In nuclear medicine, technetium-labelled flow agents are being used in combination with SPECT (single positron emission computed tomography) to assess tumors, areas of stroke and ischemia, and Alzheimer's disease (Fig. 10-14). The brain scan, once a staple of nuclear medicine, has yielded completely to CT. PET scanning allows imaging of the body's normal chemical processes and provides physiologic evaluation (Fig. 10-15, p. 360) to complement the more traditional anatomic evaluation of other modalities. Significant cost-benefit issues arise in its use and may ultimately limit its usefulness.

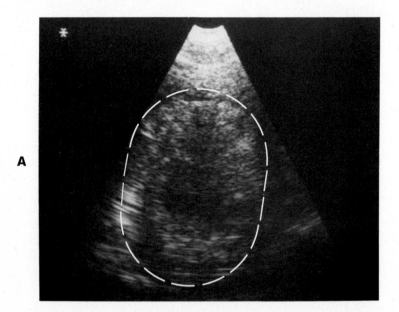

Fig. 10-13, *A.* Intraoperative ultrasound of brain tumor (glioblastoma) in a 61-year-old male showing the tumor size and location in a transverse plane for the operating surgeon. (Courtesy of Riverside Methodist Hospitals, Columbus, Ohio.)

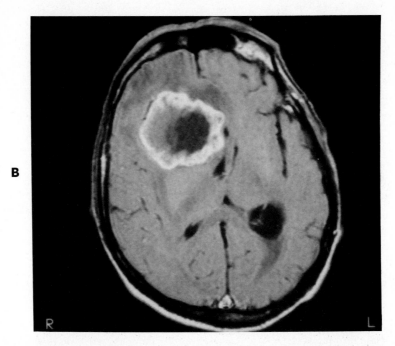

Fig. 10-13, *B.* A T1 weighted axial MRI view with contrast demonstrates the same lesion, with the *arrow* indicating the later point of entry for the operating surgeon. (Courtesy of Riverside Methodist Hospitals, Columbus, Ohio.)

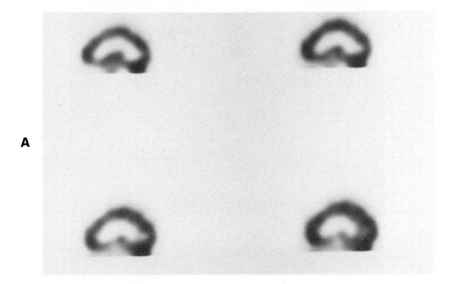

Fig. 10-14, *A.* Transaxial views of the head of a 77-year-old female seen on a SPECT scan reveal no pathology. (Courtesy of Riverside Methodist Hospitals, Columbus, Ohio.)

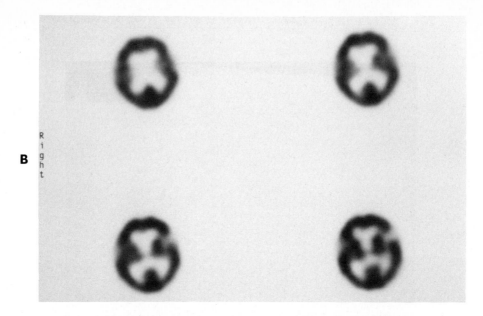

Fig. 10-14, *B.* Lateral views of the head from the same SPECT scan. (Courtesy of Riverside Methodist Hospitals, Columbus, Ohio.)

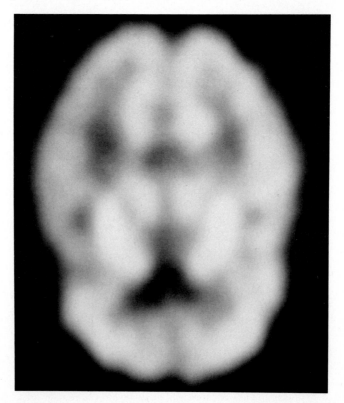

Fig. 10-15. An axial image from a PET scan demonstrating an infarct in the posterior left parieto-temporal region, with shunting of blood to hypermetabolic basal ganglia. (Courtesy of The Christ Hospital, Cincinnati, Ohio.)

CONGENITAL/HEREDITARY DISEASES
Meningomyelocele

As mentioned in Chapter 2, spina bifida is a condition in which the bony neural arch that encloses and protects the spinal cord is not completely closed. This most commonly occurs in the lumbar region, and the spinal cord and its meninges may or may not herniate through the resultant opening. Complications depend on the extent of protrusion and range from treatable to life threatening. Any opening of the sac to the exterior of the body risks meningeal infection, so surgical closure is critical. If only the meninges protrude, the condition is termed a *meningocele* (Fig. 10-16, p. 362). These are treated surgically without difficulty, and usually with an excellent prognosis. A *myelocele* is protrusion of the spinal cord, which may be treatable surgically. Supportive measures such as physical therapy may be used to correct deficits. A *meningomyelocele* is the most serious of possible conditions and consists of a protrusion of both the meninges and the spinal cord into the skin of the back (Fig. 10-17, p. 363 and 10-18, p. 364). These patients often present with severe neurologic deficit, the extent of which depends on the level of herniation. Associated neurologic difficulties include paraplegia and control of the lower limbs, bladder, and bowel. Hydrocephalus occurs in most of these patients. Medical management of bladder and bowel problems is possible, and other supportive measures are used as well for those who survive.

Hydrocephalus

CSF normally flows around the spinal cord and over the convexity of the brain before resorption into the venous sinuses. This normal circulation can be interrupted by causes including an obstruction to flow and impaired absorption; increased CSF production can also disturb the normal circulation. As a result, the ventricles distend proximal to the site of obstruction, resulting in compression atrophy of the brain tissue around the dilated ventricles. *Hydrocephalus* refers to an excessive accumulation of CSF within the ventricles and can be either congenital in nature (such as aqueduct stenosis) or acquired.

In *noncommunicating* hydrocephalus, an obstruction can result congenitally or from tumor growth, trauma, and inflammation. It interferes with or blocks the normal CSF circulation from the ventricles to the subarachnoid space. Poor resorption of CSF by the arachnoid villi results in *communicating* hydrocephalus. This can arise from a number of factors, including increased intracranial pressure caused by tumor compression, raised intrathoracic pressure impairing venous drainage, inflammation from meningitis, or following a subarachnoid hemorrhage. Hydrocephalus can also occur from overproduction of CSF, although this is the least common cause.

CT provides excellent visualization of this disorder (Fig. 10-19, p. 365). Before its advent, pneumoencephalography was used to visualize air in the ventricles and demonstrate their size. In neonates, sonography is used to demonstrate the ventricular system through the infant's fontanelles, which permit passage of the beam until their eventual closure. Treatment may consist of surgery and use of a *shunt,* an artificial passageway to divert excess fluids. Placed between the ventricles and either the internal jugular vein, the heart, or the peritoneum, it drains excess CSF. Radiographs are taken to demonstrate shunt placement after insertion, and CT is used to follow-up on a periodic basis to evaluate patency.

Text continued on p. 366.

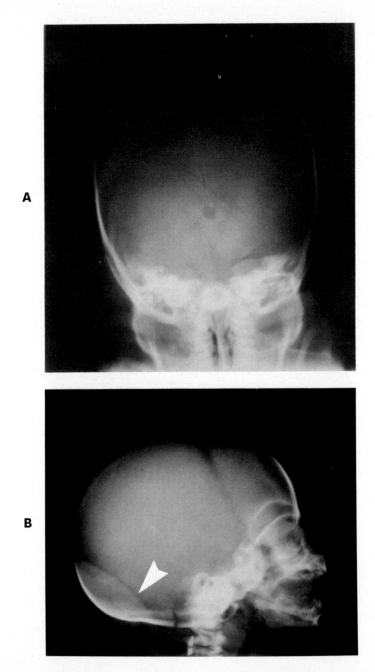

Fig. 10-16, *A.* Circular defect seen in the middle of the occipital bone of this newborn is the site of a meningocele. *B.* A lateral skull radiograph demonstrates the soft tissue density associated with the meningocele superimposed over the occipital bone. (Courtesy of the American College of Radiology, Reston, Virginia.)

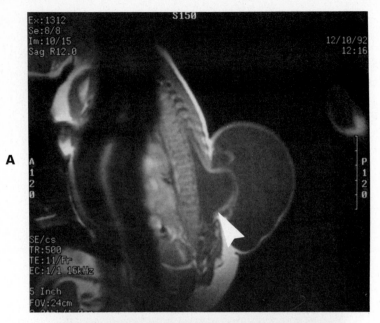

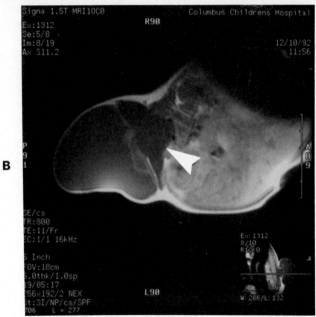

Fig. 10-17, *A.* A T1 weighted sagittal MRI view without gadolinium in this newborn readily demonstrates a meningomyelocele, with the *arrow* indicating the herniated spinal cord. *B.* A T1 weighted axial MRI view without gadolinium of the same patient similarly demonstrates the meningomyelocele, with the *arrow* indicating the herniated spinal cord. (Courtesy of Children's Hospital, Columbus, Ohio.)

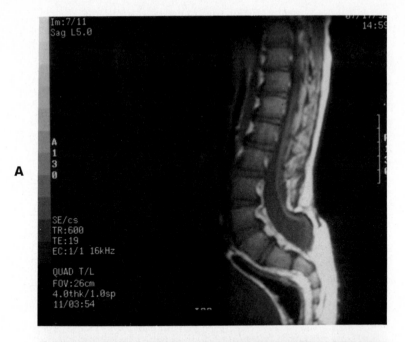

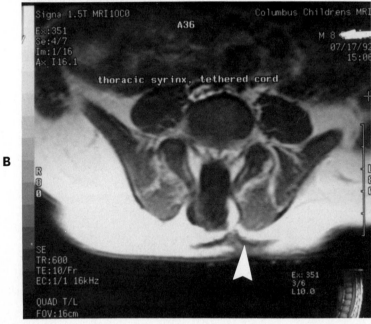

Fig. 10-18, *A.* A T1 weighted sagittal MRI view without gadolinium in this infant demonstrates a surgically repaired meningomyelocele. *B.* A T1 weighted axial MRI view without gadolinium similarly demonstrates the surgically repaired meningomyelocele, with the *arrow* pointing to the surgical site. (Courtesy of Children's Hospital, Columbus, Ohio.)

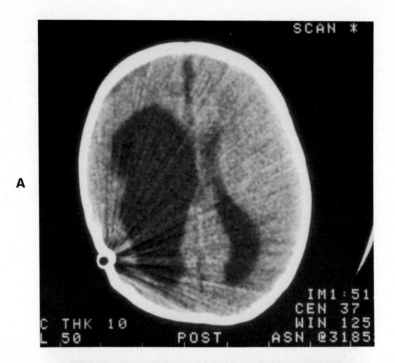

A

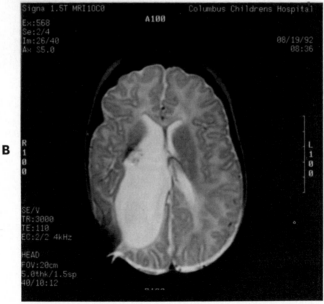

B

Fig. 10-19, *A.* Hydrocephalus as seen on this transverse CT view of a 6-month-old female with only mild dilatation of the left ventricle. Streaking artifacts originate from the shunt being checked for placement. *B.* A T2 weighted axial MRI view without gadolinium demonstrates the hydrocephalus in the same patient. (Courtesy of Children's Hospital, Columbus, Ohio.)

INFLAMMATORY DISEASE
Meningitis

An inflammation of the meningeal coverings of the brain and spinal cord is termed *meningitis*. It can be caused by bacteria, viruses, or other organisms that reach the meninges from elsewhere in the body via blood or lymph, as a result of trauma and penetrating wounds, or from adjacent structures (e.g., the mastoids) that become infected. Bacterial infection is the most common cause of meningitis (Fig. 10-20).

CSF is under increased pressure in cases of meningitis and can contribute to hydrocephalus. While radiologic imaging can show the changes associated with meningitis, the primary means of diagnosing it is the increased intracranial pressure detectable via the results of a spinal tap. Other signs and symptoms of meningitis include headache, neck stiffness, and fever. Antibiotics in particular have been greatly successful against many forms of meningitis.

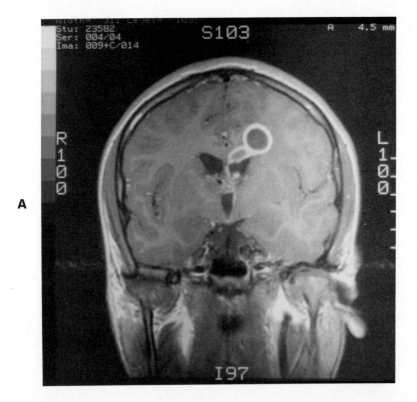

Fig. 10-20, *A.* A T1 weighted coronal MRI view with gadolinium demonstrates a ring lesion that communicates with the left lateral ventricle in this 17-year-old male, creating meningitis as a result of transplantation into the brain of a bacterial (staph) infection. (Courtesy of Riverside Methodist Hospitals, Columbus, Ohio.)

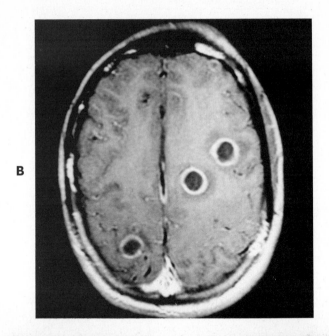

B

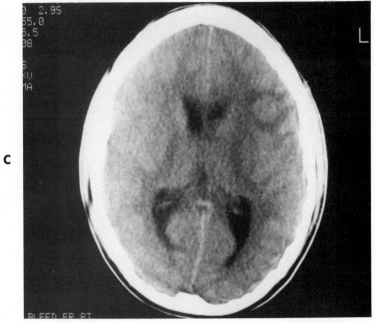

C

Fig. 10-20, *B.* A T1 weighted axial MRI view with gadolinium of the same patient demonstrates the presence of multiple infectious lesions. *C.* An axial CT view of the same patient demonstrates the presence of an infectious lesion as well as slightly widened ventricles, as characteristic with meningitis. (Courtesy of Riverside Methodist Hospitals, Columbus, Ohio.)

Encephalitis

An infection of the brain tissue is termed *encephalitis*. Usually viral in nature (Fig. 10-21), it may also occur subsequent to conditions such as chickenpox, smallpox, influenza, measles, and others. A condition even more serious than meningitis, individuals who acquire encephalitis may develop permanent neurologic disabilities. In some instances it may even be fatal because there is no specific treatment for it.

Degenerative Disk Disease

Gradual, degenerative changes of the spine associated with aging can result in rupture of the annulus fibrosus of the intervertebral disk. Pressure may be placed on the spinal cord by the nucleus pulposus spreading beyond its normal confines (Fig. 10-22). Pain is felt along the course of adjacent nerve roots, and muscles supplied are weakened. The most common locations for this to occur are in the cervical and lumbar regions. Compression of the nerve root may be demonstrated through myelography, CT, and MRI. Treatment is, at least initially, conservative and includes bed rest, possible traction, and pain relief. Surgical alternatives include laminectomy and spinal fusion.

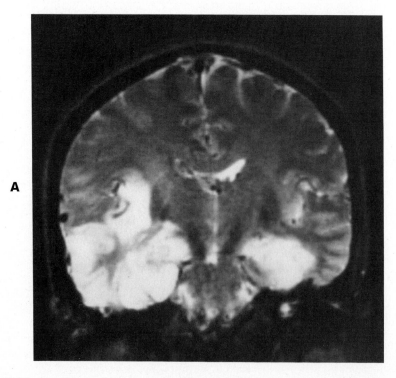

Fig. 10-21, *A.* A T2 weighted coronal MRI view demonstrates the infectious response in the brain of this young male with herpes encephalitis. (Courtesy of Riverside Methodist Hospitals, Columbus, Ohio.)

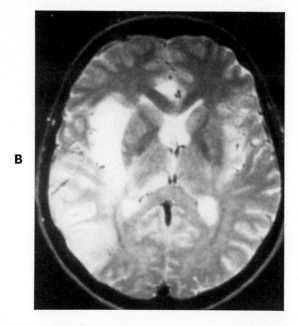

B

Fig. 10-21, *B.* A T2 weighted axial MRI view demonstrates the extent of the infectious process in the same patient with herpes encephalitis. (Courtesy of Riverside Methodist Hospitals, Columbus, Ohio.)

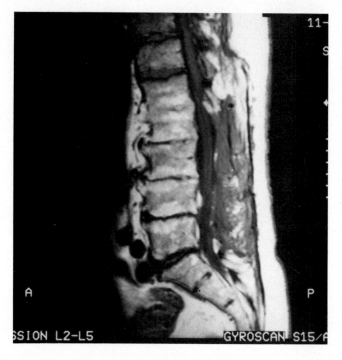

Fig. 10-22. T1 weighted sagittal MRI view of the spine in this 75-year-old male readily demonstrates severe degenerative disk disease as well as fusion of L1 and L2. (Courtesy of Riverside Methodist Hospitals, Columbus, Ohio.)

Cervical Spondylosis

Osteoarthritic conditions may also affect the vertebral column, leading to nerve disorders caused by chronic nerve root compression. These osteoarthritic changes of the neck are referred to as *cervical spondylosis* and are readily visible radiographically. Osteophytes (spurs) form in the articular facets of the cervical vertebrae and compress the nerves located in the intervertebral foramina. They may also compress the spinal cord (Fig. 10-23). MRI excels at visualization of spinal cord compression as a result of cervical spondylosis. As with degenerative disk disease, treatment is conservative at first but may include laminectomy and decompression procedures.

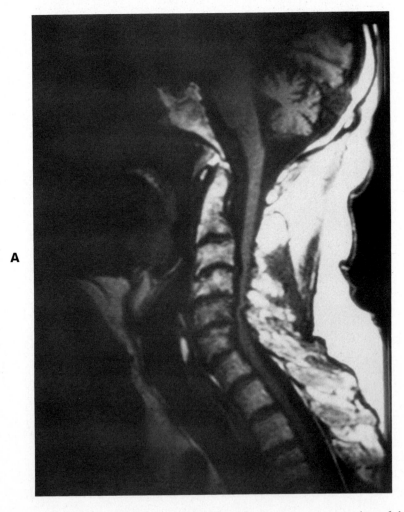

A

Fig. 10-23, *A.* A T1 weighted sagittal MRI view demonstrates compression of the spinal cord in this elderly male with cervical spondylosis. CSF is dark adjacent to the gray spinal cord. (Courtesy of Riverside Methodist Hospitals, Columbus, Ohio.)

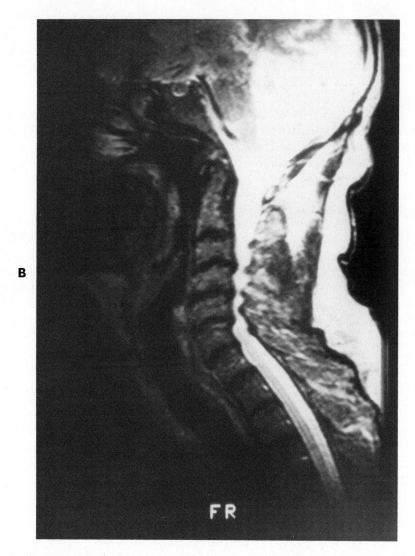

Fig. 10-23, *B.* A T2 weighted sagittal MRI image indicates the constriction of CSF flow (white) at C2 through C5. (Courtesy of Riverside Methodist Hospitals, Columbus, Ohio.)

TRAUMATIC DISEASE

The anatomy surrounding the delicate brain generally protects it well under normal conditions. The diploic arrangement of the calvarium, the mechanical buffering action of CSF, and the tough dura mater all work to prevent brain injury. Despite this protection, sufficient force to the skull can cause injury to the brain. Head trauma is the major neurologic cause of mortality and morbidity in individuals under 50 years of age.

Head trauma can result in skull fractures, brain injury, or a combination of the two. As noted in Chapter 2, the role of plain film radiography in evaluation of head trauma is rather limited, as CT allows rapid assessment of the nature of any brain injury. Assessment of the state of the brain following head injury is more crucial than that of the skull. Routine skull radiography on trauma victims may be delayed to allow treatment of the complications of brain injury readily diagnosed by CT. Skull fractures visualized by either modality are often seen with accompanying hematomas, as described on p. 373. If patients sustains an open skull fracture, they are at risk for development of meningitis or brain abscesses. Regardless of the imaging modality used, the technologist must constantly observe a patient with a head injury while performing an examination. Any change noted in the patient's condition should be reported immediately.

Brain Trauma

In addition to brain injury from a penetration wound (as could happen with a fracture), it can also occur from an acceleration and rapid deceleration of the head, which is termed a *closed head injury*. With head trauma, the brain is traumatically shaken within the cranium and subjected to forces of compression, acceleration, and deceleration. Brain tissues are injured from compression, tension, and shearing, with the latter perhaps most important (Fig. 10-24). The superficial cerebrum in the frontal, temporal, and occipital regions is most often affected.

Following a blow to the head, an individual may experience a temporary loss of consciousness and reflexes. This widespread paralysis of brain function is known as a *concussion* and is characterized by headache, vertigo, and vomiting. Higher mental functions may be impaired for several hours, with the patient remembering little of the events surrounding the concussion. There is a strong tendency toward spontaneous and complete recovery because of the lack of structural damage to the brain. Recovery generally occurs in less than 24 hours. Treatment is conservative once assessment (usually by CT) has ruled out any hemorrhage or fracture. Bed rest and possible admission to the hospital are the usual means of dealing with concussion.

A brain *contusion* can also result from a direct blow to the head. This refers to a bruising of brain parenchyma, which is more serious than a concussion. A contusion formed on the side of the head where the trauma occurs is called a *coup lesion*, while one formed on the opposite side of the skull in reference to the site of trauma is a *contre coup lesion*. Contusions are characterized by neuron damage, edema, and *punctate* (pinpoint punctures or depressions) hemorrhaging. On CT, contusions appear as small, ill-defined foci of increased density (Fig. 10-25, p. 374). Subdural or epidural hematomas can occur in conjunction with a contusion and result in increased intracranial pressure that can be life threatening. Signs seen in the patient with a contusion include drowsiness, confusion, and agitation. Hemiparesis and unequal pupil size may also be seen. CT plays a major role in the diagnosis of hematomas resulting from contusions, providing ready visualization of

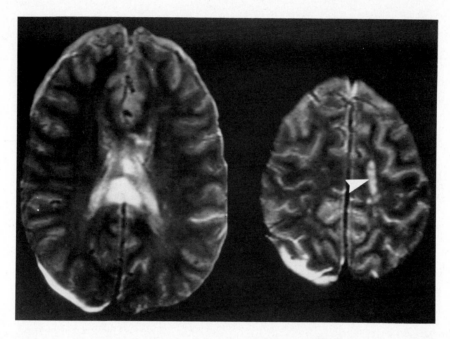

Fig. 10-24. A T2 weighted MRI image demonstrates a shearing injury of the corpus callosum (*arrow*) and a small subdural hematoma on the lateral margins of the brain in this young male who fell and failed to regain consciousness. (Courtesy of Riverside Methodist Hospitals, Columbus, Ohio.)

hemorrhagic blood as described in the following section. Treatment is generally conservative, centering on prevention of shock, control of edema, and drainage of any hematoma present.

Persistence of loss of consciousness for more than 24 hours is known as a *coma*. This is usually a serious condition and may be fatal. Over half of all comas result from trauma to the head, or circulatory problems associated with hypertension, sclerosis, thrombosis, tumor or abscess formation, or insufficient flow to the brain. Other causes include metabolic reasons such as lack of insulin (i.e., diabetic coma) and uremic poisoning from disturbed kidney metabolism. Diagnosis related to a coma may involve use of CT and/or MRI and is centered at determining, if possible, the cause of the coma. Treatment then rests on success in attacking the cause.

Hematomas of the Brain

As noted, brain trauma can result in hemorrhaging of blood from a ruptured artery or vein. Although venous bleeding occurs more slowly than arterial, both types of hemorrhage and resultant edema of the brain cause an increase in the intracranial pressure. Because the skull's structure does not allow for expansion, the increased pressure displaces the brain toward its opening, the foramen magnum. This trauma to the brain results in serious neurologic consequences or even death if not treated promptly. CT plays the major imaging role in diagnosis of the hemorrhaging.

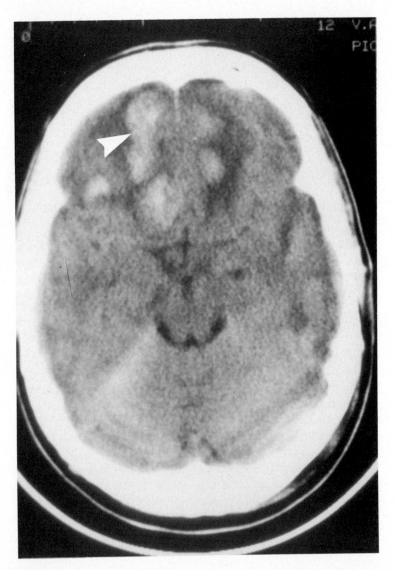

Fig. 10-25. An axial CT scan demonstrates hemorrhagic contusions of the brain as a result of a car accident for this young male. (Courtesy of Riverside Methodist Hospitals, Columbus, Ohio.)

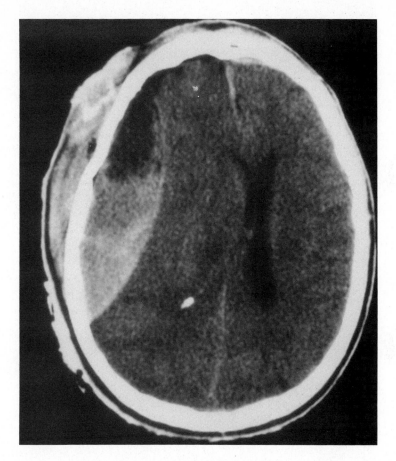

Fig. 10-26. A noncontrast axial CT view of this young male injured in an auto accident readily demonstrates a large epidural hematoma. (Courtesy of Riverside Methodist Hospitals, Columbus, Ohio.)

A *hematoma* is a collection of blood; four primary types of cerebral hematomas have been identified. The highest mortality rate is associated with an *epidural (extradural) hematoma* (Fig. 10-26). Even when promptly recognized and treated, it has a mortality rate of up to 30%. An epidural hematoma results from a torn artery, usually the middle meningeal artery, with blood pooling between the bony skull and the dura mater. Most commonly the artery or its branches are torn by a fracture of the thin, squamous portion of the temporal bone. In more than 80% of cases, the skull fracture is visible radiographically. As an arterial bleed, it accumulates rapidly and quickly causes neurologic symptoms, including early coma. It is seen on CT scans as an increased density, generally occupying a small area with a sharply convex appearance. Often it is accompanied by a fracture of the skull and/or facial bones. If not diagnosed and surgically treated quickly, the outcome is fatal as a result of brain displacement and herniation.

A *subdural hematoma* is positioned between the dura mater and the arachnoid meningeal layers (Figs. 10-27 and 10-28, *A, B,* and *C*). It usually follows blunt trauma to the frontal or occipital lobes of the skull and results from tearing of subdural veins connecting the cerebral cortex and dural sinuses. As a venous hemorrhage, it bleeds much slower than an epidural hematoma. In an acute stage, it is seen on CT as a curvilinear area of increased density on portions or all of the cerebral hemispheres. It pushes the brain away from the skull and causes a mass effect (i.e., brain shift across midline), with accompanying shift of the ventricles. In a subaccute stage (up to several days old), it appears on CT as a decreased or isodense fluid collection. In a chronic state (2 to 3 weeks old), the surface of the hematoma becomes concave. Delayed coma can occur with a subdural hematoma.

A *subarachnoid hematoma* accumulates between the arachnoid layer and the thin pia mater that invests the brain. It occurs most frequently at the vertex where the greatest brain movement occurs in trauma, and results from tearing of small vessels. In most head trauma cases, a subarachnoid hemorrhage is usually limited to one or two sulci, where it has a dense appearance (Fig. 10-29, p. 378). Less commonly, the rupture of a major cerebral vessel results in subarachnoid hematoma.

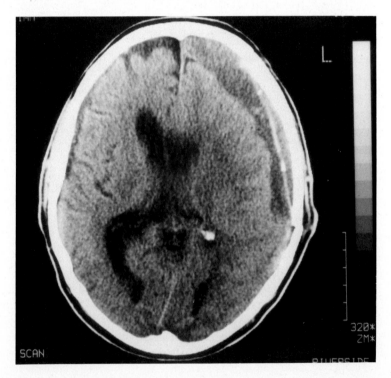

Fig. 10-27. CT demonstration of a large subdural hematoma outside the brain tissue in the left frontoparietal area of this 76-year-old male. (Courtesy of Riverside Methodist Hospitals, Columbus, Ohio.)

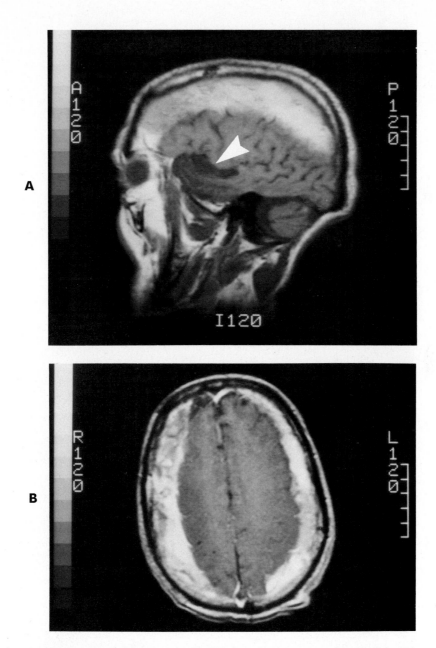

Fig. 10-28, *A.* A T1 weighted sagittal MRI view demonstrates a large subdural hematoma as well as a temporal lobe infarct (*arrow*). The white vs. gray appearance of the hematoma distinguishes subacute (fresh) from older blood. *B.* A T1 weighted axial MRI view with gadolinium demonstrates a large, bilateral subdural hematoma in this 67-year-old male. (Courtesy of Riverside Methodist Hospitals, Columbus, Ohio.)

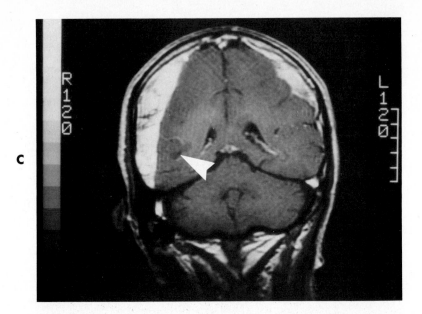

Fig. 10-28, C. A T1 weighted coronal MRI view with gadolinium demonstrates the same bilateral subdural hematoma. The *arrow* indicates the right-sided temporal lobe infarct. (Courtesy of Riverside Methodist Hospitals, Columbus, Ohio.)

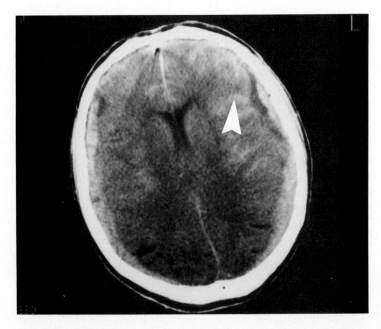

Fig. 10-29. CT demonstration of subarachnoid hematoma as indicated by the sulci opacified by blood in this 69-year-old male. Also seen is extensive bilateral subdural hematoma. (Courtesy of Riverside Methodist Hospitals, Columbus, Ohio.)

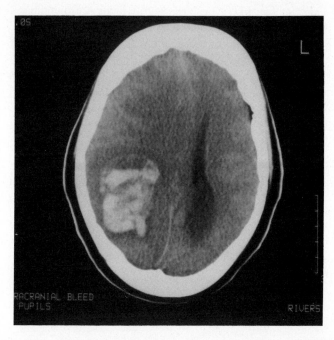

Fig. 10-30. A massive intracerebral hematoma that occurred spontaneously in this 63-year-old female. The patient expired within a few hours after the bleed began. (Courtesy of Riverside Methodist Hospitals, Columbus, Ohio.)

An *intracerebral hematoma* can result from trauma (Fig. 10-30), ruptured hemangiomas, or stroke (CVA) and creates bleeding within the brain. Common sites following trauma are the frontal, temporal, and occipital lobes of the brain. Small parenchymal vessels tear as a result of coup and contrecoup forces. An intracerebral hematoma is seen on CT as an increased density within the brain causing significant mass effect and may have an accompanying subarachnoid component. These hematomas develop edema around them as time passes and are slowly resorbed if the patient survives.

Diagnosis of hematomas is made primarily through clinical history and neurologic signs and symptoms. As noted, CT plays a major role in ready visualization of bleeding. Angiography may be used to visualize any defects in the cerebral vasculature. Treatment is often conservative unless active bleeding or significant mass effect is present, in which event an opening in the skull may be created surgically to allow drainage of blood and prevent complications. Prevention of infection and meningitis is important in the case of a fractured skull.

Herniated Nucleus Pulposus

A *herniated nucleus pulposus* (h.n.p.), or herniated disk, may result from either degenerative disease or trauma. A weakened or torn annulus fibrosus is subject to rupture, which allows the nucleus pulposus to ooze out and compress spinal nerve roots. Symptoms include a sudden and severe onset of pain in the distribution of the compressed nerve root in combination with weakened muscles, although at times symptoms may be more insidious. The image modality of choice has become MRI (Fig. 10-31), largely supplanting the roles of myelography and CT in diagnosis of disk disease. Bed rest, traction, physical therapy, and analgesics are used as treatment. If these fail to relieve pain, surgical laminectomy with spinal fusion is usually performed. Chemonucleolysis was a procedure formerly used to dissolve part of the diseased disk. Although still used in some places, it has largely fallen out of favor because of complications. Aspiration of the disk is a relatively new technique that holds promise for relief of this condition.

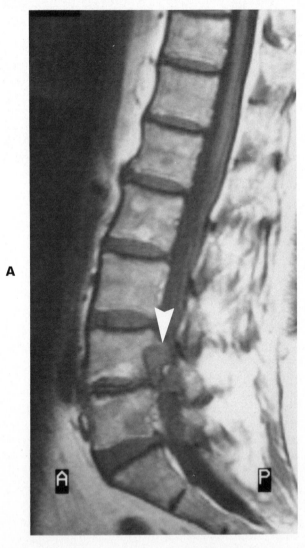

Fig. 10-31, *A.* Herniated nucleus pulposus at L4/L5 interspace seen on a T1 weighted sagittal MRI view of the lumbar spine. (Courtesy of Riverside Methodist Hospitals, Columbus, Ohio.)

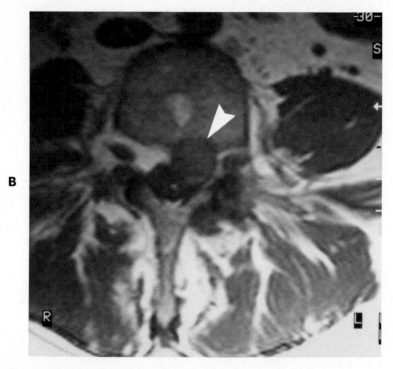

Fig. 10-31, *B.* The axial view of the same herniated nucleus pulposus demonstrates disk herniation to the left of midline on this T1 weighted MRI image. (Courtesy of Riverside Methodist Hospitals, Columbus, Ohio.)

NEOPLASTIC DISEASES

Primary tumors of the brain comprise about 10% of the deaths from cancer and may be difficult to classify as purely benign or malignant. In many cases, the location of the brain neoplasm is of equal or greater importance than its malignancy or benignancy because of the complications produced by mass effect. Edema accompanying a tumor causes an increase in intracranial pressure, which causes headaches, vomiting, blurred vision, and/ or seizures. Hemorrhage and brain stem herniation can occur, resulting in death as brain stem function (e.g., control of respiration) fails.

Other characteristics of primary brain tumors include a greater incidence in males and a relative infrequency of metastasis. In children, brain tumors often tend to occur in the posterior fossa, while the anterior portion of the cerebrum is a more prevalent site in adults. In addition, primary brain tumors are among the most common neoplasms found in children, whereas metastases to the brain from other areas is more common in adults.

Two categories of brain tumors exist: glial and nonglial. Glial tumors generate from the non-nervous system (i.e., supporting tissues of the brain and spinal cord). Gliomas account for about half of all primary brain tumors. Their growth is accomplished through infiltration, making them difficult to surgically treat through resection. Nonglial

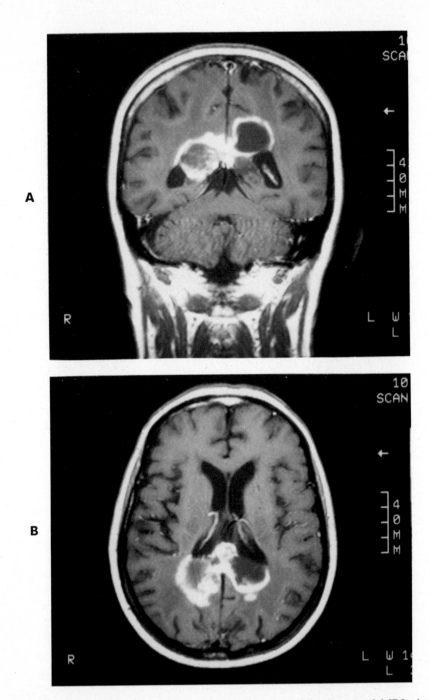

Fig. 10-32, *A.* A "butterfly" glioma seen in this T1 weighted coronal MRI view with gadolinium in a 54-year-old female. *B.* A T1 weighted axial MRI view with gadolinium of the same "butterfly" glioma. (Courtesy of Riverside Methodist Hospitals, Columbus, Ohio.)

tumors grow through expansion and are more treatable surgically. Meningiomas are the most frequently occurring nonglial tumor. MRI and CT are the modalities of choice in imaging brain tumors of all types. Beside surgical intervention, radiation therapy and chemotherapy also play an important role in treatment of brain tumors.

Gliomas

The most common type of primary brain tumor is the *glioma* (Fig. 10-32). Although derived from glial cells, their precise classification is unsettled. Tumors may contain different types of cells in the same tumor. Gliomas commonly occur in the cerebral hemispheres and posterior fossa, and affected patients may present with seizures. Nearly half of all gliomas are the malignant glioblastoma variety (Fig. 10-33, p. 384). Other types of glioma include benign astrocytomas, oligodendrogliomas, and ependymoma. In terms of imaging results, gliomas are evaluated based on the associated edema (Fig. 10-34, p. 385), mass effect, and the amount of contrast enhancement. As these three factors increase, so does the aggressiveness of the associated tumor. Surgical biopsy generally provides the final diagnosis of the exact type of glioma.

Astrocytomas account for about a third of all gliomas (Fig. 10-35, p. 386) and are composed of astrocytes. These are star-shaped neuroglial cells with many branching processes. Astrocytomas are white, usually slow-growing, infiltrative tumors that are the relatively benign. Early detection leads to a good prognosis. An *astroblastoma* is somewhat less benign, but a *glioblastoma multiforme* (an advanced astrocytoma) is highly malignant. An *oligodendroglioma* is a slow-growing, astrocytic tumor that is usually histologically relatively benign (Fig. 10-36, p. 387). It typically calcifies so that its appearance in a punctate or stippled pattern on a skull radiograph is virtually diagnostic. *Ependymoma* is a firm, whitish tumor that arises from the ependyma, the lining of the ventricles (Fig. 10-37, pp. 388–389). Typically it derives from the roof of the fourth ventricle, but it may also appear from the central canal of the spinal cord.

Medulloblastoma

Like astrocytic tumors, *medulloblastomas* are soft, infiltrating tumors of neuroepithelial tissue. These rapidly growing tumors are highly malignant and most often occur in the cerebellum of children and young adults (Fig. 10-38, pp. 389–390), usually extending from the roof of the fourth ventricle. They are rarely seen in adults. Tumor dissemination throughout the subarachnoid space often blocks the flow of CSF, causing hydrocephalus. Shunting is used to relieve the hydrocephalus. Surgical excision of the tumor as possible followed by radiation therapy to the entire CNS and chemotherapy have improved the 5-year survival rate to over 50%. Recurrence is unfortunately common with this tumor.

Meningioma

A *meningioma* is a slow-growing, generally benign tumor that originates in the arachnoid tissue. It is the most common nonglial tumor and occurs more frequently in women than in men (Fig. 10-39, pp. 390–391). Arising from the arachnoid villi, it is most often found in relation to the intracranial venous sinuses. It does not invade the brain but compresses it with its growth. Resultant neurologic deficits are generally less in proportion to the tumor size than with gliomas. Surgical removal is the method of treatment for a symptomatic mengioma.

Text continued on p. 391.

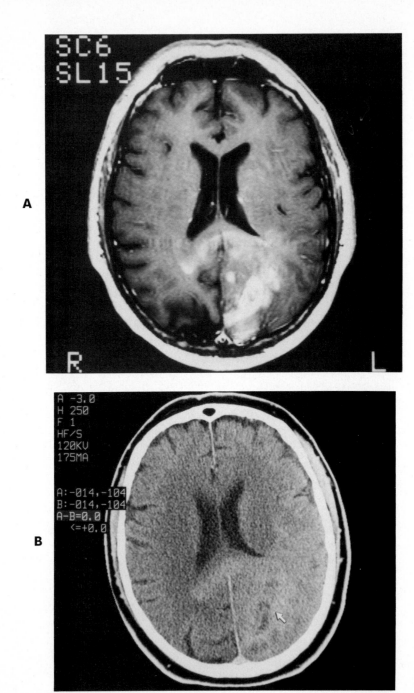

Fig. 10-33, *A.* A T1 weighted axial MRI view with gadolinium demonstrates a glioblastoma multiforme in a 70-year-old male. *B.* CT study of the brain without contrast demonstrates an intraparenchymal hemorrhage post-biopsy in the same patient with the glioblastoma multiforme. (Courtesy of Riverside Methodist Hospitals, Columbus, Ohio.)

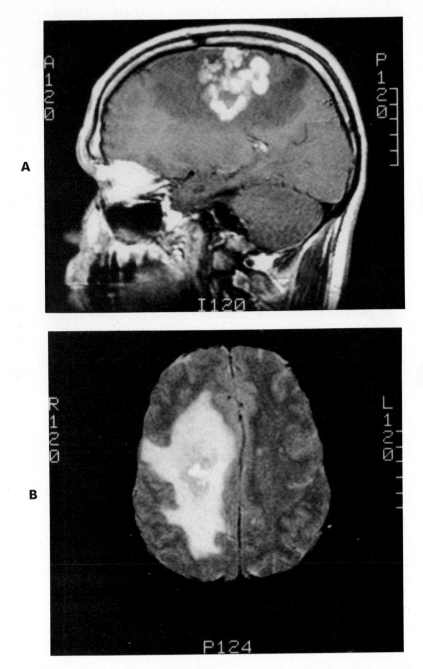

Fig. 10-34, *A.* A T1 weighted sagittal MRI view with gadolinium of a large glioma with surrounding edema in a 25-year-old male. *B.* A T2 weighted axial MRI view without gadolinium of the same glioma in the right parietal region, again with edema (white on T2) surrounding the tumor. (Courtesy of Riverside Methodist Hospitals, Columbus, Ohio.)

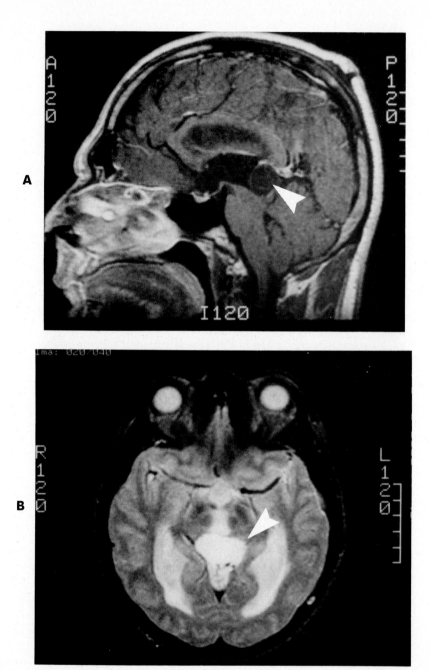

Fig. 10-35, *A.* A T1 weighted sagittal MRI view with gadolinium demonstrates a pineal gland astrocytoma in this 32-year-old male. *B.* A T2 weighted axial MRI view demonstrates the same pineal gland astrocytoma. (Courtesy of Riverside Methodist Hospitals, Columbus, Ohio.)

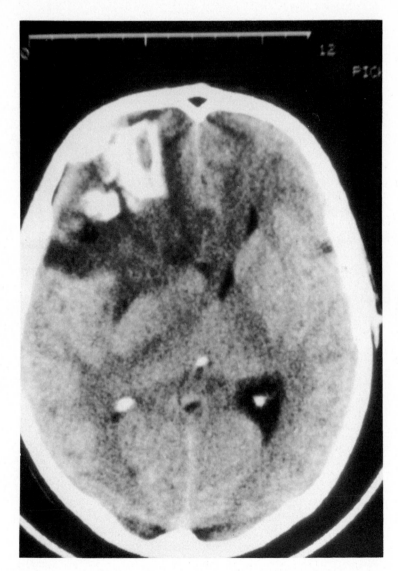

Fig. 10-36. An axial CT view without contrast demonstrates the presence of an oligo-dendroglioma and surrounding edema. (Courtesy of Riverside Methodist Hospitals, Columbus, Ohio.)

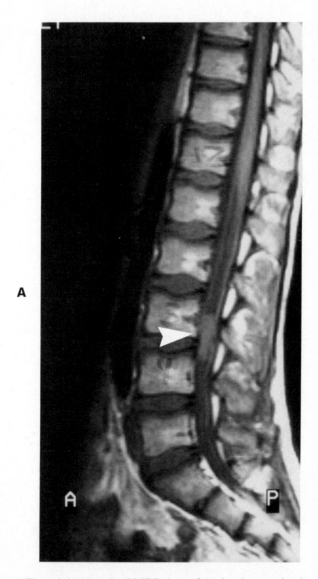

Fig. 10-37, *A.* A T1 weighted sagittal MRI view of the lumbosacral spine demonstrates an ependymoma at L3/L4 interspace in this young male. (Courtesy of Riverside Methodist Hospitals, Columbus, Ohio.)

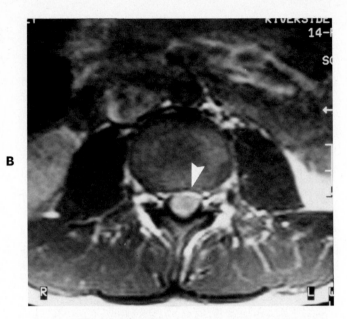

Fig. 10-37, *B.* A T1 weighted axial MRI view with gadolinium demonstrates the same ependymoma. (Courtesy of Riverside Methodist Hospitals, Columbus, Ohio.)

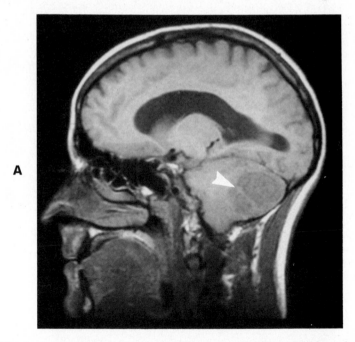

Fig. 10-38, *A.* A T1 weighted sagittal MRI view without gadolinium demonstrates a medulloblastoma in the cerebellum of this 25-year-old male. (Courtesy of Riverside Methodist Hospitals, Columbus, Ohio.)

Continued.

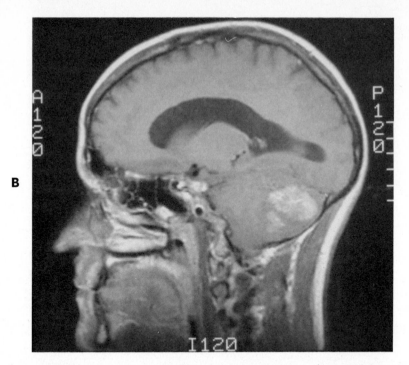

Fig. 10-38, *B.* A T1 weighted sagittal MRI view with gadolinium demonstrates the medulloblastoma, illustrating more of its actual size. (Courtesy of Riverside Methodist Hospitals, Columbus, Ohio.)

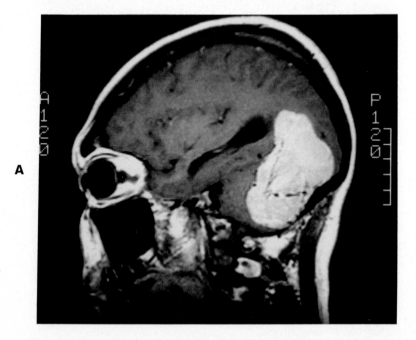

Fig. 10-39, *A.* A T1 weighted sagittal MRI view with gadolinium of a large meningioma in the posterior occipital area with marked hydrocephalus in this 31-year-old female. (Courtesy of Riverside Methodist Hospitals, Columbus, Ohio.)

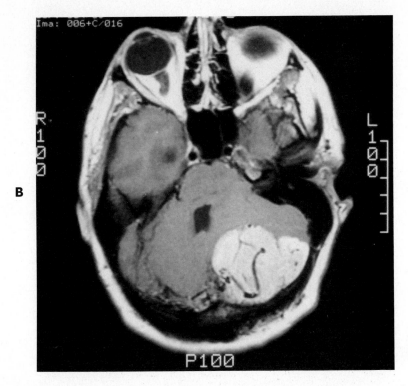

Fig. 10-39, *B.* A T1 weighted axial MRI view with gadolinium of the same meningioma. Displacement of the fourth ventricle is seen, as well as a distortion of the vascular structures within the meningioma. (Courtesy of Riverside Methodist Hospitals, Columbus, Ohio.)

Pituitary Adenoma

A *pituitary adenoma* (macroadenoma) is a usually benign tumor of the pituitary gland. Hormones produced by the pituitary are affected, with one type of adenoma resulting in giantism if developed before puberty and acromegaly if occurring in adults. Pituitary adenomas grow out of the sella turcica. As they grow, they compress structures such as the optic chiasm, causing visual problems. A common radiographic demonstration of this growth is an enlargement and erosion of the sella turcica on a lateral skull radiograph. Angiography might demonstrate a displacement of the sylvian triangle, but generally only after the adenoma has assumed a considerable size. The *sylvian triangle* is an anatomic landmark created by the middle cerebral artery and its branches. MRI is the modality of choice in visualizing pituitary adenomas (Figs. 10-40, pp. 392–393, and 10-41). Generally, they are treatable through surgical extraction, possibly followed by radiation therapy.

Text continued on p. 394.

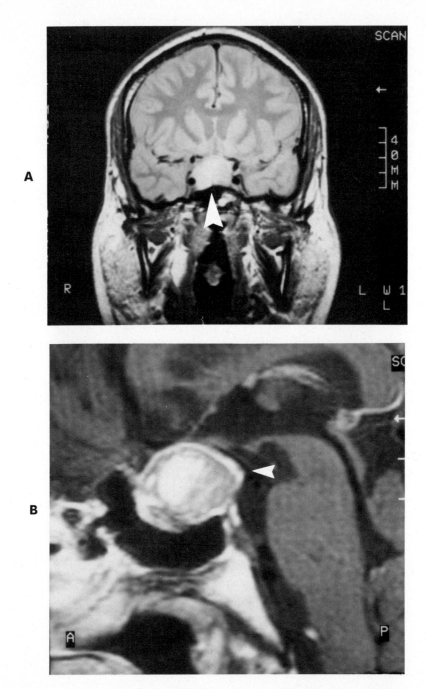

Fig. 10-40, *A.* A T1 weighted coronal MRI view demonstrates a suprasellar macroadenoma of the pituitary in this 37-year-old male. *B.* A T1 weighted sagittal MRI high resolution scan with gadolinium demonstrates the same suprasellar macroadenoma of the pituitary. (Courtesy of Riverside Methodist Hospitals, Columbus, Ohio.)

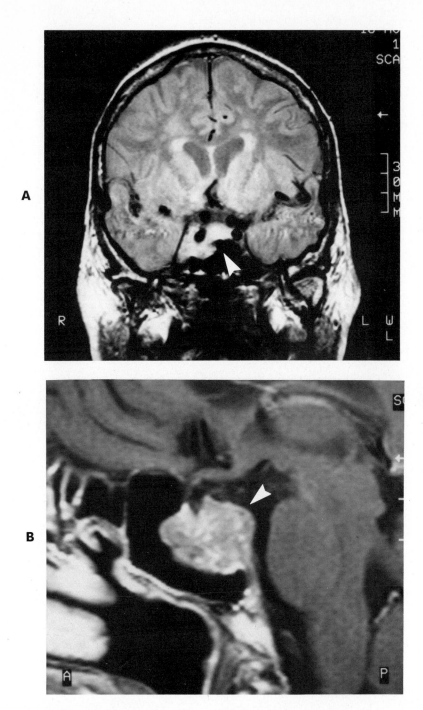

Fig. 10-41, *A.* Large pituitary adenoma extending downward into the right cavernous sinus in a 79-year-old female as seen on this MRI T2 weighted coronal scan. *B.* A high-resolution T1 weighted sagittal MRI view of the same pituitary adenoma with gadolinium. (Courtesy of Riverside Methodist Hospitals, Columbus, Ohio.)

Craniopharyngioma

A *craniopharyngioma* is a cystic, benign tumor growing from remnants of the development of the pituitary gland. It usually arises above the sella and extends upward into the third ventricle (Fig. 10-42). Occasionally they are seen within the sella and cause erosion of it. Calcification of the wall of the cyst is common and readily identifiable on plain films of the skull. Like with a pituitary adenoma, angiography may reveal displacement of the sylvian triangle if the tumor is large. Although treated surgically, excision is often difficult because of location and proximity to structures such as the optic nerves. Radiation therapy is used to enhance the effects of surgery.

Tumors of Nerve Sheath Cells

Three tumors of the peripheral nerve sheath include *acoustic neurilemoma*, *neuroma* (Fig. 10-43), and *schwannoma* (Fig. 10-44). They account for up to one-tenth of all intracranial tumors. The most common site of occurrence is the eighth cranial (i.e., the acoustic) nerve. They can be found, however, on other cranial nerves, especially the trigeminal, and on spinal nerve roots and peripheral nerves. CT is useful in demonstrating a funnel-shaped increase in the internal auditory canal. Surgical excision of the tumor is the method of treatment, although the tumor can recur.

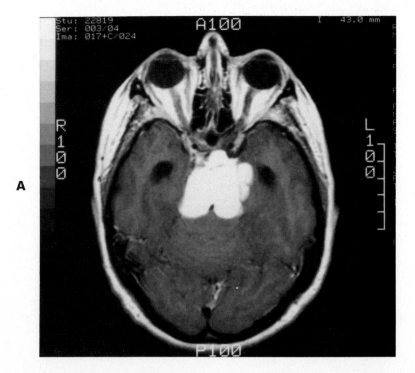

Fig. 10-42, *A.* A T1 weighted axial MRI view with gadolinium demonstrates a mass, later confirmed by biopsy to be a craniopharyngioma in this 53-year-old female. (Courtesy of Riverside Methodist Hospitals, Columbus, Ohio.)

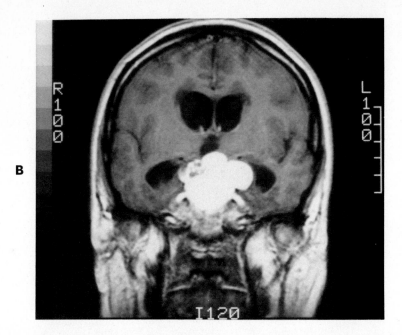

Fig. 10-42, *B.* A T1 weighted coronal MRI view with gadolinium demonstrates the relative size of the craniopharyngioma in the same patient. (Courtesy of Riverside Methodist Hospitals, Columbus, Ohio.)

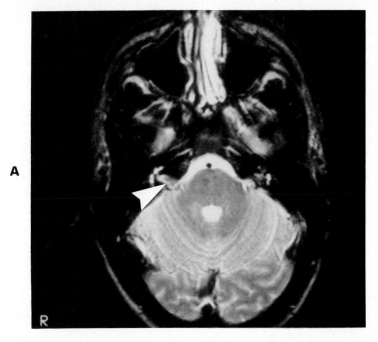

Fig. 10-43, *A.* A T2 weighted axial MRI view of a right acoustic neuroma that is not readily visible without gadolinium in this 24-year-old male. (Courtesy of Riverside Methodist Hospitals, Columbus, Ohio.)

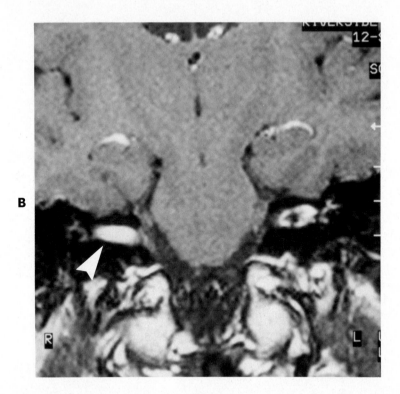

Fig. 10-43, *B.* A high resolution, T1-weighted coronal MRI view with gadolinium readily reveals the acoustic neuroma. Compare the appearance of the tumor with the appearance of the normal vasculature and anatomy on the left side. (Courtesy of Riverside Methodist Hospitals, Columbus, Ohio.)

Metastases from Other Sites

Secondary metastases from another site can involve any intracranial structure and accounts for about one-fourth of all brain tumors (Fig. 10-45, p. 398). Brain metastasis usually arises from lung carcinoma. Other significant causes include breast cancer and malignant melanoma. Signs and symptoms of brain metastasis are similar to those for other brain tumors. Patients with metastases from other sites usually present with signs of increased intracranial pressure, especially headache and ataxia; those with primary brain tumors are more likely to present with seizures. Diagnosis and follow-up are done with MRI and CT. Treatment with chemotherapy is performed, but the prognosis is generally quite poor.

Spinal Tumors

Primary tumors of the spinal cord are less common than those of the brain. They are commonly divided into extradural and intradural groups, with the latter further divided into extramedullary (outside the spinal cord) and intramedullary (within the spinal cord). The most common types of primary spinal neoplasms include *meningiomas* (Fig. 10-46, p. 399)

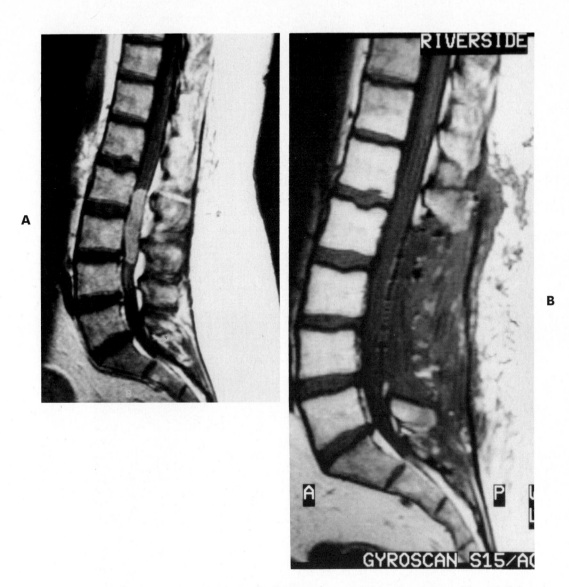

Fig. 10-44, *A.* A T1 weighted sagittal MRI view of the lumbar spine with gadolinium shows a schwannoma at L3/L4 before surgery in this 27-year-old female. *B.* A T1 weighted sagittal MRI view of the same lumbar spine without gadolinium after surgery demonstrates apparent total excision of the tumor has been accomplished. Note also the excision of the spinous processes from the surgical site. (Courtesy of Riverside Methodist Hospitals, Columbus, Ohio.)

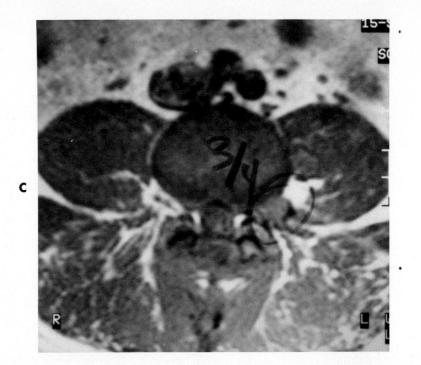

Fig. 10-44, *C.* A T1 weighted axial MRI view with gadolinium of the L3/L4 interspace demonstrates some residual tumor is present in the left neural foramina. (Courtesy of Riverside Methodist Hospitals, Columbus, Ohio.)

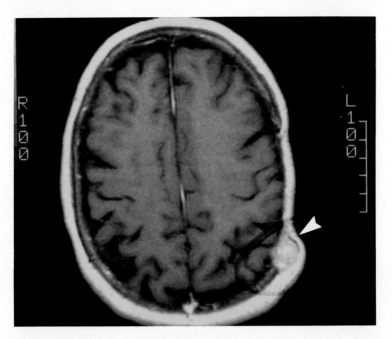

Fig. 10-45. Brain metastases from renal cell carcinoma as seen in this T1 weighted axial MRI view with gadolinium status after craniotomy in this 59-year-old female. (Courtesy of Riverside Methodist Hospitals, Columbus, Ohio.)

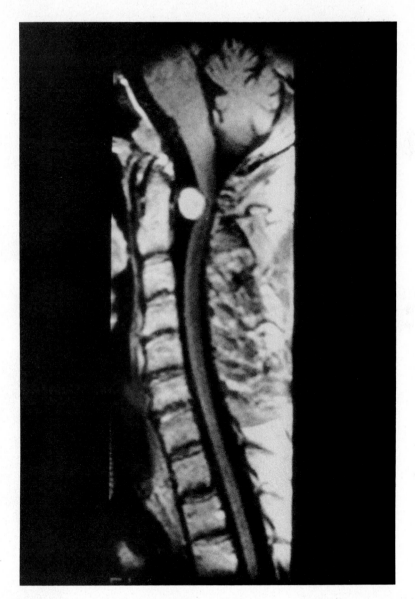

Fig. 10-46. A T1 weighted sagittal MRI view of the spine with gadolinium demonstrates the presence of a meningioma in this 45-year-old female suffering from ataxia. (Courtesy of Riverside Methodist Hospitals, Columbus, Ohio.)

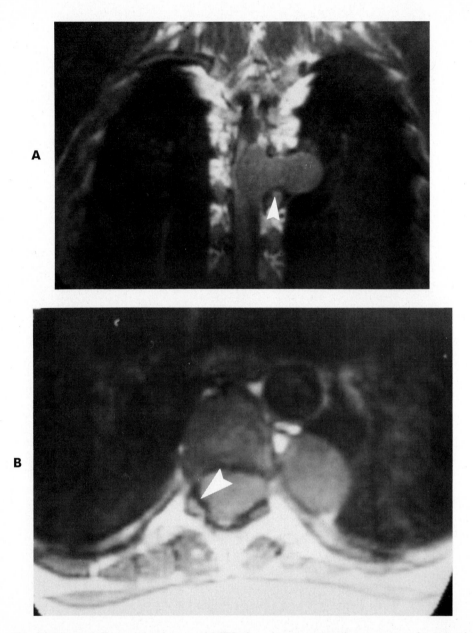

Fig. 10-47, *A.* A T1 weighted coronal MRI view demonstrates the presence of a "dumb-bell" neurofibroma showing clear compression of the spinal cord of this young female with back pain and leg weakness. *B.* An axial T1 weighted MRI image similarly demonstrates the lesion and compression of the spinal cord (*arrow*) into a narrow space. (Courtesy of Riverside Methodist Hospitals, Columbus, Ohio.)

and *neurofibromas* (Fig. 10-47), both of which are extramedullary tumors. The most common intramedullary tumors are astrocytoma and ependymoma.

Symptoms of these tumors may be similar to those of a herniated nucleus pulposus in that spinal tumors also compress the nerve roots, leading to pain and muscular weakness. MRI has essentially replaced myelography in evaluating spinal cord tumors. Radiation and chemotherapy are the primary means of treating spinal tumors because many are not surgically resectable.

▼ QUESTIONS

1. Under normal conditions, the central nervous system within the cranial vault is well protected from damage by all of the following *except* the:
    a. cauda equina
    b. cerebrospinal fluid
    c. diploe
    d. dura mater

2. The correct order of meninges from outermost to innermost is:
    a. arachnoid, pia, dura
    b. dura, arachnoid, pia
    c. dura, pia, arachnoid
    d. pia, arachnoid, dura

3. The blood-brain barrier prevents passage of unwanted substances into the CNS through the cerebral:
    a. arteries
    b. capillaries
    c. dura mater
    d. veins

4. Which of the following statements are true in relation to imaging of the CNS?
    1. A calcified pineal gland can be seen on plain skull films more often than not.
    2. CT plays a greater role in evaluation of head trauma than that of plain films.
    3. MRI has rapidly emerged as the modality of choice for many CNS conditions.
    a. 1, 2
    b. 1, 3
    c. 2, 3
    d. 1, 2, 3

5. Erosion of the sella turcica is most commonly associated with neoplasms of the:
    a. meninges
    b. pineal gland
    c. pituitary
    d. pons

6. Protrusion of both the spinal cord and meninges into the skin of the back is a:
    a. meningocele
    b. meningomyelocele
    c. myelocele
    d. spinal hydrocephalus

7. Hydrocephalus refers to excess accumulation of CSF in the ventricles before it is reabsorbed in the:
    a. arachnoid villi
    b. dural sinuses
    c. sella turcica
    d. subarachnoid space

8. The most typical cause of meningitis is:
    a. bacterial infection
    b. trauma
    c. tumor compression
    d. viral infection

9. A contusion formed on the side of the head where trauma occurs is called a:
    a. concussion
    b. contre coup lesion
    c. coup lesion
    d. spondylosis

10. Which of the following statements are true of brain trauma?
    1. Punctate hemorrhaging of the brain is characteristic of contusions.
    2. Recovery to concussion generally occurs in less than 24 hours.
    3. Widespread paralysis of brain function following a head blow is a contusion.
       a. 1, 2   **c.** 2, 3
       b. 1, 3   **d.** 1, 2, 3

11. Which type of hematoma has the highest mortality rate associated with it?
    a. epidural   **c.** subarachnoid
    b. intracerebral   **d.** subdural

12. The type of hematoma particularly common to the Circle of Willis as a result of trauma is:
    a. epidural   **c.** subarachnoid
    b. intracerebral   **d.** subdural

13. Demonstration of acute cerebral bleeding leading to a hematoma is best done by:
    a. angiography   **c.** MRI
    b. CT   **d.** plain films

14. Osteophytes are associated with:
    a. cervical spondylosis   **c.** meningiomas
    b. herniated nucleus pulposus **d.** meningoceles

15. The imaging modality of choice for demonstration of herniated nucleus pulposus has become:
    a. CT   **c.** myelography
    b. MRI   **d.** ultrasonography

16. Which of the following statements are true of neoplastic disease in the CNS?
    1. Location of the neoplasm is of equal or greater significance than malignancy.
    2. Metastatic lesions from elsewhere are more common in adults than children.
    3. Primary brain tumors account for nearly fifty percent of all cancer deaths.
       a. 1, 2   **c.** 2, 3
       b. 1, 3   **d.** 1, 2, 3

17. Which of the following is characteristic of a glial brain tumor as compared to one of nonglial type?
    a. easier treated through surgery   **c.** infiltrative in nature
    b. grows through expansion   **d.** meningioma most common type

18. Which of the following gliomas is considered malignant?
    a. astrocytoma   **c.** glioblastoma
    b. ependymoma   **d.** oligodendroglioma

19. Which of the following neoplastic conditions are highly malignant and often occur in the cerebellum of children?
    a. astrocytoma   **c.** meningioma
    b. medulloblastoma   **d.** pituitary adenoma

20. The most common nonglial tumor:
    a. compresses the brain through growth
    b. is considered to be a meningioma
    c. is generally benign in nature
    d. occurs more frequently in women
    e. two of the above
    f. all of the above (except e)

21. Pituitary adenomas tend to grow directly out of the:
    a. cerebrum
    b. cerebellum
    c. foramen magnum
    d. sella turcica

22. A cystic, benign tumor that grows from the embryologic remnants of the pituitary gland is a(n):
    a. acoustic neurilemoma
    b. craniopharyngioma
    c. meningioma
    d. pituitary adenoma

23. The most common site for tumors of the peripheral nerve sheath (e.g., schwannoma) is on which cranial nerve?
    a. 4
    b. 6
    c. 7
    d. 8
    e. none of the above

24. Brain metastasis usually arises from carcinoma of the:
    a. breast
    b. kidneys
    c. lung
    d. prostate

25. The symptoms caused by spinal tumors would most closely resemble those of:
    a. contre coup lesion
    b. craniopharyngioma
    c. herniated nucleus pulposus
    d. pituitary adenoma

ANSWER KEY

CHAPTER 1

1. c
2. d
3. b
4. b
5. b
6. b
7. c
8. b
9. b
10. d
11. d
12. c
13. d
14. c
15. b

CHAPTER 2

1. b
2. b
3. b
4. a
5. d
6. a
7. c
8. b
9. b
10. c
11. c
12. d
13. b
14. c
15. b

16. a
17. c
18. a
19. c
20. d

CHAPTER 3

1. c
2. d
3. c
4. b
5. c
6. c
7. a
8. d
9. c
10. d
11. a
12. d
13. c
14. d
15. d
16. b
17. b
18. a
19. c
20. d
21. d
22. d
23. b
24. b
25. c

CHAPTER 4

1. c
2. a
3. d
4. a
5. c
6. c
7. b
8. c
9. c
10. a
11. e
12. c
13. c
14. d
15. c
16. c
17. c
18. b
19. d
20. a
21. d
22. d
23. c
24. b
25. a

CHAPTER 5

1. b
2. d
3. b
4. b
5. d

6. e
7. d
8. d
9. d
10. c
11. d
12. d
13. d
14. c
15. e
16. c
17. a
18. a
19. c
20. b

CHAPTER 6

1. d
2. a
3. c
4. a
5. b
6. c
7. d
8. e
9. d
10. b
11. d
12. d
13. c
14. a
15. b
16. a

17. b
18. d
19. b
20. a

22. a
23. b
24. d
25. c

22. b
23. e
24. a
25. a

5. c
6. b
7. a
8. a
9. c
10. a
11. a
12. c
13. b
14. a
15. b
16. a
17. c
18. c
19. b
20. f
21. d
22. b
23. d
24. c
25. c

CHAPTER 7

1. b
2. a
3. b
4. d
5. d
6. d
7. d
8. b
9. a
10. a
11. b
12. d
13. d
14. d
15. d
16. d
17. c
18. a
19. b
20. b
21. c

CHAPTER 8

1. d
2. c
3. c
4. a
5. b
6. e
7. b
8. b
9. d
10. a
11. e
12. a
13. c
14. a
15. b
16. c
17. c
18. b
19. d
20. c
21. b

CHAPTER 9

1. c
2. a
3. a
4. a
5. d
6. d
7. b
8. b
9. b
10. d
11. d
12. a
13. b
14. b
15. b

CHAPTER 10

1. a
2. b
3. b
4. d

GLOSSARY

Abruptio Placentae · Condition in which a normally implanted placenta prematurely separates from the uterus.

Absorption Atelectasis · Type of atelectasis that occurs when air is completely absorbed from alveoli beyond an obstructed bronchus.

Achalasia · A neuromuscular abnormality of the esophagus which results in failure of the lower esophageal sphincter to relax.

Achondroplasia · A hereditary, congenital disturbance which causes inadequate bone formation and results in a peculiar form of dwarfism.

Acquired Immune Deficiency Syndrome (AIDS) · An acquired viral infection which paralyzes normal human immune mechanisms.

Acromegaly · A disease marked by progressive enlargement of the head, hands, and feet caused by abnormal secretion of growth hormone.

Acute · Having a quick onset and lasting a short period of time with a relatively severe course.

Additive Pathologies · A radiographic term used to describe diseases that are more difficult than normal to penetrate.

Adenocarcinoma · Carcinoma derived from glandular tissue.

Adenomatous Polyp · A saccular projection into the bowel lumen.

Air-bronchogram Sign · Radiographic sign seen in various respiratory diseases where air-filled bronchi become visible when surrounded by non-aerated alveoli.

Alimentary Tract · Extending from the mouth to the anus, the major portion consists of the gastrointestinal system, which digests and absorbs food.

Anemic · Condition in which level of hemoglobin in blood is less than 12 grams per 100 ml.

Anencephaly · Congenital absence of the cranial vault.

Aneurysm · A localized ballooning or outpouching of a vessel wall as a result of weakening due to atherosclerotic disease, trauma, infection, or congenital defects.

Ankylosing Spondylitis · A form of rheumatoid arthritis of unknown etiology that affects the spine in a progressive fashion, eventually fusing the spine into a rigid block of bone.

Anomaly · Any marked deviation from the norm, especially as a result of congenital or hereditary defects.

Anthracosis · Pneumoconiosis caused by inhalation and deposition of coal dust.

Appendicitis · An inflammation of the appendix.

Arthritis · Inflammation in which lesions are confined to the joints.

Asbestosis · Pneumoconiosis caused by inhalation and deposition of asbestos dust.

Ascites · An accumulation of fluid in the peritoneal cavity.

Aspiration Pneumonia · Pneumonia caused by entrance of foreign particles (e.g., vomitus) aspirated into the lower respiratory tract.

Astrocytoma · A glioma composed of astrocytes, which are star-shaped neuroglial cells with many branching processes.

Asymptomatic · Showing or causing no identifiable symptoms.

Atelectasis · Loss of air in a lung resulting from a partial or total collapse of a lung.

Atheroma · A mass of plaque occurring in atherosclerosis.

Atherosclerosis · A common form of arteriosclerosis in which deposits of fibro-fatty plaque or thickenings form within the intima or intermedia of large and medium-sized arteries.

Autoimmune Disorder · Diseases in which antibodies form against and injure the patient's own tissues, in contrast to the normal process in which antibodies form in response to foreign antigens.

Autosome · The 22 pairs of chromosomes found in a typical cell, other than the sex chromosomes.

Avulsion Fracture · A fracture in which a fragmented bone is pulled away from the shaft, usually occurring around a ligament or tendon, and often with muscle-tearing, as is associated with a sprain or dislocation.

Benign · Refers to a localized and generally noninvasive lesion.

Bicornuate Uterus · A uterus with paired uterine horns extending to the uterine tubes.

Bleb · A flaccid vesicle.

Blood-brain Barrier · The special functioning of the cerebral capillaries that prevents the passage of unwanted substances into the brain.

Blow-out Fracture · A fracture of the orbital floor resulting from a direct blow to the front of the orbit, with the force of the blow transferred to the orbital walls and floor.

Bone Cyst · A benign lesion consisting of a wall of fibrous tissue filled with fluid.

Bowel Sounds · The normal sounds of the bowel in motion as heard on auscultation.

Boxer's Fracture · A fracture of the fifth metacarpal bone as a result of a blow to or with the hand.

Bradycardia · A very slow heart rate.

Bronchial Adenoma · A glandular tumor, either benign or malignant, situated in the submucosal tissues of large bronchi.

Bronchiectasis · Chronic dilatation of the bronchi, with inflammation and destruction of bronchial walls and cilia.

Bronchitis · Inflammation of one or more bronchi.

Bronchogenic Carcinoma · Carcinoma of the lung that arises from the epithelium of the bronchial tree.

Bruise · Bleeding into the tissue spaces as a result of capillary rupture; also known as a contusion.

Bulla · A large vesicle, usually 2 cm or more in diameter, filled with air.

Bursitis · Inflammation of the bursae of the tendons, with the subdeltoid bursa as the most common site.

CAD · Coronary artery disease, resulting from deposition of atheromas in the arteries supplying blood to the heart muscle.

CVA · Cerebrovascular accident, generally resulting from a loss of blood supply to the brain or from a cerebral bleed.

Callus · An unorganized meshwork of woven bone formed following a fracture, ultimately replaced by hard, adult bone.

Cancellous · Refers to the spongy, latticelike structure of bone filled by bone marrow.

Cancer · A general term used to denote various types of malignant neoplasms.

Cantor Tube · A single-lumen, mercury-weighted gastric tube used for intestinal intubation and decompression.

Carcinoma · A malignant growth comprised of epithelial cells that tends to invade surrounding tissues and give rise to metastases.

Cardiomegaly · The appearance of an enlarged heart, as indicative of many cardiovascular disorders.

Celiac Disease · A malabsorption syndrome that occurs as a result of sensitivity to gluten, an agent found in wheat products.

Cervical Spondylosis · Degenerative joint disease affecting the cervical vertebrae, vertebral discs, and surrounding ligaments and connective tissue.

Chest Tube · Tube inserted through the chest wall between the ribs to allow for drainage of air and/or fluid from the thoracic cavity.

Chip Fracture · An avulsion fracture consisting of a small fragment or chip of bone from the corner of a phalanx or other long bone.

Cholecystitis · An acute inflammation of the gallbladder most frequently caused by obstruction.

Cholelithiasis · The presence of gallstones.

Chondrosarcoma · A malignant bone tumor composed of atypical cartilage.

Chronic · Presenting slowly and persisting over a long period of time.

Chronic Obstructive Pulmonary Disease (COPD) · Designation applied to conditions which result in pulmonary obstruction, most commonly chronic bronchitis and pulmonary emphysema.

Cirrhosis · Liver condition in which the parenchyma and architecture are destroyed and replaced by fibrous tissue and regenerative nodules.

Closed Fracture · A fracture that does not produce an open wound.

Clubfoot · Deformity of the foot involving the talus.

Coarctation · A narrowing or compression.

Coccidiomycosis · Systemic, fungal infection caused by a fungus that thrives in semi-arid soil and is particularly endemic in the southwestern United States and northern Mexico.

Colles' Fracture · A fracture through the distal 1 inch of the radius in which the distal fragment is displaced posteriorly.

Colonic Atresia · Congenital failure of development of the distal rectum and anus to a variable extent, frequently accompanied by fistula formation to the genitourinary system.

Coma · A state of unconsciousness from which the patient cannot be aroused.

Comminuted Fracture · A fracture in which the bone is splintered or crushed.

Communicating (external) Hydrocephalus · Type of hydrocephalus caused by poor resorption of cerebrospinal fluid (for a variety of reasons) by the arachnoid villi.

Compact · Refers to the dense, outer portion of bone.

Complete Noncomminuted Fracture · A fracture in which the bone separates into two fragments.

Compound Fracture · A fracture in which the bone ends penetrate the soft tissue and skin.

Compression Atelectasis · Type of atelectasis that occurs when pleural effusions, pneumothoraces, or other space-occupying lesions cause collapse.

Compression Fracture · A fracture produced by compression.

Concussion · Brief loss of consciousness as a result of a blow to the head.

Congenital · Existing at, and usually before, birth and resulting from genetic or environmental factors.

Congenital Megacolon · Hirschprung's disease, consisting of an absence of neurons in the bowel wall, typically in the sigmoid colon.

Congestive Heart Failure · Condition existing when the heart is unable to propel blood at a sufficient rate and volume to prevent congestion of subcirculatory systems.

Consolidation · The process of tissue or fluid accumulation.

Contre Coup Lesion · A contusion formed on the opposite side of the skull in reference to a trauma site.

Contusion · An injury in which the tissue is bruised but not broken.

Corpus Luteum Cyst · A cyst that develops in the yellow endocrine body formed in the ovary in the site of a ruptured ovarian follicle.

Coup Lesion · A contusion formed on the side of the head in which trauma occurs.

Craniopharyngioma · A cystic, benign tumor that usually grows above the sella and upward into the third ventricle of the brain.

Craniosynostosis · Premature or early closure of the sutures of the skull.

Crohn's Disease · A chronic granulomatous inflammatory disease of unknown etiology involving any part of the gastrointestinal tract, but commonly involving the terminal ileum.

Crossed Ectopy · A condition in which one kidney lies across the body midline and is fused to the other kidney.

Cryptococci · Yeastlike organisms of a fungal origin.

CVP Line · Specialized catheter inserted usually via the subclavian vein to the level of the right atrium to compensate for loss of peripheral infusion sites or to allow for fluid infusion in significant amounts.

Cystadenoma · Adenoma associated with cystoma.

Cystadenocarcinoma · Malignant neoplasm of the ovary; generally occurs in females over the age of 40 years.

Cystic Fibrosis · Congenital disorder affecting exocrine gland function, with respiratory effects including excessive secretions, obstruction of the bronchial system, infection, and tissue damage.

Cystitis · Inflammation of the bladder as a result of its infection.

Degenerative · Refers to deterioration of the body usually associated with the aging process.

Degenerative Disk Disease · The gradual, degenerative changes to the spine associated with aging.

Delayed Union · Refers to a fracture that does not heal in the usual amount of time.

Depressed Fracture · A fracture of the skull in which a fragment is depressed inward.

Dermoid Cysts (Cystic Teratomas) · Cystic masses arising from unfertilized ova, containing hair, fat, or bone, and located in an ovary.

Diagnosis · The name of a disease an individual is believed to have.

Diastole · The phase of the heart cycle in which the myocardium is relaxing.

Diploe · The spongy bone tissue found between the two tables of the cranial bones.

Disease · Any abnormal disturbance of the normal function or structure of a body part, organ, or system that may display a variety of manifestations.

Dislocation · The displacement of any part out of contact with its normal articulation.

Dissecting Aneurysm · An aneurysm resulting from hemorrhage that causes longitudinal splitting of the arterial wall.

Diverticula · A pouch or sac of variable size occurring normally or created by herniation of a mucous membrane through a defect in its muscular coat.

Diverticulitis · Inflammation of a diverticula.

Diverticulosis · The presence of diverticula in the absence of inflammation.

Dobhoff Tube · An enteral tube used to deliver a liquid diet directly to the duodenum.

Dominant · In relation to hereditary diseases, refers to a disease transmitted by a single gene from either parent.

Dysphagia · Difficulty in swallowing.

Ectopic Kidney · A kidney that is out of its normal position, usually found lower than normal.

Emphysema · A lung condition characterized by an increase in the air spaces distal to the terminal bronchioles and with destruction of alveolar walls.

Empyema · An accumulation of pus in the pleural cavity.

Encephalitis · Inflammation of the brain.

Enchondroma · A benign growth of cartilage arising in the metaphysis of a bone.

Endemic · Term given to disease of high prevalence in an area where the causative organism is commonly found.

Endometriosis · A condition in which endometrial tissue implants in aberrant pelvic locations.

Endoscopy · The use of lighted instruments with optic connections to visualize disease of the esophagus and stomach, or rectum and distal colon (e.g., sigmoidoscopy).

Endotracheal Tube · Tube inserted via the nose or mouth into the trachea for purposes of airway management, suctioning, or mechanical ventilation.

En Face · A radiographic descriptor referring to visualization of a pathology in a "head-on" or "straight-on" fashion, as compared to a profile-like image.

Ependymoma · A glial tumor that is firm and whitish and arises from the ependyma, the ventricle lining.

Epidemiology · The investigation of disease in large groups.

Epidural Hematoma · A hematoma positioned between the bony skull and the dura mater.

Epiphrenic Diverticulum · A pulsion diverticulum of the distal esophagus just above the hemidiaphragm.

Erythrocytes · Red blood cells.

Esophageal Atresia · Congenital lack of esophageal development past some point, commonly associated with tracheoesophageal fistula.

Esophageal Varices · Varicose veins of the esophagus that occur in patients with portal hypertension.

Etiology · The study of the cause and origin of disease.

Ewald/Edlich tube · A large bore gastric tube used to evacuate the contents of the stomach.

Ewing's Sarcoma · A primary malignant bone tumor arising in medullary tissue, occurring more often in cylindrical bones.

Exostosis · A benign bone growth, projecting outward from the bony cortex.

Expectoration · Expulsion of mucus or phlegm from the throat.

Fat Pad Sign · A radiographic indicator of a nonvisualized, underlying fracture of the bones of the elbow that displays as a tear-shaped radiolucency adjacent to the anterior and sometimes posterior surface of the distal humerus.

Fecalith · A hardened ball of stool that forms in the intestine.

Fibroadenoma · Adenoma containing fibrous tissue.

Fibrocystic Disease · A benign, generally bilateral breast condition characterized by various-sized cysts located throughout the breasts.

Filling Defect · An area of total or relative radiolucency within a column of barium.

Fistula · An abnormal, tubelike passage from one structure to another.

Foley Catheter · A catheter that is placed through the urethra and retained in the urinary bladder by a balloon which is inflated with air or fluid.

Follicular Cyst · A cyst arising from the ovum.

Fracture · The breaking or rupturing of bone caused by mechanical forces either applied to the bone or transmitted directly along the line of a bone.

Fusiform Aneurysm · An arterial aneurysm in which the entire circumference of the vessel wall is affected.

Gallstone Ileus · A condition in which gallstones erode from the gallbladder, creating a fistula to the small bowel that may cause a bowel obstruction.

Gastritis · Inflammation of the stomach mucosa.

Gastroenteritis · General grouping of a number of inflammatory disorders of the stomach and intestines.

Glioma · A tumor composed of tissue that represents neuroglia, commonly occurring in the cerebral hemispheres of the posterior fossa.

Glomerulonephritis · An inflammatory reaction of the renal parenchyma caused by streptococcal infection.

Gouty Arthritis · An inherited, metabolic disorder with excess amounts of uric acid produced and deposited in the joint and adjacent bone, most commonly in the metatarsophalangeal joint of the great toe.

Greenstick Fracture · A fracture in which the cortex breaks on one side without separation or breaking of the opposing cortex.

Growth-Plate Fracture · A fracture that involves the end of a long bone of a child, and that may be limited to growth-plate cartilage or extend into the metaphysis, epiphysis, or both.

Harris Tube · A single lumen gastric tube using mercury as a weight that is used as a decompression and diagnostic aid.

Heartburn · Burning symptoms experienced substernally as a result of the reflux of gastric acids into the esophagus.

Hemangioma · A benign tumor of dilated blood vessels.

Hematoma · A localized collection of blood in an organ, space, or tissue due to a break in the wall of a blood vessel.

Hemothorax · Pleural effusion containing blood.

Hepatitis · An inflammation of the liver resulting from a variety of causes.

Hepatoma · A primary malignant tumor of the liver.

Hepatomegaly · Enlargement of the liver as might be seen with viral hepatitis.

Hereditary · Genetically transferred from either parent to child and derived from ancestors.

Hernia · The protrusion of a part of an organ (e.g., bowel loop) through a small opening in the wall of a cavity.

Herniated Nucleus Pulposus · Herniation of the nucleus pulposus of the disc through a rupture in the anulus fibrosus.

Herpes · An inflammatory skin disease caused by a virus.

Hiatal Hernia · Protrusion of any structure, especially some portion of the stomach, into the thoracic cavity through the esophageal hiatus of the diaphragm.

Hickman Catheter · Specialized catheter inserted via the subclavian vein to allow for multiple tapping for injection of various agents, especially tissue-toxic chemotherapeutic agents.

Hirschprung's Disease · An absence of neurons in the bowel wall, typically in the sigmoid, preventing relaxation of the colon and normal peristalsis; congenital megacolon.

Histoplasmosis · Systemic, fungal infection caused by a fungus that thrives in soil, especially that fueled by bird or bat excreta; especially endemic to the Ohio and Mississippi River valleys.

Hodgkin's Disease · A malignant condition of lymphoid tissue associated with Reed Sternberg cells.

Homeostasis · The body's normal, internal resting state of equilibrium.

Horseshoe Kidney · A condition where the lower poles of the kidney are joined across midline by a band of soft tissues, resulting in a rotation anomaly on one or both sides.

Human Immunodeficiency (HIV) · The virus associated with acquired immune deficiency syndrome.

Hyaline Membrane Disease · Also known as *respiratory distress syndrome,* it is a disorder of prematurity caused by incomplete maturation of the alveoli that makes proper gas exchange difficult.

Hydrocephalus · A congenital or acquired condition resulting from accumulation of cerebrospinal fluids in the ventricles of the brain and leading to ventricular enlargement, compression of brain tissue, and increased intracranial pressure.

Hydronephrosis · An obstructive disease of the urinary system that causes a dilatation of the renal pelvis and calyces with urine.

Hypernephroma · The most common malignant tumor of the kidney.

Hyperparathyroidism · Abnormally increased activity of the parathyroid glands, causing excess hormone production, which overstimulates osteoclasts, which are responsible for bone removal.

Hyperplasia · Overdevelopment.

Hypertrophic Pyloric Stenosis · A congenital anomaly of the stomach in which the pyloric canal is greatly narrowed because of hypertrophy of the pyloric sphincter.

Hypoplasia · Less than normal development.

Iatrogenic · Pertains to any adverse condition in a patient occurring as a result of medical treatment.

Idiopathic · No identifiable causative factor.

Imperforate Anus · Congenital disorder characterized by lack of an anal opening to the exterior.

Incarcerated Hernia · A hernia in which the bowel is trapped by tissues that prevent it from being reduced, possibly causing an obstruction.

Incidence · A statistical measure that refers to the number of new cases of a disease found in a given time period.

Incompetency (Valvular) · Regurgitation of blood through the heart valves as a result of improper closure.

Incomplete Fracture · A fracture in which only part of the bony structure gives way, with little or no displacement.

Infection · An inflammatory process caused by exposure to some disease-causing organism.

Inflammatory · Refers to the body process of destroying, diluting, or walling off a localized injurious agent.

Inguinal Hernia · Hernia in which a bowel loop protrudes through a weakness in the inguinal ring, with descension into the scrotum.

Insufficiency (Valvular) · Regurgitation of blood through the heart valves.

Intraaortic Balloon Pump · Specialized catheter with a balloon at its distal end; inflation and deflation from a pump provides mechanical support of the left ventricle and the systemic circulation.

Intracerebral Hematoma · Bleeding within the brain tissue, commonly in the frontal lobe, which results from trauma or a ruptured hemangioma.

Intrathoracic Stomach · Condition in which all of the stomach slides above the diaphragm into the thoracic cavity.

Intussusception · The prolapse of a segment of bowel into a distal segment.

Involucrum · A shell or sheath of new supporting bone laid down by periosteum around a sequestrum of necrosed bone.

Jaundice · Yellowish discoloration of the skin and whites of the eyes caused by bilirubin accumulation in the body tissues.

Kaposi's Sarcoma · A sarcoma present in the connective tissues of about one fourth of all AIDS patients.

Le Fort Fracture · Bilateral, horizontal fractures of the maxillae, subcategorized as Le Fort I, II, or III fractures, depending on the extent of injury.

Left Ventricular Failure · Congestive heart failure that results when the left ventricle cannot pump an amount of blood equal to the venous return in the right ventricle.

Legionnaire's Disease · Severe, bacterial pneumonia named for its outbreak at an American Legion Convention in Pennsylvania in 1976.

Leiomyoma · A benign tumor derived from smooth muscle.

Lesion · General term used to describe the various types of cellular change that can occur in response to a disease.

Leukemia · A malignant disease of the leukocytes and their precursor cells in the blood and bone marrow.

Leukocytes · White blood cells.

Levacuator Tube · A wide double-lumen tube used for evacuation of gastric contents and irrigation of stomach.

Levin Tube · A gastroduodenal catheter of a small enough caliber to allow transnasal passage, often termed a *nasogastric tube*.

Linear Fracture · A fracture that extends lengthwise through a bone.

Malabsorption Syndrome · Group of diseases of various causes in which there is interference with normal digestion and absorption of food to the small bowel.

Malignant · Refers to a lesion that grows, spreads, and invades other tissues.

Malrotation · Unnatural position of the intestines caused by failure of normal rotation during embryologic development.

Malunion · Union of fragments of a fractured bone in a faulty position, impairing normal function or cosmetic appearance.

Manifestation · Observable changes resulting from cellular changes in the disease process.

Mantoux Text · Injection of purified protein derivative (PPD) under the skin for purposes of diagnosing tuberculosis.

Mastitis · Inflammation of the breast, most often caused by staphylococcus bacteria.

Mechanical Obstruction · Refers to a bowel obstruction that occurs as a result of blockage of the bowel lumen.

Mediastinal Emphysema (Pneumomediastinum) · The presence of air or gas in the mediastinum as a result of leakage of air from the bronchial tree.

Medical Jaundice · Jaundice that occurs due to hemolytic disease, in which excessive amounts of red blood cells are destroyed, or when the liver is damaged as a result of cirrhosis or hepatitis.

Medulloblastoma · Soft, infiltrating tumors of neuroepithelial tissue that are highly malignant.

Meningioma · A hard, usually vascular tumor which occurs mainly along meningeal vessels and the superior longitudinal sinus.

Meningitis · Inflammation of the meninges caused by bacteria or virus.

Meningocele · Hernial protrusion of the meninges through a defect of the skull or vertebral column.

Meningomyelocele · Protrusion of the spinal cord and meninges through a defect of the vertebral column, as is commonly associated with spina bifida.

Metabolic · Pertaining to the normal physiologic function of the body.

Metastasis · The spread of cancer cells.

Miliary Tuberculosis · Type of tuberculosis caused by hematogenous spread of the disease, with a characteristic appearance similar to millet seeds, which are small, white grains.

Milk of Calcium · A semiliquid sludge seen radiographically in the gallbladder; it results from the settling of bile caused by an obstruction at the neck of the gallbladder.

Miller-Abbott Tube · A double-lumen intestinal tube with an inflatable balloon at the distal end, used in the treatment of bowel obstructions.

Monteggia Fracture · A fracture in the proximal third of the ulnar shaft with dislocation of the radius.

Morbidity Rate · The incidence of illness in the population sufficient to interfere with an individual's normal daily routine.

Morphology · The form and structure of disease.

Mortality Rate · The number of deaths from a particular disease averaged over a population.

Multiple Myeloma · A malignant neoplasm of plasma cells characterized by skeletal destruction, pathologic fractures, and bone pain.

Mycoplasma Pneumonia · The most common form of primary atypical pneumonia, occurring most frequently in young adults.

Myelocele · Protrusion of the spinal cord through the normally closed bony neural arch of the spine.

Mycobacterium Avium · A type of tubercle bacillis that may cause tuberculosis; rare in humans, but most common in chickens and swine.

Necrosis · Tissue death.

Neoplastic · Pertaining to new, abnormal tissue growth.

Nephroblastoma (Wilm's Tumor) · A rapidly developing malignancy of the kidneys, usually affecting children before age 5.

Nephrocalcinosis · A condition characterized by precipitation of calcium in the tubules of the kidney, resulting in renal deficiency.

Nephroptosis · Prolapse of a kidney.

Nephrosclerosis · Intimal thickening of predominantly the small vessels of the kidney as a result of reduced blood flow through arteriosclerotic renal vasculature.

Nephrostomy Tube · A tube inserted through the abdominal wall into the renal; pelvis to drain urine.

Neurofibroma · A tumor of peripheral nerves caused by abnormal proliferation of Schwann cells.

Neurogenic Bladder · A bladder dysfunction caused by interference with the nerve impulses concerned with urination.

Nidus · An area of sclerosis with a radiolucent center associated with an osteoid osteoma.

Noncommunicating (Internal) Hydrocephalus · Type of hydrocephalus where obstruction occurs congenitally, from tumor growth, trauma and inflammation; interferes or blocks normal CSF circulation.

Nonunion · Complication of a fracture when healing does not occur and fragments do not join.

Nosocomial · Refers to diseases acquired in or from a health care environment.

Oligodendroglioma · A glioma, it is a slow-growing astrocytic tumor that is usually relatively benign.

Oligohydramnios · The presence of too little (less than 300 ml) amniotic fluid at term, generally associated with renal disorders in the fetus.

Osteoarthritis · Noninflammatory degenerative joint disease occurring mainly in older persons, producing gradual deterioration of the joint cartilage.

Osteoblasts · The bone-forming cells responsible for bone growth, ossification, and regeneration.

Osteochondroma · A benign tumor of adult bone capped by cartilage.

Osteoclastoma (Giant Cell Tumor) · A tumor that is usually benign and characterized by osteolytic areas, most commonly found around the knee and wrist of young adults.

Osteoclasts · Cells which are associated with absorption and removal of bone.

Osteogenesis Imperfecta · A congenital disease in which the bones are abnormally brittle and subject to fractures.

Osteoid Osteoma · A benign tumor of bonelike structure developing on a bone and sometimes other structures.

Osteomalacia · A condition marked by softening of the bones, caused by lack of calcium in the tissues and a failure of bone tissue to calcify.

Osteomyelitis · Infection of bone, most often caused by staphylococcus, which may localize or spread to the bone to involve the marrow and other bone tissues.

Osteopetrosis · A hereditary disease characterized by abnormally dense bone, likely as a result of faulty bone resorption.

Osteophytes · An osseous outgrowth (spur).

Osteoporosis · Metabolic bone disorder resulting in demineralization of bone, most commonly seen in women past menopause.

Osteosarcoma · A primary malignancy of bone usually arising in the metaphysis, most commonly around the knee.

Paget's Disease · A metabolic disorder of unknown etiology, most common in the elderly, characterized by an early, osteolytic stage and a late, osteoblastic stage.

Pancreatitis · Acute or chronic, asymptomatic or symptomatic, inflammation of the pancreas caused by autodigestion by pancreatic enzymes.

Paraesophageal Hiatal Hernia · A hiatal hernia in which the stomach or adjacent structures herniate above the diaphragm, while the gastroesophageal junction remains below the diaphragm.

Paralytic Ileus · A failure of bowel peristalsis, often seen following abdominal surgery, that may result in bowel obstruction.

Patent Ductus Arteriosis · Abnormal persistence of an open ductus arteriosis after birth, resulting in recirculation of arterial blood through the lungs.

Pathologic Fracture · A fracture which occurs in abnormal bone weakened by a disease process.

Pathology · The study of structural and functional manifestations of disease.

Palliative · Treatment designed to relieve pain without the goal of curing the disease.

Peau d'Orange Appearance · Appearance of multiple small depressions on the skin surface as a result of hair follicles becoming visible from skin edema, as might occur with breast cancer.

Pedunculated Polyp · A polyp attached to the bowel wall by a narrow stalk.

Pelvic Inflammatory Disease (PID) · A bacterial infection of the female genital system, most often caused by bacteria.

Penetrating Fracture · A type of incomplete fracture resulting from penetration by a sharp object, frequently with comminution at the site of injury.

Peptic Ulcer · Ulceration of the mucous membrane of the esophagus, stomach, or duodenum by action of acidic gastric juice.

Phlebitis · Inflammation of a vein, often associated with venous thrombosis.

Placenta Previa · The condition in which the placenta develops in the lower half of the uterus, encroaching or on, and completely or partially covering, the internal cervical os.

Platelike Atelectasis · Radiograhic appearance seen in atelectasis in which one or more linear opacities are seen, usually at the lung bases and parallel to the diaphragm.

Pleural Effusion · A collection of excess fluid in the pleural cavity.

Pleurisy · Inflammation of the pleura with exudation into the pleural cavity and on its surface.

Pneumatocele · A thin-walled, air-containing cyst that is a characteristic radiographic lesion seen in staphylococcal pneumonia.

Pneumococcal Pneumonia · The most common bacterial pneumonia, generally affecting an entire lobe of a lung.

Pneumoconioses · A group of occupational diseases characterized by permanent deposits of particulate matter in the lungs and by resultant pulmonary fibrosis.

Pneumocystitis Carinii Pneumonia · Life-threatening infection of the lungs most commonly associated with AIDS.

Pneumonia · The most frequent type of lung infection, resulting in an inflammation of the lung with compromised pulmonary function.

Pneumoperitoneum · The presence of air or gas in the peritoneal cavity.

Pneumothorax · An accumulation of free air or gas in the pleural space that compresses the lung tissue.

Polycystic Kidney Disease · A familial kidney disorder in which innumerable tiny cysts that are present congenitally gradually enlarge during aging to compress and eventually destroy normal tissues.

Polycystic Ovaries · Ovaries that contain multiple small cysts.

Polydactyly · The presence of more than five digits.

Polyhydramnios · An excess of amniotic fluid; it may be associated with anencephaly or gastrointestinal disturbances in the fetus.

Polyp · A small mass of tissue arising from mucous membrane to project inward into the lumen of the bowel.

Pott's Fracture · A fracture of the lower part of the fibula involving both malleoli with dislocation of the ankle joint.

Prevalence · A statistical measure that refers to the number of cases of a disease found in a given population.

Prognosis · The prediction of course and outcome for a given disease.

Pseudocyst · An abnormal or displaced space resembling a cyst.

Pseudopneumothorax · A radiographic artifact produced by a wrinkle in the skin that mimics a pneumothorax.

Pseudopolyps · Islands of unaffected mucosa that are visible when surrounded by the affected mucosa of ulcerative colitis.

Pulsion Diverticulum · A diverticulum created by herniation of the mucous membrane through the muscular coat of the esophagus as a result of pressure from within.

Punctate · Pinpoint punctures or depressions; commonly used in reference to the appearance of a type of hemorrhaging.

Pyelonephritis · Bacterial infection of the kidney and its pelvis.

Pyogenic Arthritis · Joint inflammation that occurs secondary to other infections.

Pyuria · The presence of pus in the urine created by its drainage from renal abcesses into the kidney's collecting tubules.

Recessive · In relation to hereditary disease, refers to a disease transmitted by both parents to an offspring.

Reflux Esophagitis · The backward flow of gastric acids into the esophagus.

Regeneration · Process in which damaged tissues are replaced by new tissues that are essentially identical to those replaced.

Regional Enteritis · A chronic granulomatous inflammatory disease of unknown etiology involving any part of the gastrointestinal tract, but commonly involving the terminal ileum.

Renal Agenesis · The absence of the kidney on one side, with an unusually large kidney on the other side.

Renal Colic · Severe, agonizing pain that refers along the course of a ureter toward the genital and loin regions in response to the movement of a renal calculus.

Renal Failure · The end result of a chronic process that gradually results in lost kidney function.

Reticuloendothelial System · Specialized cells found in the liver, bone marrow, and spleen, whose function is phagocytosis.

Rheumatoid Arthritis · A chronic, systemic disease primarily of joints, characterized by an overgrowth of synovial tissues and articular structures, and progressive destruction of cartilage, bone, and supporting structures.

Rh Factor · Blood factor first discovered in the blood of the rhesus monkey; contained by approximately 85% of the population who are said to be ''Rh positive.''

Rickets · Osteomalacia that occurs before growth-plate closure, caused by deficiency of vitamin D, especially in infants and children.

Right Ventricular Failure · Congestive heart failure that results when the right ventricle cannot pump as much blood as it receives from the right atrium, slowing venous blood flow.

Saccular Aneurysm · A localized sac affecting only a part of the circumference of an arterial wall.

''Sail sign'' · Radiographic appearance of an enlarged thymus in an infant, so described because of its characteristic sail-like appearance.

Sarcoma · A type of tumor, often highly malignant, composed of a substance like embryonic connective tissue.

Schatzki's Ring · A ring of mucosa that protrudes into the lumen of the esophagus, thought to develop as a defense mechanism against gastric reflux.

Scoliosis · Abnormal lateral curvature of the spine.

Seminoma · A malignant neoplasm of the testis, usually occurring in males between the ages of 30 and 40 years.

Sequestrum · A piece of dead, devascularized bone that separates from living bone during the process of necrosis.

Sessile Polyp · A polyp with a wide base attached directly to the bowel wall.

Shunt · An artificial passageway used to drain excess fluids (e.g., from the ventricles into the internal jugular vein, the heart, or the peritoneum in the case of excess CSF).

Sign · An objective manifestation of disease perceptible to the managing physician, as opposed to subjective symptoms perceived by the patient.

Silicosis · Pneumoconiosis caused by inhalation of silica dust, as is common among miners, grinders, and sand blasters.

Sinusitis · Inflammation of a sinus, which may be purulent or nonpurulent, acute or chronic.

Situs Inversus · Complete reversal of the viscera of the thorax and abdomen.

Sliding Hiatal Hernia · A hiatal hernia in which a portion of the stomach and gastroesophageal junction are both situated above the diaphragm.

Somatic Cells · Those body cells other than the germ cells of the egg in the female and spermatozoa in the male.

Spina Bifida · A developmental anomaly characterized by incomplete closure of the vertebral canal, through which the choriomeninges may or may not protrude.

Spiral (Oblique) Fracture · A fracture in which the bone has been twisted apart, usually resulting from a rotary-type injury.

Spondylolisthesis · Forward displacement of one vertebra over another (commonly occurring at the L5/S1 junction), usually caused by a developmental defect in the pars interarticularis.

Spondylolysis · A condition marked by a cleft or breaking down of the body of a vertebra between the superior and inferior articular processes.

Staghorn Calculus · A large renal calculus that assumes the shape of the pelvicalyceal junction, resembling the horn of a stag.

Staphylococcal Pneumonia · Pneumonia caused by infection with staphylococcus that localizes in and/or around the bronchi.

Strangulated Hernia · Herniation in which the bowel loop passes through a constriction tight enough to cut off its blood supply, leading to necrosis of that portion of the bowel without prompt surgical intervention.

Strangulation · A constriction that cuts off blood supply.

Stress Fracture · A fracture that occurs at a site of maximal strain on a bone, usually connected with some unaccustomed activity (also known as march, stress, or insufficiency fractures).

Subarachnoid Hematoma · A hematoma that accumulates between the brain's arachnoid layer and its pia mater.

Subcutaneous Emphysema · The presence of air or gas in the subcutaneous tissues of the body.

Subdural Hematoma · A hematoma positioned between the dura mater and the arachnoid meningeal layer.

Subluxation · An incomplete or partial dislocation.

Subtractive Pathology · A radiographic term used to describe diseases that are easier than normal to penetrate.

Supernumerary Kidney · A relatively rare anomaly consisting of the presence of a third, small rudimentary kidney.

Surgical Jaundice · Jaundice that occurs as a result of biliary system blockage, which prevents bile from entering the duodenum.

Swan-Ganz Catheter · Specialized, multilumen catheter inserted usually via the subclavian vein for positioning outside the pulmonary artery for purposes of evaluating cardiac function.

Sylvian Triangle · An anatomic landmark in cerebral angiography, created by the middle cerebral artery and its branches.

Symptom · Any subjective evidence of a disease as perceived by a patient.

Syndactyly · A webbing or fusion of digits.

Syndrome · A group of signs and symptoms that occur together and characterize a specific abnormal disturbance.

Systole · The phase of the heart cycle in which the myocardium is contracting.

Tendinitis · Inflammation of a tendon.

Tenosynovitis · Inflammation of a tendon and its sheath.

Tension Pneumothorax · A pneumothorax in which air enters the pleural space but cannot leave because the tissues surrounding the opening into the pleural cavity act as valves; it results in a complete lung collapse and a mediastinal shift to the opposite side of the pneumothorax.

Teratoma · A neoplasm comprised of different types of tissue, none of which is native to the area where it occurs, commonly found in the ovary or testis.

Tetrology of Fallot · A combination of four congenital cardiac defects: pulmonary stenosis, ventricular central defect, overriding aorta, and hypertrophy of the right ventricle.

Thrombocytes · Platelets.

Thrombophlebitis · The presence of inflammation and blood clots within a vein.

TNM System · A recognized, standard system for clinical classification of cancer.

Torus Fracture · A fracture in which the cortex folds back upon itself, with little or no displacement of the lower end of the bone.

Toxic Megacolon · An acute dilatation of the colon from paralytic ileus, particularly susceptible to rupture.

Toxoplasma Gondii · intracellular parasites of sporozoa origin which affect tissue and organs of mammals and birds.

Trabecula · The spongy substance found within a bone; it gives a characteristic appearance to bony detail.

Traction Diverticulum · A localized bulging of the full thickness of the esophageal wall, caused by adhesions from an external lesion.

Transient Ischemic Anemia (TIA) · A temporary episode of neurologic dysfunction that can precede a cerebrovascular accident.

Transitional Vertebra · A vertebra that assumes the characteristics of the vertebrae on each side of a major spine division.

Transposition · Displacement of a viscus to the opposite side.

Transposition of Great Vessels · Congenital malformation of the cardiovascular system in which the aorta arises from the right ventricle and the pulmonary artery from the left ventricle.

Transverse Fracture · A type of complete, noncomminuted fracture that occurs at right angles to the axis of the bone.

Traumatic · Pertaining to the effects of a wound or injury, whether physical or psychic.

Tripod Fracture · A fracture of the zygoma at its three sutures: frontal, temporal, and maxillary.

Tuberculosis · Any of the infectious diseases of man and animals caused by mycobacterium tuberculosis, generally affecting the lungs in the human body.

Ulcerative Colitis · A chronic, recurrent ulceration of the colon mucosa of unknown etiology.

Unicornuate Uterus · A uterus whose uterine cavity is elongated and has a single uterine tube emerging from it.

Uremia · The retention of urea in the blood, as characteristic of renal failure.

Ureteral Stent · A tube used to maintain patency of the ureter with the proximal end placed in the renal pelvis and the distal end placed in the urinary bladder.

Ureterocele · Cystlike dilatation of the terminal portion of the ureter as a result of stenosis of the ureteral meatus.

Urethral Valves · Congenital presence of mucosal folds that protrude into the posterior urethra, which may cause significant obstruction to urine flow.

Uterus Didelphys · Complete duplication of the uterus, cervix, and vagina.

Venous Thrombosis · The formation of blood clots within a vein.

Ventricular Pacing Electrodes · Either temporary or permanent, they provide electrical pacing of the heart in situations in which the normal electrical system of the heart is misfiring.

Vesicoureteral Reflux · The backward flow of urine out of the bladder and into the ureters.

Viral Pneumonia · Pneumonia caused by a virus, spread by an infected person to a nonimmune individual.

Virulence · The ease with which an organism overcomes body defenses.

Volvulus · An intestinal obstruction caused by a twisting of the bowel about its mesenteric base.

Wound · An injury of soft body parts associated with rupture of the skin.

Zenker's Diverticulum · A pulsion diverticulum located at the pharyngoesophageal junction.

BIBLIOGRAPHY

American College of Radiology: *Index for radiological diagnoses,* ed 3, Reston, Virginia, 1986, The American College of Radiology.

American Joint Committee on Cancer: *Manual for staging of cancer,* ed 3, New York, 1988, JB Lippincott.

Atlas: *Magnetic resonance imaging of the brain and spine,* New York, 1991, Raven Press.

Bontrager, KL: *Textbook of radiographic positioning and related anatomy,* ed 3, St Louis, 1993, Mosby.

Bradley W and Brant-Zawadzki M: *The Raven MRI teaching,* Vols. I - III, New York, 1991, Raven Press.

Cawson RA et al: *Pathology: the Mechanisms of disease,* ed 2, St Louis, 1989, Mosby.

Chey WY: *Functional disorders of the digestive tract,* New York, 1983, Raven Press.

Chopra S and May R: *Pathophysiology of gastrointestinal diseases,* Boston, 1989, Little, Brown, and Co.

Crowley LV: *Introductory concepts in pathology,* Chicago, 1972, Mosby.

Crowley LV: *Introduction to human disease,* ed 2, Boston, 1988, Jones and Bartlett.

Gitnick G: *Gastroenterology,* New York, 1983, John Wiley and Sons.

Greenberger N: *Gastrointestinal disorders: a pathophysiologic approach,* ed 3, Chicago, 1986, Mosby.

Hatfield P and Wise R: Radiology of the gallbladder and bile ducts, In *Golden's Diagnostic Radiology,* Baltimore, 1976, Williams and Wilkins.

Heptinstall R: *Pathology of the kidney,* ed 3, Volumes I - III, Boston, 1983, Little, Brown and Co.

Hinshaw HC and Murray J: *Diseases of the chest,* ed 4, Philadelphia, 1980, WB Saunders.

Hudson L, et al: *Respiratory infections,* New York, 1986, Churchill Livingstone.

Jariwalla G, and Fry J: *Respiratory diseases,* Lancashire, UK, 1985. MTP Press Limited.

Lapides J: *Fundamentals of urology,* Philadelphia, 1976, WB Saunders.

Lieberman J: *Inherited diseases of the lung,* Philadelphia, 1988, WB Saunders.

Latchaw R: *MR and CT imaging of the head, neck, and spine,* vols 1 and 2, *Year Book* St Louis, 1991, Mosby.

Levine D: *Care of the renal patient,* ed 2, Philadelphia, 1991, WB Saunders.

Mulvihill M: *Human diseases: a systemic approach,* ed 3, East Norwalk, Connecticut, 1991, Appleton and Lange.

Norris H: *Pathology of the colon, small intestine, and anus,* ed 2, New York, 1991, Churchill Livingstone.

Pomeranz, S: *Craniospinal MRI,* Philadelphia, 1991, WB Saunders.

Purtilo D and Purtilo R: *A survey of human diseases,* ed 2, Boston, 1989, Little, Brown, and Co.

Scheld WM Whitley, RJ, and Durack D: *Infections of the central nervous system,* New York, 1991, Raven Press.

Sheldon H: *Boyd's introduction to the study of disease,* ed 10, Philadelphia, 1988, Lea and Febiger.

Sherlock S: *Diseases of the liver and biliary system,* ed 8, Boston, 1989, Blackwell Scientific Publications.

Sleisenger M and Fordtran J: *Gastrointestinal disease: pathophysiology, diagnosis, management,* ed 3, vols I and II, Philadelphia, 1983, WB Saunders.

Snively WD and Beshear D: *Textbook of pathophysiology,* Philadelphia, 1972, JB Lippincott.

Swash M and Kennard C: *Scientific basis of clinical neurology,* New York, 1985, Churchill Livingstone.

Taussig MJ: *Processes in pathology,* Oxford, 1979, Blackwell Scientific Publications.

Tattersfield AE and McNicol M: *Respiratory disease,* New York, 1987, Springer-Verlag.

Walton J: *Brain's diseases of the nervous system,* ed 9, New York, 1985, Oxford University Press.

INDEX

A

Abdomen, 147-218; *see also* Gastrointestinal system
  computed tomography of, 160-162
  congenital/hereditary anomalies of, 165-172
  degenerative diseases of, 186-188
  imaging considerations for, 153-154, 157-160
  inflammatory diseases of, 173-186
  magnetic resonance imaging of, 160-162
  neoplastic diseases of, 212-215
  neurogenic diseases of, 197-199
  traumatic diseases of, 205-208
Abdominal tubes, 162-164
Abruptio placentae, 302
Abscess, lung, 127-129
Absorption atelectasis, 132-135
Achalasia, 197, 198, 199
Achondroplasia, 15
Acoustic neurilemoma, 394-396
Acoustic neuroma, 394-396
Acquired immune deficiency syndrome (AIDS), 342-343
Acromegaly, 39, 40-41
Acromioclavicular joint dislocation, 64, 66
Adenocarcinoma(s)
  colon, 214-215
  endometrial, 295
  gastric, 212
  prostate, 305
  renal, 275, 279
Adenomas
  bronchial, 139
  pituitary, 391-393
Adenomatous polyps, 212-213
Agglutination, 337
Air-bronchogram sign in hyaline membrane disease, 112
Albers-Schönberg disease, 16
Alimentary tract, 150-151; *see also* Gastrointestinal system
Amniotic fluid disorders, 302
Anemia, hemoglobin levels in, 337
Anencephaly, 22
Aneurysms, 329-330
Angiography, 319
  central nervous system, 358
  renal, 248
Ankylosing spondylitis, 27, 29, 30
Annulus fibrosus, 351
Anthracosis, 125, 126-127
Anus, imperforate, 172
Aorta, coarctation of, 319-321

Appendicitis, 184, 185
Artery(ies), 312-313
Arthritis, 23-33
  ankylosing spondylitis, 27, 29, 30
  gouty, 32-33
  osteoarthritis, 28,31
  pyogenic, 24-25
  rheumatoid, 25-27
Asbestosis, 125
Ascites in cirrhosis of liver, 229-230
Aspiration pneumonia, 117-118
Astrocytomas, 383, 386
Atelectasis, 132-135
Atheroma formations, 326
Atherosclerosis, 326-327
Atherothrombic brain infarction (ABI), 328-329
Atria, left and right, 310-311
Autoantibodies, 4
Autoimmune disorders, 4
Autosomes, 3

B

Basilar skull fractures, 58-59
Battered child syndrome, 66-67
Bicornuate uterus, 291
Biliary tree; *see* Hepatobiliary system
Bladder 242-244; *see also* Urinary system
  carcinoma of, 280-283
  diverticula of, 261-262
  neurogenic, 267
  trabeculated, 262
Blood 336-339
Blood-brain barrier, 351
Bone(s), 10-13
Bone cyst, simple, 76-77
Bony callus in fracture healing, 42-43
Bowel
  large, 152-153
    imaging considerations for, 153-155
  malrotation of, 171-172
  obstructions of, 164, 188-196
  small, 212
Brain 348-352; *see also* Central nervous system (CNS)
  embolism to, 328-329
  hematomas of, 373-379
  hemorrhage in, 328-329
  metastases to, 388, 396
  trauma to, 372-373
Breast(s) 288; *see also* Female reproductive system

Breast(s)—cont'd
  carcinoma of, 299-301
  fibroadenoma of, 296-297
  fibrocystic, 298
  inflammation of, 292
  masses of, 296-297
  mastitis, 292
Bronchial adenomas, 139
Bronchiectasis, 118-119
Bronchitis, chronic, 122-123
Bronchogenic carcinoma, 139-141
Bursitis, 29, 32
C
Calcifications
  pancreatic, 274-275
  urinary tract, 269-275
Calculi
  renal, 269-275
  staghorn, 270-271
Callus
  bony, in fracture healing, 42-43
  provisional, in fracture healing, 42
Cancer, 7-8
  colon, 214-215
Cantor tube, 164
Capillaries, 309, 312-313
Carcinoma, 7
  bladder, 280, 282-283
  breast, 299-301
  bronchogenic, 139-141
  cervical, 294
  gallbladder, 237-238
  pancreatic, 238-239
  prostate, 305
  renal, 275, 279-280
  testicular, 306
Cardiac cycle, 312-313
Cardiomegaly, 316
Cardiovascular system, 309-335
  aneurysms in, 329-330
  congenital/hereditary diseases of, 319-323
    coarctation of aorta as, 319-321
    patent ductus arteriosus as, 319, 320
    septal defects as, 321
    tetralogy of Fallot as, 323
    transposition of great vessels as, 322
  congestive heart disease in, 324-325
  degenerative disease of, 326-329
  imaging considerations for, 314-319
    controllable, 314-316
    uncontrollable, 317
  valvular disease in, 323-324
  venous thrombosis in, 331-332
Catheter(s)
  abdominal, 162-164
  central venous pressure, 107-108, 109
  Foley, 164, 253
  Hickman, 109-110
  intra-aortic balloon pump, 110
  Swan-Ganz, 108-109
Celiac disease, 181

Cellular necrosis, 4
Central nervous system (CNS), 348-401
  congenital/hereditary diseases of, 361-365
    hydrocephalus as, 361-365
    meningomyelocele as, 361, 362-364
  imaging considerations for, 353-360, 383
  inflammatory diseases of, 366-371
    cervical spondylosis as, 370-371
    degenerative disk disease as, 368-369
    encephalitis as, 368-369
    meningitis as, 366-367
  neoplastic diseases of, 381-389
    craniopharyngioma as, 394-395
    gliomas as, 382, 383-389
    medulloblastoma as, 383, 390-391
    meningioma as, 383, 390-391
    metastatic, 396
    nerve sheath cell tumors as, 394-396
    pituitary adenomas as, 391,392-393
    spinal tumors as, 396-410
  traumatic diseases of, 372-381
    brain trauma as, 372-373
    hematomas of brain as, 372-379
    herniated nucleus pulposus as, 379-381
Central venous pressure (CVP) lines, 107-109
Cerebrovascular accident (CVA), 328-329
Cervical spondylosis, 370-371
Cervix; see also Female reproductive system
  carcinoma of, 294
Chemical pneumonia, 117-118
Chest tubes, 105-109
Cholangiography
  percutaneous transhepatic, 223-224
  T-tube, 2224-225
Cholangiopancreatogram, endoscopic retrograde, 224-225
Cholecystitis, 231-232
Cholelithiasis, 230-232
Chondrosarcoma, 81-83
Choriocarcinomas, testicular, 305
Chronic obstructive pulmonary disease (COPD), 122-123
Circle of Willis, 351, 352
Circulatory vessels, 336-339
Cirrhosis of liver, 228-230
Coarctation of aorta, 319-321
"Cobblestone" appearance in regional enteritis, 183, 185
Coccidiomycosis, 126-127, 128
Colic, renal, 270, 273
Colitis, ulcerative, 184-186
Colon
  atresia of, 165-170
  cancer of, 214-215
  diverticuli of, 204-205
  polyps of, 212-213
Colostomy, 159, 160
Coma, 373
Communicating hydrocephalus, 361
Compression atelectasis, 153
Computed radiography of respiratory system, 97-98
Computed tomography (CT)
  of abdomen, 160-162
  of central nervous system, 353, 358
  of gastrointestinal system, 160-162

Computed tomography (CT)— cont'd
  of hemopoietic system, 339-340
  for hepatobiliary system disorders, 225-227
  of respiratory system, 93, 95-96
  of urinary system, 248
Concussion, brain, 372
Congenital/hereditary disorders, 3, 4
  of abdomen, 165-172
  of cardiovascular system, 319-323
  of central nervous system, 361-365
  of gastrointestinal system, 165-172
  of respiratory system, 111-113
  of skeletal system, 14-22
  of urinary system, 254-263
Congestive heart disease, 324-325
Contre coup lesion in brain trauma, 372
Contusion, 7
  brain, 372, 374
Cor pulmonale in emphysema, 123
Coronary artery disease (CAD), 326-328
Corpus luteum cysts, 292
Coup lesion in brain trauma, 372
Cranial anomalies, 21-22
Craniopharyngioma, 394-395
Craniosynostoses, 22,
Craniotubular dysplasias, 17
Crohn's disease, 183-184
Curative treatment, 7
Cyst(s)
  bone, simple, 76-77
  corpus luteum, 292
  dermoid, 292
  follicular, 292
  ovarian, 292-293
  renal, 275, 276-293
Cystadenocarcinoma of ovary, 293-294
Cystic fibrosis, 111-112
Cystic teratomas of ovary, 293
Cystitis, 266-267
Cystography
  imaging considerations for, 248, 252
  voiding, imaging considerations for, 248

D

Degenerative diseases, 6
  of abdomen, 186-188
  of cardiovascular system, 326-329
  of gastrointestinal system, 186-188, 189-193
  of urinary system, 267-275
Degenerative disk disease, 368-369
Dermoid cysts of ovary, 292
Diastole, 312
Digital radiography of respiratory system, 97-99
Disease(s), 1, 3-8; *see also* Congenital/hereditary disorders
Disk(s), intervertebral, 351, 353
  degenerative disease of, 368-369
  herniated, 379-380
Dislocation(s), 64-66
  of hip, congenital, 17-18
Dissecting aneurysm, 330
Diverticula
  bladder, 260, 262
  ureteral, 259

Diverticular disease, 199, 201-205
Diverticulitis, 199, 201-205
Dobhuff tube, 163
Dominant inheritance, 3-4
"Double bubble sign" in duodenal atresia, 166-168
Duodenum
  atresia of, 165-170
Dysphagia, 181

E

Echocardiography, 318
Ectopic kidney, 256, 258, 259
Ectopic pregnancy, 302
Edlich tube, 162-163
Ejaculatory ducts, 303
Electrodes, ventricular pacing, 110-111
Embolism to brain, 328-329
Emphysema, 123-124
  mediastinal, 103-104
  subcutaneous, 103, 105
Encephalitis, 368-369
Endocardium, 312
Endochondroma, 75
Endometriosis, 292
Endometrium, carcinoma of, 295-296
Endoscopic retrograde cholangiopancreatogram (ERCP),
    224-225
Endoscopy in GI tract examination, 154-160
Endotracheal (ET) tube, 106-107
Enteral tube, 163
Enteritis, regional, 183-184, 185
Epididymides, 303
Epididymo-orchitis, 306
Epiphrenic diverticulum, 199, 203
Erythrocytes, 336-337
Esophagitis, reflux, 173-174
Esophagus, 155-156
  atresia of, 165-167
  diverticuli of, 199, 201-205
  foreign bodies of, 205, 206
  imaging considerations for, 155-156
  strictures of, 173-174
  tumors of, 209-210
  varices of, 174-175
Ewald tube, 162-163
Exostosis, 73
Extracorporeal shock wave lithotripsy (ESWL),
    248-251

F

Fat pad sign, elbow, 54-55, 56
Female reproductive system, 287-288; *see also* Pregnancy
  congenital abnormalities of, 291
  imaging considerations for, 288-291
  inflammatory diseases of, 291-292
  neoplastic diseases of, 292-301
    breast masses as, 296
    carcinoma as
      breast, 299-301
      cervical, 294
    cystadenocarcinoma as, 293-294
    endometrial adenocarcinoma as, 295-296
    fibrocystic breasts as, 298

Female reproductive system—cont'd
  neoplastic diseases—cont'd
    ovarian cystic masses as, 292-293
    uterine masses as, 295
Fibroids, uterine, 295
Fluoroscopy
  of cardiovascular system, 319
  in GI tract examination, 153-160
Foley catheter, 164, 253
Follicular cysts, 292
Foot malformations, 17
Foreign bodies of esophagus, 205, 206
Fracture(s), 39-63
  avulsion, 44, 49
  blow-out, 60, 62
  Boxer's, 54
  butterfly, 43
  chip, 44
  Colle's, 53-54
  comminuted, 43, 45
  complete noncomminuted, 43-44, 46
  cranial
    cerebral, 57-59
    visceral, 59-61
  delayed union of, 43
  fatigue, 52-53
  greenstick, 44, 50-51
  growth plate, 52
  incomplete, 44, 50-51
  LeFort, 60
  malunion of, 43
  mandibular, 60
  maxillary, 60
  Monteggia, 54
  multiple, 44, 49
  nonunion of, 43
  oblique, 43-44
  pathologic, 44, 48
  penetrating, 52
  Pott's, 54-55
  rib, 101
  Smith's, 54
  spiral, 43-44, 46
  splintered, 43
  stress, 52
  torus, 51
  transverse, 44, 47
  tripod, 62-63
  of vertebral body
    compression, 70
    Hangman's, 70
Fungal disease of respiratory system, 126-127, 128
Fusiform aneurysm, 329
G
Gallbladder 221, 231-232, 237-238; *see also* Hepatobiliary
        system
  carcinoma of, 237-238
  inflammatory disorders of, 231-232
Gallstone ileus, 232-233
Gallstones, 230-232
Gastric tubes, 162

Gastroenteritis, 176, 179-180
Gastrointestinal system
  computed tomography of, 160-162
  congenital/hereditary anomalies of, 165-172
    atresia as, 165-170
    hypertrophic pyloric stenosis as, 171
    imperforate anus as, 172
    malrotation as, 171, 172
  degenerative diseases of, 186-188, 189-193
    herniation as, 186-188
    hiatal hernia as, 188, 189-192
  imaging considerations for, 153-160
  inflammatory diseases of, 173-186
    appendicitis as, 184, 185
    esophageal strictures as, 173-174
    esophageal varices as, 173-174
    gastroenteritis as, 176
    malabsorption syndrome as, 176, 177-178, 181-182
    peptic ulcer as, 174, 176-178
    regional enteritis as, 183-184
    ulcerative colitis as, 184-186
  magnetic resonance imaging of, 160-162
  neoplastic diseases of, 209-215
    colon cancer as, 214-215
    colonic polyps as, 212-213
    esophageal tumors as, 209-210
    gastric tumors as, 210-211
    small bowel neoplasms as, 212
  neurogenic diseases of, 197-199
  traumatic diseases of, 205-208
    abdominal trauma as, 205-206, 207
    foreign bodies in esophagus as, 205, 206
Giant cell tumor, 78-79
Glioblastomas, 382, 383-384
Gliomas, 382, 383-389
Glomerulonephritis, acute, 265-266
Gouty arthritis, 32-33
H
Hand malformations, 17
Harn's tube, 164
Heart, 309-313
  congestive disease of, 324-325
  valves of, disease of, 323-324
Heartburn, 173-174
Hemangioma of liver, 235-236
Hematocrit, 337
Hematomas of brain, 373-379
Hemocytoblasts, 337
Hemopoietic system, 336-347
  acquired immune deficiency syndrome, 342-343
  imaging considerations for, 339-341
  neoplastic diseases of, 343-346
    Hodgkin's disease as, 345-346
    leukemia as, 345, 346
    multiple myeloma as, 343-344
Hepatitis, viral, 230
Hepatobiliary scans, 225-228
Hepatobiliary system, 219-241
  imaging considerations for, 222-228
    for computed tomography, 225-227
    for contrast studies, 223-225

Hepatobiliary system—cont'd
   imaging considerations for—cont'd
      for diagnostic medical sonography, 225-226
      for hepatobiliary scans, 225-228
      for plain film, 222-223
   inflammatory diseases of, 229-234
      cholelithiasis as, 230-232
      cirrhosis of, 228-230
      pancreatitis as, 232-234
      viral hepatitis as, 230
   metabolic diseases of, 234-235
   neoplastic diseases of, 235-239
      carcinoma as
         of gallbladder, 237-238
         of pancreas, 238-239
      hemangioma as, 235-236
      hepatoma as, 235-237
Hepatoma, 235-237
Hernia
   hiatal, 188, 189-192
   incarcerated, 188, 189
   inguinal, 186-187
   strangulated, 186
Herniated nucleus pulposus, 379-381
Herniation, 186-188
Hiatal hernia, 188, 189-192
Hickman catheter, 109-110
Hip, dislocation of, 64-65
   congenital, 17-18
Hirschsprung's disease, 199, 200
Histoplasmosis, 126-127, 128
Hodgkin's disease, 345-346
Homeostasis, 6
Horseshoe kidney, 256, 257
Human immunodeficiency virus (HIV), 342
Hyaline membrane disease, 112-113
Hydrocephalus, 361, 365
Hyperparathyroidism, 37-39
Hyperplasia, prostatic, 304-305
Hypertrophic pyloric stenosis, 171

I

Iatrogenic reactions, 2
Idiopathic disease, 2
Ileus, gallstone, 232-233
Imperforate anus, 172
Incarcerated hernia, 188, 189
Infection, 6
Inflammatory diseases, 4-6
   of abdomen/gastrointestinal system,
      173-186
   of central nervous system, 366-371
   of female reproductive system, 291-292
   of hepatobiliary system, 229-234
   of respiratory system, 113-133
   of skeletal system, 23-33
   of urinary system, 264-267
Inguinal hernia, 186-187
Intervertebral disk(s), 351, 353
   degenerative disease of, 379-380
   herniated, 379-380
Intestines; *see* Bowel

Intra-aortic balloon pump (IABP), 110
Intravenous urography, 245-247

J

Joint(s)
   dislocations of, 64-66
   inflammation of, 29, 32

K

Kaposi's sarcoma in AIDS, 342-343
Kidney(s) 242-244; *see also* Urinary system
   agenesis of, 254
   anomalies of, 254-261
      fusion, 256-258
      numerical, 254-255
      position, 256, 258
      size, 254-255
   carcinoma of, 275, 276-278
   crossed ectopy of, 256, 258
   cysts of, 275, 279-280
   ectopic, 256, 258, 259
   failure of, 268-269
   horseshoe, 256, 257
   hyperplasia of, 255
   hypoplasia of, 255
   malrotation of, 256, 258
   polycystic, 261, 262
   supernumerary, 255

L

Large bowel, 152-153
   imaging considerations for, 153-155
Legg-Perthes disease, 67-68
Legionnaires' disease, 115, 116
Leiomyomas, 295
Leukemia, 345-346
Leukocytes, 337, 338
Levacuator tube, 163
Levin tubes, 162
Lithotripsy, extracorporeal shock wave, 248-251
Liver; *see also* Hepatobiliary system
   cirrhosis of, 228-230
   hemangioma of, 235-236
   hepatoma of, 235-237
   viral hepatitis and, 230
Lung(s)
   abscess of, 127-129
   disease of, chronic obstructive, 122-123
   edema of, in emphysema, 123
   metastases to, 142-143
Lymphadenogram, 340
Lymphatic system, 338-339
Lymphocytes, 338-339
Lymphoma, 339

M

Magnetic resonance imaging (MRI)
   of abdomen, 160-161
   of central nervous system, 353, 356-357, 359, 363-373
   of gastrointestinal system, 160-161
   of hemopoietic system, 340, 341
Malabsorption syndrome, 176, 177-178,
      181-182

Male reproductive system, 303-306
 imaging considerations of, 304
 neoplastic diseases of, 304-306
Malignant neoplasm, 7
Malrotation
 of intestines, 171,172
 of kidneys, 256-258
Mammography, 290
Mastitis, 290
Mediastinum, 101-105
Megacolon
 toxic, 184
Meningiomas
 cranial, 383, 390-391
 spinal, 398, 399
Meningitis, 366-367
Meningocele, 361, 362
Meningomyelocele, 361, 362-364
Metabolic diseases, 6
 of hepatobiliary system, 234-235
 of skeletal system, 33-39, 40-41
 of urinary system, 267-275
Metastasis(es), 7
 to bone, 83
 pulmonary, 142-143
Miliary tuberculosis, 120-122
Miller-Abbott tube, 163-164
Multiple myeloma, 343-344
Mycoplasma pneumonia, 115
Myocardium, 311-312

N

Nasoenteric decompression tube, 163-164
Necrosis, cellular, 4
Neoplasms, benign and malignant, 7
Neoplastic diseases, 7-8
 of abdomen/gastrointestinal system, 209-215
 of central nervous system, 381-391
 of female reproductive system, 292-301
 of hemopoietic system, 343-346
 of hepatobiliary system, 235-239
 of respiratory system, 139-143
 of skeletal system, 73-83
 of urinary system, 275-283
Nephrocalcinosis, 268
Nephroptosis, 267
Nephrosclerosis, 267
Nephrostomy tube, 252-253
Nephrotomography, 250
Nerve sheath cells, tumors of, 394-395, 397-398
Neurilemoma, acoustic, 394-396
Neurofibromas, spinal, 400-401
Neurogenic bladder, 267
Neuroma, acoustic, 394-396
Noncommunicating hydrocephalus, 361
Nuclear cardiology, 318-319
Nucleus pulposus, 351, 353
 herniated, 379-381

O

Osteitis deformans, 36-37
Osteoarthritis, 28, 31
Osteoblasts, 11-13

Osteochondroma, 73-74
Osteoclastoma, 78-79
Osteogenesis imperfecta, 14
Osteogenic sarcoma, 78, 80, 81
Osteoid osteoma, 77-78
Osteoma, 74-75, 77-78
 osteoid, 77-78
Osteomalacia, 35
Osteomyelitis, 4, 23, 24
Osteoporosis, 33-34, 68
Osteosarcoma, 79, 80, 81
Ovary(ies), 297-288; *see also* Female reproductive
  system
 cystadenocarcinoma of, 293-294
 cystic masses of, 292-293
 polycystic, 292-293
Ovulation, 288

P

Paget's disease, 36-37
Palliative treatment, 7
Pancreas, 221-222, 232-234, 238-239; *see also* Hepatobil-
  iary system
 calcification of, 274-275
 carcinoma of, 238-239
Pancreatitis, 232-234
Paralytic ileus, 188, 196-198
Patent ductus arteriosus, 319, 320
Pectus excavatum, 101, 102-103
Pelvic inflammatory disease (PID), 291-292
Pelvis, renal, 259
Peptic ulcer, 174, 176-178
Percutaneous transhepatic cholangiogram, 223-224
Perfusion scans of respiratory system, 97
Periosteum, 13
Pituitary adenoma, 391-393
Placenta previa, 302
Platelets, 339
Pleural effusion, 130-131
Pleurisy, 128, 130
Pneumatocele, 114, 116
Pneumococcal pneumonia, 113-115
Pneumoconioses, 1124-127
Pneumocystis carinii pneumonia, 342-343
Pneumomediastinum, 103-104
Pneumonia(s), 113-116, 117-118
 bacterial, 113-115
 chemical, 117-118
 mycoplasma, 115
 pneumococcal, 113-115
 Pneumocystis carinii, in AIDS, 342-343
 staphylococcal, 114, 116
 streptococcal, 114-115
 viral, 118
Pneumothorax, 133-138
Polycystic kidney disease, 261, 262
Polycystic ovaries, 292-293
Polyps, colon, 212-213
"Porcelain" gallbladder in carcinoma, 237,238
Positron emission tomography (PET)
 of cardiovascular system, 319
 of central nervous system, 358, 360
Pregnancy, disorders during, 302

Prostate gland, 303
  carcinoma of, 305
  hyperplasia of, 304-305
Provisional callous in fracture healing, 42
Pyelography, retrograde, 248
Pyelonephritis, 264-265
Pyloric stenosis, hypertrophic, 171
Pyuria in pyelonephritis, 264
R

Recessive inheritance, 4
Reflux esophagitis, 173-174
Regeneration, tissue, 4
Regional enteritis, 183-184, 185
Renal angiography, 248
Renal pelvis, 259
Reproductive system, 286-308
Respiratory distress syndrome, 112-113
Respiratory system, 86-146
  computed tomography of, 93, 95-96
  congenital/hereditary diseases of, 111-113
    cystic fibrosis as, 112-113
    hyaline membrane disease as, 112-113
  digital radiography of, 97-99
  imaging considerations for, 88-111
    for bony structures, 100-101, 102, 103
    for chest tubes/lines/catheters, 105-111
    exposure factors as, 89
    for mediastinum, 101-105
    position as, 89, 90, 91
    projection as, 89, 90, 91
    for soft tissues, 99-100
    for standard chest radiograph, 89, 90, 91
  inflammatory diseases of, 113-133
    bronchiectasis as, 118-119
    chronic obstructive pulmonary disease as, 122-123
    fungal diseases as, 126-127, 128
    lung abscess as, 127-129
    pleural effusion as, 130-131
    pleurisy as, 128-130
    pneumoconioses as, 124-127
    pneumonias as, 113-116, 117-118
    sinusitis as, 131-133
    tuberculosis as, 119-122
  neoplastic diseases of, 139-143
    bronchial adenomas as, 139
    bronchogenic carcinoma as, 139-141
    metastases, 142-143
  perfusion scans of, 97
  traumatic diseases of, 132-138
    atelectasis as, 132-135
    pneumothorax as, 133-138
  ventilation scans of, 97
Reticuloendothelial system, 337
Rh factor, 336
Rickets, 35
S

Sarcoma, 7
  Ewing's, 79-81, 82
  Kaposi's in AIDS, 342-343
  osteogenic, 79, 80, 81
Scoliosis, 17, 19

Seminomas, testicular, 305
Septal defects, 321
Shoulder joint, dislocation of, 64-66
Silicosis, 125
Single positron emission computed tomography (SPECT) of
        central nervous system, 358, 359-360
Sinusitis, 131-133
Skeletal system, 10-85
  congenital/hereditary diseases of, 15-23, *24, 25*
    achondroplasia as, 15-16, *17*
    congenital hip dislocation as, 19-20
    cranial anomalies as, 23, *24-25*
    foot malformations as, 19
    hand malformations as, 19
    osteogenesis imperfecta as, 15, *16*
    osteopetrosis as, 15-16, 17
    vertebral anomalies as, 17, 19, 20-21
  imaging considerations for, 13
  inflammatory diseases of, 23-33
    arthritis as, 23-33; *see also* Arthritis
    osteomyelitis as, 4, 23-24
    tuberculosis as, 23, 25
  metabolic diseases of, 33-39, 40-41
    acromegaly, 39, 40-41
    hyperparathyroidism as, 37-39
    osteomalacia as, 35
    osteoporosis as, 33-34
    Paget's disease as, 36-37
  neoplastic diseases of, 73-83
    chondrosarcoma as, 81-82
    endochondroma as, 75
    Ewing's sarcoma as, 79-81, 82
    metastases from other sites, 83
    osteochondroma as, 73-74
    osteoclastoma as, 78-79
    osteoid osteoma as, 77-78
    osteoma as, 74-75
    osteosarcoma as, 79, 80, 81
    simple bone cyst as, 76-77
  traumatic diseases of, 39-73
    battered child syndrome as, 66-67
    dislocations as, 64-66; *see also* Dislocation(s)
    fractures as, 39-63; *see also* Fracture(s)
    Legg-Perthes disease as, 67-68
    vertebral column injuries as, 68-73
Small bowel
  tumors of, 212
Somatic cells in congenital diseases, 3
Sonography; *see* Ultrasound
Spina bifida, 20-21
Spinal cord, 405; *see also* Central nervous system
        (CNS)
Spondylitis, ankylosing, 27, 29, 30
Spondylolisthesis, 70-71
Spondylolysis, 70-71, 72
Staghorn calculi, 270-271
Staging of cancer, 7-8
Staphylococcal pneumonia, 114, 116
Stomach, 147, 148-149
  imaging considerations for, 160-162
  intrathoracic, 188-189
  tumors of, 210-212

Streptococcal pneumonia, 114-115
''String sign'' in regional enteritis, 183-184
Stroke, 328-329
Subarachnoid hematoma, 380
Subcutaneous emphysema, 103, 105
Subdural hematoma, 380-381
Swan-Ganz catheter, 108-109
Systole, 312

T

T-tube cholangiography, 224-225
Tendinitis, 29
Tenosynovitis, 29
Teratomas
  cystic, of ovary, 293
  testicular, 306
Testes
  masses of, 306
Tetralogy of Fallot, 323
Thrombosis, venous, 331-332
Tissue regeneration, 4
TNM staging system, 7-8
Toxic megacolon, 184
Trabeculae, of bladder, 262
Transient ischemic attack (TIA), 328-329
Traumatic diseases, 6-7
  of abdomen/gastrointestinal system, 205-208
  of central nervous system, 372-381
  of respiratory system, 132-138
  of skeletal system, 39-73
Tuberculosis, 23, 25, 119-122
Tube(s)
  abdominal, imaging considerations for, 162-164
  Cantor, imaging considerations for, 164
  Dobhuff, imaging considerations for, 163
  Edlich, imaging considerations for, 162-163
  enteral, imaging considerations for, 163
  Ewald, imaging considerations for, 162-163
  gastric, imaging considerations for, 162
  Harris, imaging considerations for, 164
  Levacuator, imaging considerations for, 163
  Levin, imaging considerations for, 162
  Miller-Abbott, imaging considerations for, 163-164
  nasoenteric decompression, imaging considerations for, 163-164
  nephrostomy, imaging considerations for, 252-253
Tumor(s)
  esophageal, 209-211
  gastric, 210-211
  giant cell, 78-79
  of nerve sheath cells, 394-395, 397-398
  small bowel, 212
  Wilms', 280, 281

U

Ulcerative colitis, 184-186
Ulcers, peptic, 174, 176-178
Ultrasound
  diagnostic medical, for gallbladder disease, 225-226
  of female reproductive system, 288-290, 302
Unicornuate uterus, 291
Uremia in renal failure, 269

Ureteral stents, 252
Ureteroceles, 259-260
Ureter(s), see Urinary system
Urethra, see Urinary system
Urethral valves, 261, 262
Urinary system, 242-263
  congenital/hereditary diseases of, 254-263
    lower tract, 259-261
    renal, 254-259; see also Kidney(s)
  degenerative/metabolic diseases of, 310-320 *321*
    calcifications as, 268, 269-275
    nephrocalcinosis as, 268
    nephrosclerosis as, 267
    renal failure as, 268-269
  imaging considerations for, 245-253
    for computed tomography, 248
    for cystogram, 248, 252
    for extracorporeal shock wave lithotripsy, 248-251
    for intravenous urography, 245-247
    for nephrotomography, 248
    for renal angiography, 248
    for retrograde pyelography, 248
    for ultrasound, 248
    for voiding cystography, 248
  inflammatory diseases of, 264-267
    cystitis as, 266-267
    glomerulonephritis as, 265-266
    pyelonephritis as, 264-265
  neoplastic disease of, 275-283
Urinary tubes/catheters, 252-253
Urography, intravenous, 245-247
Uterine tubes; see also Female reproductive system
Uterus, 287-288; see also Female reproductive system
  anteflexed, 291
  bicornuate, 291
  masses of, 291
  retroflexed, 291
  unicornuate, 291
Uterus didelphys, 291

V

Valvular disease, 323-324
Vas deferens, 303
Vein(s), 312-313
Venography in venous thrombosis, 331-332
Venous thrombosis, 331-332
Ventilation scans of respiratory system, 97
Ventricular pacing electrode, 110-111
Vertebra
  anomalies of, 17, 19, 20-21
  transitional, 19-20
Vertebral column, trauma to, 68-73
Viral hepatitis, 230
Virulence, 6
Voiding cystography, 248

W

Wilms' tumor, 280-281

Z

Zenker's diverticulum, 199-201